ASSISTANT SECRETARY FOR HEALTH

JUARY 1974

NATIONAL INSTI-
TUTES OF HEALTH

Office of the
Director

National Cancer
Institute

National Heart and
Lung Institute

National Institute
of Allergy and
Infectious
Diseases

National Institute
of Arthritis,
Metabolism and
Digestive
Diseases

National Institute
of Child Health
and Human
Development

National Institute
of Dental
Research

National Institute
of Environmental
Health Sciences

National Institute
of General
Medical Sciences

National Institute
of Neurological
Diseases and
Stroke

National Eye
Institute

National Library
of Medicine

Fogarty Interna-
tional Center

ALCOHOL, DRUG ABUSE
AND MENTAL HEALTH
ADMINISTRATION

Office of the
Administrator

National Institute
of Mental Health

National Institute
of Drug Abuse

National Institute
on Alcohol Abuse
and Alcoholism

CENTER FOR
DISEASE CONTROL

Office of the
Center Director

National Institute
for Occupation-
al Safety and
Health

Bureau of
Epidemiology

Bureau of
Laboratories

Bureau of State
Services

Smallpox Eradica-
tion Program

Tropical Disease
Program

National
Clearinghouse
for Smoking
and Health

INTRODUCTION
TO
PUBLIC HEALTH

Daniel M. Wilner, Ph.D.
*Professor of Public Health and Professor of
Preventive and Social Medicine, University
of California, Los Angeles*

Rosabelle Price Walkley, B.A.
*Research Behavioral Scientist and Lecturer in
Public Health, University of California,
Los Angeles*

Lenor S. Goerke, M.D., M.S.P.H.
*Late Professor of Public Health and Professor
of Preventive and Social Medicine, University
of California, Los Angeles; Dean, School of
Public Health, University of California,
Los Angeles*

INTRODUCTION

TO

PUBLIC HEALTH

SIXTH EDITION

MACMILLAN PUBLISHING CO., INC.
New York
COLLIER MACMILLAN PUBLISHERS
London

Earlier editions entitled *An Introduction to Public Health,* by
Harry S. Mustard, copyright 1935, 1944, and 1953 by Macmillan
Publishing Co., Inc. Earlier edition entitled *An Introduction to
Public Health,* by Harry S. Mustard and Ernest L. Stebbins, ©
1959 by Macmillan Publishing Co., Inc. Earlier edition entitled
Mustard's Introduction to Public Health, by Lenor S. Goerke and
Ernest L. Stebbins, © copyright 1968 by Macmillan Publishing
Co., Inc. Copyright renewed 1963 by Harry S. Mustard, 1972
by Sarah H. Mustard.

MACMILLAN PUBLISHING CO., INC.
866 Third Avenue, New York, New York 10022

COLLIER-MACMILLAN CANADA, LTD.

Library of Congress Cataloging in Publication Data

Wilner, Daniel M.
    Introduction to public health.

    First-5th ed. entered under H. S. Mustard.
    1. Hygiene, Public. I. Walkley, Rosabelle Price, joint author.
II. Goerke, Lenor S., joint author. III. Mustard, Harry Stoll,
1889–1966. An introduction to public health. IV. Title. [DNLM:
1. Public health. WA 100 W744i 1973]
RA425.W749   1973   614   73-5281
ISBN 0-02 428200-6

Printing: 2 3 4 5 6 7 8   Year: 4 5 6 7 8 9 0

PREFACE

As an introduction to public health this textbook is designed to offer the student a broad perspective on the health field of the 1970's. The intention is to provide insight into a wide range of topics ordinarily not contained in a single volume.

The book is oriented to professional schools, departments, and training programs that are preparing students for careers in fields in which some knowledge of public health is considered desirable or essential—students in nursing, nutrition, dietetics, pharmacy, medical technology, x-ray technology, physical therapy, occupational therapy, dental hygiene, optometry, podiatry, and others. For public health students (who receive in-depth instruction in the various areas presented in the book) as well as for professional health practitioners, this volume can serve as a useful source and reference book. Many of the "new careers" that are burgeoning in the health industry have a strong overlay of public health and, for students training for these careers, the book provides relevant background information.

A basic thought underlying the book is that, whatever careers students are preparing for, knowledge about this nation's health system will put their jobs in better perspective once they become professional health practitioners. Thus, the sixth edition (75 per cent revised from the preceding edition) is particularly concerned with (a) objectives of major health and health-related programs in the United States; (b) their general sponsorship and financial backing; (c) their personnel requirements, qualifications, and opportunities; and (d) certain health trends that began earlier in this century and are continuing through the 1960's and 1970's. In the latter connection, a special effort has been made to describe and discuss recent developments for which students need clarifying perspective.

These new developments occur, for example, in *health care* (activities in the chronic disease field and in financing, organizing, and delivery of health services), in *health manpower* (career expansion in the nursing profession; the physician's assistant movement; "new careers"; and current trends in pharmacy, nutrition, and laboratory technology), in *mental health care* (community mental health centers), and in *environmental health* (the ecology movement and its import for health). In short, the health field—a most dynamic segment of American professional life—is undergoing exciting changes that, within a decade, will see vast transformations in the activities and concerns of health professionals.

The sixth edition is organized into four sections. Section I discusses several principal health problems of the 1970's; the broad organization of health services; and the basic, direct-service, and

clinical professions of nursing, medical, and related health manpower categories. Section II describes, in detail, the complexities of
contemporary medical care, mental health care, and environmental
health. Section III covers health-status measurement, communicable
and chronic diseases, the health of mothers and children, and some
basic concerns regarding population growth and family planning.
Section IV discusses community health research; covers community
health education concepts, including personal health maintenance;
and gives attention to principal problems and trends in nutrition,
laboratory, and pharmacy services. Some tables and other illustrative
materials have been included to assist the student in grasping the
essence of health trends, although care has been taken to avoid needless or irrelevant items.

A number of grateful acknowledgments are in order: to our
predecessors in the preparation of previous editions of the book, to
the sources of data for the many facts reported in the present edition,
and to the individuals who assisted in the preparation of the volume
itself.

We therefore wish to acknowledge the trail blazed in the past by
two distinguished public health pioneers and statesmen—Harry S.
Mustard, M.D., who initiated the first edition; and Ernest L. Stebbins,
M.D., who coauthored the fourth and fifth editions. We also acknowl-
edge the work of several individuals who participated in the prepara-
tion of the fifth edition: Virginia A. Clark, Ph.D.; David P. Discher,
M.D.; Arnold I. Kisch, M.D.; Jean L. Mickey, Ph.D.; Audrey J. Naylor,
M.D.; Harriett B. Randall, M.D.; Charles L. Senn, M.S.; Walter H.
Smartt, M.D.; Guy W. Steuart, Ph.D.; J. Albert Torribio, M.S.W.;
Arthur J. Viseltear, Ph.D.; Marsden Wagner, M.D.; and Telford H.
Work, M.D.

A debt is owed to various sources of data and illustrative materials used in the present edition: to the Office of the Secretary, Department of Health, Education, and Welfare; to the offices of the administrators of the three major organizations constituting the Public Health
Service (Health Services and Mental Health Administration, National
Institutes of Health, and Food and Drug Administration); and to the
Environmental Protection Agency. Finally, a good picture of the contemporary state and local health scene was obtained from dozens of
state and local health departments, from state and local mental health
agencies, from comprehensive health planning agencies, and from
regional medical programs across the country. A special note of
acknowledgment is due the California and Los Angeles County
official public health agencies.

Preparation of the sixth edition was made possible by the fine
secretarial work of Margaret Weichel, our secretary of many years.
Diana Springer assisted in the typing of a portion of the manuscript.

Finally, we were fortunate to have as research and editorial assistants two exceptional persons who quickly grasped the mission of the book and who materially aided us in its preparation: Ellen Gold and Darlene Johnson.

D.M.W.
R.P.W.
L.S.G.

A few weeks after completion of the sixth-edition manuscript we were deeply saddened by the sudden death of Lenor S. Goerke, our friend and colleague of more than a dozen years. As founding dean of a school of public health, he was a pioneer in public health training and education of several thousand students from diverse backgrounds. This textbook is a fitting embodiment of Professor Goerke's broad view of the field and a reminder of his insistence that knowledge about the American health system is a prelude to and accompaniment of influence in it.

D.M.W.
R.P.W.

CONTENTS

SECTION IV
SELECTED PUBLIC HEALTH
SUPPORTIVE SERVICES

SECTION

I

THE
FRAMEWORK
OF
PUBLIC HEALTH

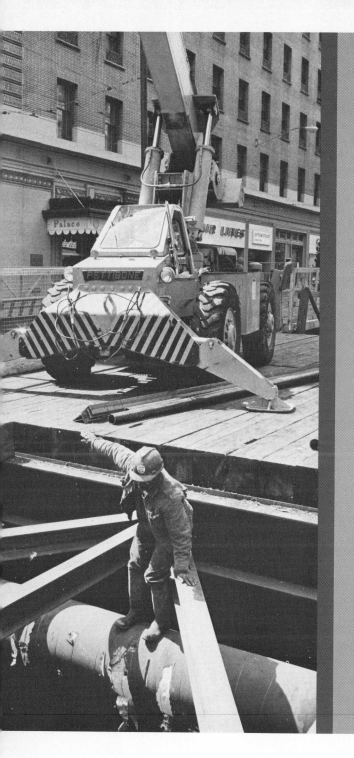

1

**PUBLIC HEALTH
IN THE 1970's**

CHAPTER OUTLINE

Background of Today's Public Health

Major Public Health Problems of the 1970's

The Environment
Chronic and Communicable Diseases
Delivery of Health and Mental Health Services
Psychiatric Problems and the Addictive Diseases

Significant Forces Influencing Public Health

Health Awareness and Health Habits
New Mores and New Freedoms
Economically and Culturally Deprived Populations
The Consumer Movement in Health

Background of Today's Public Health

The public health field has as its chief concern the health needs of populations. In all periods of its development there has been involvement in (a) the search for understanding of the causes of disease, (b) the development of technical means for protecting the population against disease, the targets being the environment as well as disease-producing organisms, and (c) the organization of health programs to bring technology to bear on the central health problems of the nation or the community.

In different periods of time these concerns expressed themselves in different ways, always reflecting the social pressures and influences of the day. In past periods, as civilization progressed, the main health problems related to the means of achieving sanitation, the growing of food, and the conditions of work. Since the beginning of the seventeenth century there have been impressive biologic and medical accomplishments that gradually unfolded the knowledge of today about the cause, prevention, and treatment of many diseases. The struggle against infectious disease—not completely won by any means—is particularly striking in its achievements, and all persons alive today are in one way or another its beneficiaries.

In the United States, in the period 1900–1945, the public health field had much narrower interests than it has today. It restricted itself largely to control measures for communicable diseases and to systems for reporting these conditions; to health "education" about selected illnesses; to surveillance and control of the handling of water, food, and milk; to recording of vital statistics; and to the operation of clinics for detection and treatment of tuberculosis, venereal disease, and, for the poor, prenatal and well-baby clinics.

In the several decades following World War II, all this has changed. Public health is no longer the concern only of the 1,800 local and 50 state health departments—as important as their func-

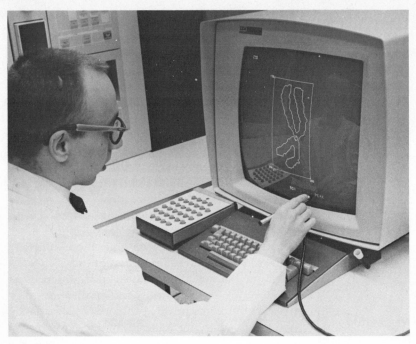

Courtesy of Health Sciences Computing Facility, University of California, Los Angeles.

tions continue to be. Public health is no longer only the concern of doctors, nurses, dentists, and other specialized health professionals. Public health today is *everybody's* concern, and has become in the United States an issue of the highest public and political salience.

Public health today includes such familiar topics as the *costs* of medical care and the complex problems of *planning* for the best of health care for the general population as well as for special groups such as inner-city dwellers and the elderly. It includes consideration of the *hospitals* of the future, needed to fulfill the promises of existing technical knowledge. It includes consideration of the *chronic diseases*, e.g., heart disease and cancer, that have replaced communicable diseases as the main causes of death.

Public health today also includes *all* the hazards to health residing in the environment — the microbiologic, physical, and chemical dangers in the atmosphere, in water supplies, and in the soil. It includes problems of *population growth*, the rate of which is a matter of international crisis. Public health, finally, includes the *social and behavioral aspects of life* — endangered by contemporary stresses, addictive diseases, and emotional instability.

Looking backward, it is easy to forget that the important health accomplishments of the past sometimes took years, decades, and even generations to accomplish. Today there is much significant progress in the health field emerging from the nation's experimental laboratories and clinical treatment settings. There are, for example, advances in physiology, biochemistry, virology, the development of vaccines, and specific medical-surgical accomplishments such as kidney dialysis and transplants and emergency coronary care.

Health news, however, is not uniformly good. Many headlines and much personal experience introduce a discouraging note regarding the health affairs and mental health status of the American people. Some morbidity and death rates are at or close to their all-time highs, particularly for the chronic diseases. Infant mortality is higher in the United States than in many other countries in the world and is particularly high in the inner-city ghetto. Several environmental health hazards are far from solution. The delivery of health services is in a turmoil, the quality of care is uneven, and prices are high, with plenty of complaints on all scores. In other words, there seems to be confusion about what is known for sure that works in *curing* chronic disease, in *preventing* some illness, in *subduing* environmental hazards, and in the overall *provision* of health services.

Considering technologic advances in so many facets of American life, it is sometimes hard to imagine why progress is not quicker in the health field. It would appear that technology alone is not sufficient. The scientific and medical aspects of the diseases afflicting advanced societies today are unbelievably complex, and probably require more allocation of resources—money and scientific manpower—than are assigned at present.

Matters are no less complex when one considers the social forces affecting today's health scene. The health status of Americans is affected in direct and indirect ways by the state of the economy (i.e., affluence and recession), the social organization of the health effort, national fears and anxieties (e.g., regarding war and peace), changing mores and life-styles, etc. National health affairs—in fact, health status itself—must be thought about in the broadest social perspective. In this way the significance of one's own health role can be understood, either as a highly skilled professional, as a well-trained technical specialist, or as an informed citizen. In this way also links can be forged connecting the likely events of the 1970's and 1980's with earlier public health periods, particularly the span between World War II and the present, when new ideas in the health field were being tried out in such profusion.

Major Public Health Problems of the 1970's

THE ENVIRONMENT

Since the mid-1940's there has been successive fouling of the environment at such an accelerated rate that some observers despair of seeing the situation righted before the year 2000—if ever. At least three factors have had significant effect on the environment and the aspects of health that are dependent on it. These are accelerated economic growth, the expansion of population, and the growth of poverty areas (the ghetto).

Economic development in the United States has taken place since 1945 at a rate far exceeding any in past history. The technical developments in that growth made enormous demands on the nation's energy supply, and the products and by-products of this expansion upset important ecologic balances. All of this took place at a pace so fast as to outrun normal ecologic safeguards of slower times. Efforts to control almost all pollution sources have the same scenario. The act of environmental polluting is normally an unanticipated and disregarded by-product of ordinary business pursuits. Therefore, the solution of America's environmental problems is complicated because it runs head-on into what is possibly the most cherished of American goals—growth and economic development.

Population growth in all its complexities also has adverse effects on the environment. Considering the size of the earth, it may be hard to believe that there are at present too many people on it. However, ruinous population growth is a real possibility in view of the near-geometric rate of prevailing expansion. In the world's *urban* areas there is no doubt that quality of life is affected by population congestion. In the United States, the drift to cities from rural places began during World War I and picked up again in World War II. It has continued to the point where, in 1970, about two thirds of the American population lived in metropolitan areas which, altogether, occupied less than 10 per cent of the land area of the nation. One glance at America's cities reveals congestion and its consequences and, in combination with economic activity, shows the potentials of environmental hazards: the wastes generated, the noise emitted, the power requirements increased, the water endangered, and the air polluted.

All large cities in the United States (and some smaller cities and rural places, too) have *slums*. The large urban slums are most often inhabited by impoverished minorities—principally Negroes, Puerto Ricans, and Mexican-Americans—and possess many attributes of the "classical" ghetto. The ghetto is the product of racial pressures which affect housing and employment, the encapsulated welfare system which affects below-poverty-line populations, and the countless social aspects of schooling, crowding, and nutrition. As a hazardous environment, the ghetto operates diffusely, but no less inexorably, on its inhabitants. It is the site of much illness and death among infants and mothers, of much hard narcotics use and its attendant misery, of much recorded venereal disease, and of much illegitimacy. If *health* is poorer there, so is the health *care* rendered. There are fewer physicians, dentists, hospitals, and nursing homes serving ghetto areas than are found in better-off sections of cities.

CHRONIC AND COMMUNICABLE DISEASES

In the United States, the period since 1900 has seen a steady rise in incidence and mortality of chronic illness, but a sharp decline in communicable or infectious disease. In other parts of the world, however, incidence of disabling or killing infectious and parasitic diseases such as cholera, malaria, and trachoma (a blinding eye infection) still represent significant health problems. Even in the United States, it would be a mistake to conclude that infectious disease is no longer a matter for vigilance. Quite the contrary. While the first six months of 1972 turned up only 90 cases of diphtheria and 156 cases of typhoid fever, there were reported 29,000 cases of infectious hepatitis, 25,000 cases of measles (rubeola), and 19,000 cases of German measles (rubella). There were also 17,000 new active cases of tuberculosis, 12,000 cases of syphilis, and *360,000 cases of gonorrhea.* The fact is that the communicable disease scene is a dynamic one and continues to require close public health attention.

The chronic diseases are another story altogether, despite the fact, for example, that some neoplastic diseases (cancers) may turn out to have viral origins. The cause, prevention, treatment, and control of most chronic diseases are substantially different from those of communicable diseases. Chronic diseases (heart disease, stroke, cancer, etc.) probably are caused by many factors, have a long duration, frequently involve lengthy hospitalization, cause protracted pain and disability, and are hard to treat or control.

Aging brings in its wake a wide array of chronic diseases, and in the United States, in 1970, there were approximately 20 million individuals age 65 and older. It is a paradox that the health breakthroughs since 1900 are directly responsible for the size of the elderly population today. Without the vast improvements in the earlier period—in sanitation, nutrition, immunization, diagnosis, and the development of pharmacology—death would no doubt long since have overtaken half or more of the persons who are now in their sixties or older. Since there is much disability associated with chronic illness, there is consequently far greater use of hospital, nursing home, and rehabilitation facilities by the elderly than by younger persons. Providing quality medical care for 20 million

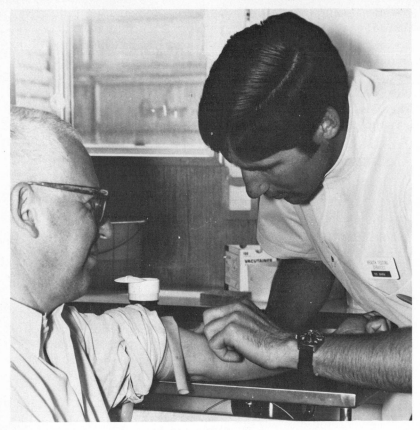

Courtesy of Health Testing Services, Berkeley, California.

elderly is a formidable task, and the problem is to some extent responsible for the present medical care crisis in the United States. The search for a solution will continue to call on the best organizational, scientific, and technical talents available.

DELIVERY OF HEALTH AND MENTAL HEALTH SERVICES

In considering the elements of a productive health and mental health care system, one needs to keep several aims in mind. The system should be one that offers high-quality care, that encourages economies in the rendering of service, and that embodies some financial scheme for making possible the obtaining of health care routinely as needed. It should be a system that develops and maintains its technical excellence (through basic, clinical and managerial research) and directs the development of needed manpower.

Public opinion polls show that Americans are convinced there is a health care crisis in the United States. The polls reveal that Americans like their own doctors, but they do not like the health care system in which their doctors work, with its delays, its discourtesies, its difficult access to care, and its actual or potential astronomic costs.

The health consumer is joined in these views by many health professionals—some doctors and many health administrators—by economists, by congressmen and senators, by the White House, and in recent years by the American business and financial community. There is near common agreement that some fundamental changes will be made in the American health system in the 1970's and 1980's. There is no precise agreement on all counts regarding the exact description of these changes but the rough outlines have emerged.

In the 1960's, it was thought by some that money alone could do the trick and ensure wide and equitable distribution of health services. "Money alone" was essentially embodied in the amendments of 1965 to the Social Security Act and resulted in Medicare and Medicaid (as described in Chapter 4). This legislation may be looked upon as a significant experiment, with some successes but also fraught with economic difficulties. Thus, real financial relief for medical care is now provided for the elderly (and their families), and in most states health services to welfare patients have for the first time been genuinely coordinated. But a major unlooked-for bad consequence has been the skyrocketing cost of medical care.

If money alone will not reach the goal, what will? The decade of the 1970's will no doubt be occupied with consideration of legislative measures bearing on national health insurance proposals and on organizational structures for the delivery of health services. *Health insurance* involves a widely prevailing mode of spreading risk, and existing private group health insurance plans and Medicare both provide good dry runs. An *organizational structure* that is promising involves a group health plan which has prepayment features, a published schedule of comprehensive benefits, and costs related to actual experience. The wise and judicious interlocking of these two concepts will no doubt go a long way to help solve America's health dilemmas, and in the long run will be equally applicable to all kinds of health care, including mental health.

PSYCHIATRIC PROBLEMS AND THE ADDICTIVE DISEASES

Psychiatric problems are among the most complex in the health field and the most resistant to treatment and cure. Two landmark events occurred in the 1950's and 1960's that altered the general treatment of persons with psychiatric problems. First was the development of ataractic drugs (tranquilizers) which made for easier management of patients with certain forms of mental illness. This resulted in decreased length of stay in state mental hospitals for the more seriously ill and in sharply reduced inpatient populations. The second event was the decentralization of mental health care through closing of a number of large mental hospitals and the development of several hundred community mental health centers. The objective of high importance in these activities was keeping the mentally ill patient close to home in his or her own community.

Two disorders affecting large groups of people which have both mental health and physical health aspects are alcoholism and drug abuse. *Alcoholism* is possibly the oldest, most baffling of man's dependency states, affecting millions of adults in the United States and destructive of family relationships, work performance, and productivity. Sociocultural origins of this affliction are not well known, and the personal-psychologic causative chain seems to defy identification. Alcoholism has serious physical effects well known to doctors and nurses. Death from cirrhosis of the liver—closely linked to alcohol consumption—is at an all-time high, and alcoholism's role in heart disease is known as a significant factor.

Drug abuse must be looked at in the light of the general pharmacologic behavior of Americans. Compared with other nations in the world, Americans are a "pill-popping" society. In 1969, more than $6.5 billion were spent by Americans on drugs and sundries: $2.5 billion on patent medicines, and most of the remainder on prescription items. Studies of drug-certifying, drug-prescribing, and legal drug-taking behavior tell of major problems in this field of strong consumer protection concern. Pill- and nostrum-taking has achieved in recent years the status of a norm and no doubt contributes to the predispositions which, several steps further removed, lay the groundwork for illicit drug-taking.

Drug addiction, while also affecting adults, does its greatest damage to the young. In the 1970's, prescription drugs that are increasingly available illegally include energizers, depressants, sleep-inducers, opiate and morphine derivatives. Nonprescription illegal drugs include heroin, the hardest of the hard drugs, as well as LSD, an experimental hallucinogenic drug. Drug problems, already widely prevalent in America, have been aggravated in recent years by involvement of soldiers and veterans of the Vietnamese War. Addictive drugs may have vicious outcomes for users, with possible irreversible psychopathologic consequences as well as the chance of overdose or drug impurity which can result in serious illness or death.

Significant Forces Influencing Public Health

HEALTH AWARENESS AND HEALTH HABITS

In the United States, awareness of health as a national problem area emerged in the 1950's and early 1960's. Health and illness are part of the human condition, and individually all must cope with their vagaries between birth and death. But as a public issue to be discussed openly, to grouse about in unison, and to vote on, health has emerged only recently. Public opinion polls mirror this high saliency and interest. Polls now regularly report health care and environmental hazards as among the leading issues "bothering" people today. Over the years everyone has heard about the "magic bullets" and the miracles of modern medicine. The news media have had a significant role in this. News agencies, newspapers in major American cities, and large-circulation magazines have health writers, editors, and columnists whose job is to sift the health news of the day for national and local interest, picking up items from medical and other health journals and from scientific conventions and meetings. They also report regularly the legislative events concerning health from Washington, D.C., and from state capitals.

Another important media influence is television (and to a lesser extent motion pictures). Since the 1950's every television season has seen one or more dramatic series dealing with health or medicine. These shows are extremely popular, with millions of people every week viewing the essential drama of health and illness, in formats running the gamut from balanced presentations of medical problems to vastly oversimplified (soap opera) solutions to complex issues.

Everyone has more personal health experience today than formerly. Thus, each individual — without exception — is exposed regularly to evidence of the polluted environment. There are few who have not had a brush with the problem of cigarette smoking or overweight, or who have not observed from closeby the consequences of alcoholism. There is hardly an individual in his forties or older who is not closely in touch with the personal health care scene, because he or she either suffers from illness or has an elderly relative who does. Since the issue of costs has great meaning in these experiences, the saliency of the personal equation in health care is very high.

While health interest of Americans is thus admittedly high, their health habits are deplorable — looked at from the point of view of what is known or strongly suspected as contributing to or preventing illness or accidents. Americans sometimes tend to neglect even sure-fire preventives, such as vaccines of known protectiveness. The failure to act on known health protective information is sometimes attributed to lack of education or "ignorance." Yet what is to be made of the fact that while socioeconomic status, age, and sex do seem to play certain special roles in health habits, almost *all* Americans fail to act in their own best interests in their daily health-related behavior.

For example, although the seven danger signals of cancer are widely publicized, not all Americans know what they are. In fact, a recent Blue Cross survey showed that 30 per cent of the persons surveyed could identify *none* of the seven signs. In the same survey, only half the respondents could identify more than one symptom of a heart attack or heart condition (one quarter were unable to identify any symptoms). Further, while 80 per cent of individuals claimed to be informed about the health gains deriving from exercise, fewer than half that number exercised regularly.

Another recent opinion poll showed a startling number of persons who reported not knowing that lung cancer was suspected of being associated with cigarette smoking. The association of cigarette smoking and lung cancer is by now one of the most widely publicized health facts in the nation. Yet in studies made in 1964 and 1965 and again in 1970, half the men in the United States and about one third of the women age 17 and older were smoking cigarettes.

Convincing evidence is beginning to accumulate regarding health habits, which, singly and in combination, can add up to substantially better health status and freedom from disability. Much (although not everything by any means) is known through science about likely relationships of personal habits to health status. Some way must be found to counteract the many forces at work—some cultural, some social, some personal-psychological—that interfere with attaining a health goal because of poor habits.

NEW MORES AND NEW FREEDOMS

The period since 1950 has seen some new themes emerge in American life that have substantial meaning for health. This is the period in which there appeared new mores and social customs that gained sanction unheard of before. There was a new freedom, particularly for younger persons, in personal and social expression and in sexual relations. The new social freedoms have stretched old notions of personal control and permissiveness. Many teen-agers, for example, are searching for—and achieving—psychologic independence earlier than in past periods. Likewise young adults, men and women alike, have opted for modes of behavioral expression unknown to the generation of their parents.

The meanings for health in these developments can be detected in many forms of personal exploration, including the use of marijuana and "mind-expanding" drugs and the tryout of new dietary forms and food habits, often bordering on food faddism. Increased sexual activity among young people also has had health consequences. Opinion polls in recent years show consistently more young men and women reporting having had sexual intercourse than in former years. While the moral consequences of the new sexual freedom may be debated, there is no debating the heavy accompanying nationwide epidemic in venereal disease, notably gonorrhea. Although the principal venereal diseases are at present normally treatable successfully with antibiotic therapy, some strains of the gonococcus are showing increased resistance to antibiotics.

Related to the new freedoms in quite another way is the unprecedented activity in the field of family planning. Until the 1950's it was the rare local health agency that would openly espouse "family planning" advice, much less offer contraceptives. In the 1970's this has changed. No city of any size in the United States is without one or more family planning centers or clinics. While some states (particularly in New England) prohibit over-the-counter or general prescription contraceptives, laws in most states have long permitted their prescription or sale. Nationally, the Office of Economic Opportunity and the Public Health Service have provided funds in recent years to stimulate local family planning services and to support relevant basic and applied research in the field.

One long-time force in liberalizing ideas about family planning and contraception in the United States has, of course, been the plight of women with more children than they wanted or could manage, given the family income. Another is the extraordinary rise in illegitimate births since 1940. The new freedoms gave these problems a philosophic base and asserted that in childbearing, as in other roles, women were to be determiners of their own fate and have the right to make personal decisions about the bearing of children. For some women the philosophic aim was to separate the sex act from conception. The result of these forces has been a persistent widespread educational campaign to bring rational decision-making into the childbearing process.

A particularly serious aspect of family planning is, of course, abortion. Here fetal life has begun and was not prevented from getting started through contraceptive methods. All traditional strictures that are called out against contraception are multiplied when considering abortion. However, even in this instance, a few states in recent years had passed substantially liberalized abortion laws, and in 1973 a landmark decision of the U.S. Supreme Court struck down anti-abortion laws across the country. It goes without saying that some physicians, nurses, and technicians feel disturbed by these trends. This is particularly true when they view the matter either in the light of personal religious principles and background or in the light of the life *preservative* focus of everything else they do. Yet mores change, and with them a host of personal predilections and philosophic values.

ECONOMICALLY AND CULTURALLY DEPRIVED POPULATIONS

No cultural change since 1950 has had such strong impact on American society as the emergence of self-identity and activism among racial minority groups (Blacks, Spanish-American-Chicanos, and Puerto Ricans). Beginning in 1954 with the Supreme Court decision banning segregation in schools—affecting mainly Negroes—there ensued a number of other court cases, legislative enactments, and executive orders that have attempted to correct inequities of opportunity in the lives of all America's ethnic minorities. Facets of life affected include education, employment, social benefits, and health.

Good health has been seen by minority group members as a quality they have had less of than other citizens largely because of their economic status—poverty. Many indicators of health status show disadvantages for inner-city minority group members. Housing and neighborhoods are dilapidated, fire-prone, run-down, and in other ways undesirable, replete with vermin and other infestation. There are higher rates of childhood communicable diseases, infant and maternal deaths, venereal disease, drug addiction, and other disorders than elsewhere.

Medical care opportunities have been fewer for minority inner-city residents than for better-off white neighbors. The plight of the inner-city resident is only partly a matter of race, although racial feelings no doubt play a substantial role. Mainly it is a matter of economics: inner-city residents do not normally have purchasing power to obtain first-class medical care.

There have been health developments that have affected, but have not yet by any means entirely corrected, the inner-city health deficits. These include the passage of Medicare (affecting the minority elderly) and Medicaid (pulling together scattered medical benefits from many welfare programs). There are also countless health and mental health programs initiated by the federal government (e.g., Office of Economic Opportunity, Children's Health Service, National Institute of Mental Health) and by city and county health agencies that have resulted in increased and improved health services to inner-city residents. In addition, a few cities and counties have also taken the initiative, since the late 1960's, in building municipal hospitals and clinics in the heart of inner cities so that they are easily accessible (e.g., the 500-bed Martin Luther King Hospital located in the Watts-Willowbrook section of Los Angeles, opened in 1972).

Since 1960, American Indians, too, have come in for increased attention in the education, employment, social service, and health fields. Living on reservations and in nearby towns, the basic health outlook of American Indians bears strong resemblance to that of inner-city residents. The health care neglect of this group has been nothing short of scandalous until recent years, despite the fact that on the reservation they are charges of the United States government.

An important characteristic of the minority-group health scene has to do with "who runs the show." Across the face of America there is a strong movement for minority-group direction of the health services that affect minority populations. The movement is analogous to the itchy desires of developing nations overseas to eliminate what is now perceived as medical colonialism. A major problem is

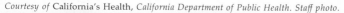

Courtesy of California's Health, *California Department of Public Health. Staff photo.*

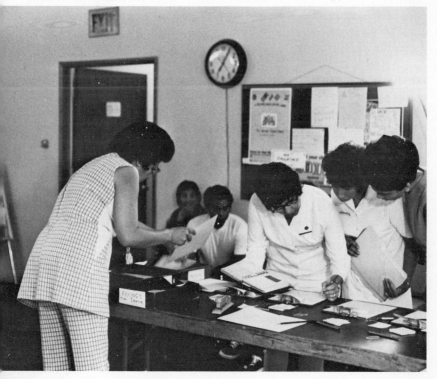

that there are too few well-trained minority group personnel to go around, so that sometimes less-qualified staff must do the job. A consequence has been the substantial beginning investment by national and local government in training minority group members for occupations in the health field. In time, no doubt, more Blacks, Chicanos, Puerto Ricans, and American Indians will be introduced into the health system in the physician, nursing, and dental professions and in various technical occupations and administrative posts. Meanwhile, aside from the relatively few minority group members with traditional training, a principal minority group force for health care in the inner city is exercised by *consumer* representatives on directing boards and committees of neighborhood health agencies.

THE CONSUMER MOVEMENT IN HEALTH

Consumerism has become a force in the health field, paralleling consumer developments in other areas. Consumerism emerges under several circumstances: when there is dissatisfaction with the ways things are run; when regulatory bodies do not regulate; when changes occur so slowly that the health system or a portion of it must be given a shove; or when too many individuals get the runaround too often at the level of direct service.

The United States Congress has the power to investigate and regulate, and in this capacity—when not bogged down in debate—it acts on behalf of the consumer. The end product of congressional investigation often is amendment to or tightening of existing laws. State and local legislatures sometimes act in the same capacity.

Governmental regulatory agencies are charged with the responsibility of acting in the public interest and on behalf of the consumer. For example, the Food and Drug Administration regulates the introduction and sale of prescription drugs. It has sometimes been criticized for not being tough enough on drug manufacturers in the testing and readying of drugs for sale.

The advent of consumer advocates, the creation of official "consumer offices," and the provision of consumer representation on various health advisory boards are relatively recent developments that may be expected to unfold further in the 1970's. The nation's best-known public consumer advocate is Ralph Nader, whose broad swath of activities frequently touches on health themes and sometimes strikes a sensitive nerve. Nader and a small army of young workers (mainly lawyers) have given visibility to problems of pollution and health services. Some of their targets have included General Motors (auto safety and air pollution), the Food and Drug Administration (drug safety), and the National Institute of Mental Health (relevance of activities to community needs).

The federal government and a number of states have established offices of consumer affairs whose job is to further consumer education and to be responsive to consumer complaints on health as well as other topics. Sometimes these offices act as ombudsmen and seek redress for complaints. Selected official health agencies are appointing consumer representatives to governing bodies and policy boards, particularly (as mentioned earlier) those agencies that provide service to minority communities. Substantial consumer participation is also a feature of official, regional, health planning bodies; and consumer membership is mandatory in community mental health centers across the nation. There are problems, to be sure, in identification and selection of "representative" consumers for advisory-group membership; and sometimes there are serious factional disputes that relate to administrative position and power, control of funds, job allocation, and other interests.

At the point of health delivery, the health consumer—as patient in the hospital, clinic, or other health institution—is often overwhelmed by the "system." To help solve this problem, health institutions are experimenting with the employment of "expediters," variously titled and often new-career employees, who function as ombudsmen. This innovation offers valuable service to the consumer by providing assistance and orientation in what sometimes is a bewildering, if not frightening, experience.

Additional Reading

Rosen, George. *A History of Public Health.* MD Publications, New York, 1957.

Sigerist, Henry E. *Civilization and Disease.* Cornell University Press, Ithaca, 1945.

Sigerist, Henry E. *A History of Medicine,* 2nd ed. Oxford University Press, New York, 1955.

Smillie, Wilson. *Public Health, Its Promise for the Future; A Chronicle of the Development of Public Health in the United States, 1607–1914.* The Macmillan Company, New York, 1955.

Winslow, Charles-Edward Amory. *The Conquest of Epidemic Disease.* Princeton University Press, Princeton, 1944.

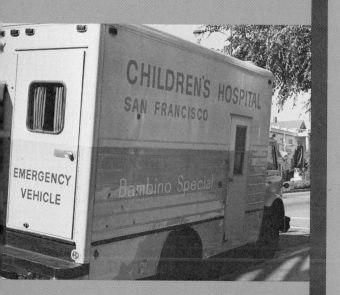

2

ORGANIZATION
OF
PUBLIC HEALTH
SERVICES

CHAPTER OUTLINE

The Need for Organization for Health

The Legal and Governmental Framework of Public Health in the United States

Constitutional Powers and Organization of the Federal Government
The Nature and Intent of Federal Health Legislation
State and Local Health Legislation

Health Roles of the United States Government

Health Programs of the Federal Government
Organization and Change in Federal Health Functions
The U.S. Department of Health, Education, and Welfare
Other Federal Agencies with Health Functions

State and Local Health Services and Organization

Basic Tasks and Range of Services
Health Department Organization
Other Official State and Local Health Agencies

Voluntary Health Agencies

History of Voluntary Health Agencies
Categories and Activities of Voluntary Health Agencies
Organization and Financing of Voluntary Health Agencies
Contributions and Problems in the Voluntary Agency Movement

Foundations

Professional Associations

International Health Agencies

The Need for International Health Work
History of International Health Organization
Principal Contemporary International Health Agencies

Courtesy of California's Health, *California Department of Public Health. Staff photo.*

The Need for Organization for Health

One of the keys to successful organization of health services resides in the increased understanding of the causes, prevention, and cure of disease. As knowledge advanced over the centuries, and the possibilities of control of disease became a reality through the efforts of countless health workers, organization for health took on new meaning and reality.

Today every nation has a ministry of health or federal health department that shapes broad health policy for its citizens and develops broad programs leading to health protection and health maintenance. At state and provincial levels there is organization for health that helps carry out nationally inspired programs. And finally, in counties and cities there are local health departments with broad responsibilities for health protection activities. At all levels, these governmental activities constitute a major force for health.

In the governmental sector there are many other organizations—in addition to health ministries and departments—that deal, for example, with health planning, with mental health, with the health care of older persons, of veterans, and of individuals on welfare. There are other agencies dealing with aspects of the environment, responsible for air pollution control, water purity and safety, and food protection. There are sometimes special agencies that license doctors, nurses, pharmacists, sanitarians, and other professional categories.

In some countries there are only governmentally organized health services (e.g., in England, where there is a national health system). In many countries, however, health concerns are not the sole province of national and local governmental agencies, as important as these are. At the broadest level of nongovernmental agencies is the work of the World Health Organization, active in health protection of the world community. Within any nation and community there is a broad panorama of voluntary and private organizations that have important relationships to health. This is particularly true, for example, in the United States, Canada, and many nations in western Europe, but less true in Latin America, Australia, and countries in Asia and Africa.

In the United States, a comprehensive view of organization for health must include the nation's vast hospital system, including many nongovernmental hospitals; the many health professions associations (to name a few: the American Medical Association, the American Nurses' Association, the American Hospital Association, the American Public Health Association); the voluntary health agencies (e.g., the American Cancer Society, the American Heart Association); the universities and colleges for the education and training of health manpower; and the philanthropic foundations concerned with health. It is a testimonial to the education, standard of living, and human concern that a nation can generate such intense health interests.

It would not be correct to claim that this multiplicity is without problems. Different organizations develop their own ideas about solutions to health problems even when long-term goals are similar or identical. Sometimes any one agency's thoughts are in opposition to others; sometimes one agency ranks its priorities differently from those of other agencies. Sometimes several are competing for public attention and for the same dollars.

It is the continuing goal of organization for health to harness and focus these diverse interests so that the many problems of health and disease can be attacked and overcome. This is the reason for the numerous attempts reported daily in the press to reshape plans and objectives, to reorganize existing agencies, and to organize new ones when necessary to meet the health problems of the day.

The Legal and Governmental Framework of Public Health in the United States

CONSTITUTIONAL POWERS AND ORGANIZATION OF THE FEDERAL GOVERNMENT

Public health activities in the United States are covered by legal provisions at all levels of government. Sometimes these laws are *enabling*, i.e., provide for the establishment of programs and organizations, and frequently specify amounts of money to carry activities forward. Sometimes the laws are *prohibitive*, i.e., specify what may and may not be done and often prescribe the range of punishments that may be invoked when the law is broken, as well as naming the agency to enforce the statutes.

At the federal level, the basis of public health is imbedded in the United States Constitution, within which both national and state governments operate. The authors of the Constitution used certain broad and general phrases which have permitted considerable latitude in interpretation with respect to matters of public health. An example of such phrasing is the basic mandate to the federal government to "promote the general welfare," which occurs in the Preamble to the Constitution.[1]* In addition, the body of the Constitution grants several powers to the federal government that have been interpreted to include health activities. Thus, the power to regulate commerce with foreign nations and among the several states (Art. I, sec. 8) has been construed as including such matters as international and interstate quarantine, sanitary supervision, and vital statistics. The power to levy taxes "to provide for the common defense and general welfare" (Art. I, sec. 8) permits, for example, federal government activity in maternal and child health and the subsidization of state and local health programs. The power to raise, support, and make rules for the regulation of the land and naval forces (Art. III, sec. 8) has given to federal agencies the reponsibility for maintaining the health of the armed forces. Still other opportunities for health activities are provided by the power to exercise exclusive legislation in federal territory (the District of Columbia, military bases, national parks, Indian reservations, etc.; Art. I, sec. 8) and by the power to make treaties (Art. II, sec. 2). Finally, an omnibus provision grants the federal government the authority "to make all Laws which shall be necessary and proper for carrying into Execution the foregoing Powers, and all other Powers vested by this Constitution in the Government of the United States, or in any Department or Officer thereof" (Art. III, sec. 8).

The powers vested in the federal government by the Constitution are considerable and permit opportunity for the exercise of leadership in developing and implementing policy (including health policy) based on changing concepts, philosophy, and community needs. Over the years, the intent, interpretation, and application of the Constitution and Bill of Rights have changed. These changes have come about through Constitutional amendments, Supreme Court decisions, unchallenged state laws and administrative law, and socially accepted practices. As a consequence, there has been an accelerated increase in the role and influence of federal law

* Throughout the book, the superscript numbers pertain to references that appear at the end of each chapter.

and administration on state and local governments in meeting health and social problems.

At the federal level, *the Congress,* a bicameral body, enacts national laws and appropriates tax monies for support of governmental activities, including those of a health and welfare nature. The *executive branch,* headed by the President and composed of many departments and special agencies, has the responsibility of carrying out the provisions of the Constitution and its amendments, all other national legislation (including that affecting health and welfare), and federal court interpretations of the laws. The *judicial branch,* composed of the Supreme Court and lower federal courts, interprets all national laws and constitutional amendments (including those affecting the health and welfare of individuals and groups). This general distribution of function—executive, legislative, and judicial—is found typically also at state and local levels.

THE NATURE AND INTENT OF FEDERAL HEALTH LEGISLATION

Changes in organization for health to meet contemporary problems take place as a consequence of activities in the governmental and private (including voluntary) sectors. In some respects governmental activity is the most vital element—sometimes the most visible—and deserves particular attention. In all activities there is considerable interplay among governments at federal, state, and local levels.

The twentieth century has been marked by an expansion not only in the quantity but also in the variety of federal health legislation generated by the United States government. Congress has enacted several general kinds of measures, including the creation of new services and programs; the training of personnel for the health professions; the support of basic and applied research on a vast array of health-related topics; and, periodically when required, the organization and reorganization of administrative structures in an effort to optimize the delivery of health services.

A basic aim of federal health and health-related legislation enacted in recent years has been to establish integrated, federal-state-local programs which will strengthen the roles of the lower-echelon governments as effective instruments of public policy. The intention is to stimulate the development of better community health programs by supporting local governments in health activities and by encouraging the growth of regional jurisdictions to solve the health and social problems of modern America.

Since national health affairs often have a decided political coloration, it is well to note the structure and climate within which national health legislation arises. While legislation is introduced and enacted in the Congress, it may originate in the executive branch, the elements and back-up being ordinarily developed by the federal department involved (for example, Health, Education, and Welfare), as well, sometimes, as by outside agencies and organizations sympathetic to the legislation. Such bills are formally introduced by congressmen friendly to the executive administration and to the intent of the proposed program. Often, and particularly when the majority political party of the Congress is not the same as the political party of the President, health legislation originates in the Congress itself. In such cases the details of the legislation and back-up are developed by the personal staffs of the congressmen involved, by the staffs of standing or special congressional committees, and sometimes with the assistance of outside agencies and organizations.

After a bill is introduced in Congress, there are various circumstances that can influence its chances of passage. One is the amount of political appeal the proposed legislation has. Another is the magnitude of the consequences the bill can be expected to have, if passed. While some legislation has a neutral character, other legislation quickly finds individuals and groups choosing up sides. For example, continuing high on the lists for the next generation, no doubt, will be the politically potent legislative attempts to cope with the national pollution crisis (air, water, waste, etc.) as well as efforts to propel forward health care strategies suitable to the needs of all people in the present day. In such cases, it comes as no surprise that much heated debate is generated attending consideration and passage or defeat of a bill.

A significant influence on the final provisions of a legislative measure comes from the need for both houses of Congress to agree on identical bills for passage. This often requires House-Senate conferring on the proposed legislation. The tenor of most legislation as a result is often tinged with adjustment and compromise.

As with all legislation, national health measures requiring expenditures of federal funds must include appropriation as well as authorization for expenditure. Authorization is, in effect, a limit on what Congress feels should be spent in connection with a health program. Appropriation is what Congress actually allocates in a given year, sometimes far below the authorization. In past periods, particularly in the 1950's and early 1960's, it was not uncommon for authorizations (and actual appropriations) to be in excess of that called for in introductory legislation. For example, final congressional appropriations for the National Institutes of Health were frequently higher than those asked for in the originating Administration bill. In tighter fiscal times, the opposite is the case, with a

TABLE 2-1. Important U.S. Federal Health Legislation and Administrative Actions

1946	Hill-Burton legislation authorizing federal assistance in the construction of hospitals and health centers.
1948	Creation of the National Heart Institute and the National Institute of Dental Research as part of a broadened National Institutes of Health.
1949	Establishment of a common system of ten regional offices of the Federal Security Agency (later to become the nucleus of the Department of Health, Education, and Welfare).
1953	Establishment of the Department of Health, Education, and Welfare as a cabinet-status agency, combining under one roof health and related activities formerly residing in many federal departments and agencies.
1956	Authorization of the National Health Survey, a continuing interview and clinical appraisal of the health of Americans.
	Establishment of the National Library of Medicine.
1958	Passage of amendments to the Food, Drug and Cosmetic Act requiring manufacturers of new food additives to submit evidence to the Food and Drug Administration that a product's safety had been tested and established before marketing.
1960	Establishment of the Division of Air Pollution in the Public Health Service.
1961	Establishment of a Division of Chronic Diseases; and a five-year program of grants in the field of juvenile delinquency.
1962	Organization of a Special Staff on Aging, later to become the Administration on Aging.
1963	Passage of the Health Professions Educational Assistance Act to help meet critical manpower shortages; the Mental Retardation Facilities and Community Mental Health Centers Construction Act; and the Clean Air Act giving assistance to state and local governments to meet the problems of air pollution.
1964	Passage of the Nurse Training Act, aiding construction of new schools of nursing and expansion of existing schools, loans for nursing students, and support for curriculum development.
	Passage of the Economic Opportunity Act and the Civil Rights Act of 1964, both with broad meaning for health aspects of urban and rural life.
1965	Establishment of the Federal Water Pollution Control Administration; establishment of the National Clearinghouse for Smoking and Health.
	Establishment of Regional Medical Programs to attack the problems of heart disease, cancer and stroke by cooperative regional arrangements among medical schools and hospitals to make available to patients the latest advances in diagnosis and treatment of these major diseases.

1966	Passage of Medicare legislation which resulted in hospital insurance and other benefits for approximately 19 million Americans 65 years of age or older. Medicaid, a corollary program for welfare recipients, became effective the same year.
	Major reorganization of the Public Health Service.
	Passage of Comprehensive Health Planning legislation that furthered the proposition that planning for the health of states and communities must involve broad cooperation among governmental agencies, nongovernmental groups and organizations as well as representatives of consumers of health services.
1967	Establishment of a Center for Community Planning (U.S. Department of Health, Education, and Welfare) to coordinate programs with Model Cities Projects of the Department of Housing and Urban Development.
	National Institute of Mental Health authorized to launch new research programs in suicide prevention, alcoholism, and drug abuse.
	Passage of the Clinical Laboratories Improvement Act authorizing establishment of minimum performance standards for all clinical laboratories engaged in interstate commerce.
1968	Vocational Rehabilitation Amendments extended appropriations for grants to states for services, innovation projects, and training.
	Juvenile Delinquency Prevention and Control Act passed providing for research, training, and assistance for diagnosis, treatment, and rehabilitation for delinquents or predelinquents.
1969	Establishment of the National Center for Family Planning to assist 5 million low-income women of childbearing age who desire family planning services but who cannot afford them.
1970	Migrant Health Amendments extended health services for migrant and other seasonal agricultural workers.
	Creation of the Environmental Protection Agency, bringing together under one roof all federal programs for controlling air and water pollution, solid wastes, pesticides, and radiation.

Not included in the above are countless executive orders on health matters, reorganizations and regroupings of existing agencies, and national conferences (including notably White House Conferences on Children and on Aging, and National Conferences on Health Manpower).

SOURCE: Adapted from U.S. Department of Health, Education, and Welfare, Office of the Secretary, *A Common Thread of Service*, 1970.

scaling-down process in evidence prior to passage and, if the bill is made into law, with final money appropriation even below the agreed upon authorization.

Despite the complexities of the legislative process, dozens of federal laws are passed annually, many with far-reaching consequences for the health of individuals, groups, and communities in the United States. The administrative superstructure (executive branch) needed to supervise and manage the developing programs and disbursement of funds is discussed in a later section of this chapter.

Table 2-1 shows some important federal legislation and administrative actions taken since 1946 that have come as responses to national health needs and which have, in turn, affected the health and lives of millions of Americans. The enactment of federal laws such as those summarized in Table 2-1 may be viewed as a significant form of "creative federalism" which extends and expands the partnership of federal, state, and local agencies. Federal programs of this nature rely on local initiative and the strength of local government and local officials to solve the more pressing social and other domestic problems that confront America in the last third of the twentieth century. In the process, the federal income tax dollar is returned to the states, regional bodies, and local governments in order that these governments can, by a concerted and well-organized effort, attack their own problems and, in doing so, improve the health and welfare of the entire nation.

STATE AND LOCAL HEALTH LEGISLATION

In the United States each state is a sovereign power, and through its state constitution has responsibility for and authority to protect the health of people within its geographic boundaries. New issues are met by adoption of specific health laws or statutes by state legislatures. State and local laws must, of course, be compatible with American constitutional provisions.

Federal-state relationships are based on (1) the principle that the states are inseparable units of one nation rather than independent governments and (2) provisions of the Constitution whereby certain powers are delegated to the federal government, certain powers are prohibited to the states, and all powers not so delegated or prohibited are reserved for the people and their states. Around these constitutional provisions the so-called states' rights issue has arisen frequently from the earliest years of the nation to the present time. The "reserved" powers of the states are not clearly defined, and from time to time controversy arises as to whether a power asserted by the federal government or by a state is valid under the

Constitution. No state may determine such issues for itself. The United States Supreme Court determines the line between federal and state powers, and its decisions have the force of national law.

The states have broad powers to organize their own government, to generate programs to meet social needs, and to raise revenues to support these programs. They also have the power to organize local governments and to authorize the levy of local taxes. The federal government intervenes in state activities when foods, drugs, and biologic products are sold in interstate commerce or when certain problems arise that are beyond the control of an individual state. A good example is the interstate pollution of common waterways by cities and industries. When cities and states pollute water or use an inequitable amount of any natural resources to the detriment or disadvantage of surrounding states, the federal government has the power to intervene for mutual protection of all population groups. Thus, when one level of government fails to meet the needs of the people, the next higher level undertakes action through policy legislation and financing of programs.

Within the broad framework just described, general health policy, philosophy, and intent are established by the state legislature in a manner similar to that followed at the national level. Legislative bills are introduced in response to need or other felt pressures and eventually, through normal legislative processes, become law. There follows implementation of the new health regulations by some executive arm, e.g., the governing body of the state health department (which is usually the state board of health). These regulations then are enforced or monitored by state or local health agencies. In the event that a city or county fails, refuses, or is otherwise unable to cope with its health problems, the state may lend assistance, or it may even assume control, as it has on occasion.

No two states have the same system of resolution of problems of health and social need, and few states are consistent in the application of their sovereign powers to specific issues. In fact, the exercise of these powers has resulted in 50 different state sanitary codes, 50 different requirements for marriage and divorce, legal adoption, education and employment of children, licensure of practitioners of the healing arts, safety of buildings, eligibility for public assistance and medical care, procedures for handling the mentally ill and retarded, and so on.

Local government has only the authority that the state delegates, and on this basis it adopts ordinances as well as supplementary rules and regulations. Through federal, state, and local governmental mechanisms, there is now some sort of legal provision in almost every community for the reporting of births and deaths, the reporting of certain communicable diseases, food and milk control,

TABLE 2-2. Selected State and Local Health Laws and Amendments Enacted or Adopted in 1969–1971

COLORADO

Passage of a law requiring women under age 55 applying for a marriage license to obtain—in addition to the test for syphilis—tests for rubella immunity, blood group, and Rh type.

CONNECTICUT

Estuaries along the shore closed to the taking of shellfish because of contamination.

FLORIDA

Compulsory certification of water and sewage treatment plant operators.

GEORGIA

Passage of laws defining alcoholism and drug dependence or abuse as illnesses and public health problems affecting the general welfare, revising all previous laws relating to the care and treatment of individuals addicted to alcohol or drugs.

ILLINOIS

Passage of an Environment Protection Act and establishing an Environmental Protection Agency, Pollution Control Board, and Institute for Environmental Quality.

INDIANA

Passage of legislation giving counties authority to enact air pollution ordinances.

Authorization for a plan for diagnostic and evaluative services to the handicapped.

NEW YORK STATE

Immunization against rubella made compulsory for schoolchildren; establishment of a board of examiners to license nursing home administrators; legalization of abortions by licensed physicians within 24 weeks of the beginning of pregnancy.

ERIE COUNTY

Regulation passed compelling each industry to inventory every emission from its smokestacks.

LOS ANGELES COUNTY

Los Angeles County Health Officer given administrative and coordinative responsibility for county alcoholic rehabilitation program.

NEW YORK CITY

Health code amendment passed requiring that with every birth certificate there be included a letter urging mothers to get postpartum care.

SEATTLE-KINGS COUNTY

Ordinances adopted for sanitation of public and semipublic swimming and wading pools.

CITY OF ST. LOUIS

Ordinance passed to institute a lead poison control program providing for screening, education, and inspection.

SOURCE: Annual reports (1969–1971) of specified state and local health departments.

and environmental sanitation. Such provisions are considered to be the minimum, basic public health laws needed to monitor and protect the health of the community. Many communities are developing laws either directly or indirectly related to health which go well beyond these minimum requirements. Financial support by the federal government to the states and by the states to local governments influences the quality and kinds of health programs and the administration of services by local health agencies.

Annually, many state and local health laws and amendments are enacted that affect residents of the state, region, and locality. These laws and amendments are embodied in the health (or health and safety) codes of the different states and localities. Some new enactments take their inspiration and cues from national legislation, and some are frank efforts to align state procedures to permit participation in federal funding. Many, on the other hand, represent the most concerned efforts to develop health legislation in the best interests of state and local residents, and sometimes appear more farsighted than the federal view of the same issues. Table 2-2 shows sample health laws and codes enacted in selected states and localities in 1969–1971.

Health Roles of the United States Government

HEALTH PROGRAMS OF THE FEDERAL GOVERNMENT

As has been seen, the health activities of the United States government are authorized by specific laws designed to achieve particular objectives. The programs are financed by appropriations passed by Congress each year, and they are administered by various federal departments and other executive bodies. The specific functions may be classified broadly as dealing with the health of the general population, with the health of special population groups, and with international health.

Functions Dealing with the General Population. Health functions that the federal government undertakes for the general population include (1) protection against hazards affecting the entire population which cannot be provided by the states; (2) collection and dissemination of national vital and health statistics and related data; (3) advancement of the biologic, medical, and environmental sciences; (4) augmentation of health facilities and certain categories of health personnel; (5) support of state and local governments in the maintenance of public health services; and (6) organization and support of disaster relief and civil defense.

Functions Dealing with Special Population Groups. The special population groups and the kinds of health measures provided for them by the federal government are (1) protection of certain classes of workers against hazardous occupations and adverse conditions of work; (2) provision of categorical and special services by state and local governments for children, the aged, the mentally ill and retarded, the economically deprived, vocationally handicapped adults, and blind persons; (3) purchase of medical care by state and local governments for certain financially dependent population groups; (4) provision of special services for farm families; (5) provision of hospital and medical care to veterans, merchant seamen, American Indians and Alaska natives, federal prisoners, narcotic addicts, persons with leprosy, members of the "uniformed services" (e.g., the Army, Navy, Coast Guard, and commissioned officers of the Public Health Service) and their dependents, and civil service employees of the government injured as a result of their employment; and (6) hospital and medical insurance for civil service employees of the federal government.

Functions Dealing with International Health. Participation of the United States government in international health activities is based on the intention to make this country's public health knowledge available to other nations, particularly those developing countries where there are still high disease and death rates owing to malnutrition, poor environmental sanitation, and inadequate health care programs. In addition, there are growing sentiment and experience that much is to be learned in international health work of direct benefit to the United States and its inhabitants. Toward this end, the federal government maintains membership in the World Health Organization and is involved in the health activities of such international organizations as the Pan-American Union, the Organization of American States, the North Atlantic Treaty Organization, and the Southeast Asia Treaty Organization. In addition, the government participates in the conduct of health programs through bilateral treaties with the governments of Canada and Mexico and certain countries in Central and South America, Africa, the Eastern Mediterranean, Southeast Asia, and the Southwest Pacific. The federal government also makes financial grants for the conduct of research in the health sciences *in* foreign countries and for fellowships for the training of health personnel *from* foreign countries.

ORGANIZATION AND CHANGE IN FEDERAL HEALTH FUNCTIONS

The health functions just described are widely distributed throughout various departments and other organizations of the

United States government. The greatest concentration of health activities resides in the Department of Health, Education, and Welfare, although there are sizable health functions carried out by several other federal agencies.

The particular placement of a given activity in government is sometimes as much a matter of historical development and organizational ties and energies as it is of rational decision-making. This phenomenon is characteristic of all complex social organizations, and the federal bureaucracy is no exception. In all branches of government, at every level—local, state, and federal—there are repeated attempts to reorganize activities into more sensible, more manageable, and more efficient entities.

Even while reorganizations go on, current health problems give rise to agencies outside the "organized" departments set up for these functions. American presidents since Woodrow Wilson have created special "offices" and special "staffs" for carrying out health functions, sometimes out of impatience with the productivity of an agency in an older organizational setting, or with an eye to upgrading the importance of the health activity in question. For example, as will be seen, important programs in environmental health were regrouped in 1970 into the Environmental Protection Agency, drawing on elements in the Public Health Service and other existing agencies. There was created in 1971 a Special Action Office for Drug Abuse Prevention—with direct responsibility to the White House—in recognition of the crisis nature of the drug problem in the United States. Federal agencies for health may be expected to be in flux for at least a generation in the face of changing priorities that depend upon new modes of organizing health care, new medical advances, and new environmental developments.

THE U.S. DEPARTMENT OF HEALTH, EDUCATION, AND WELFARE

Created in 1953, the U.S. Department of Health, Education, and Welfare took over the functions and components of the Federal Security Agency (established in the depression years of the 1930's), which was then abolished. The purpose of the new department was to improve the administration of those agencies of the federal government that have major responsibility in promoting the general welfare in the fields of health, education, and social security.

The programs of the Department of Health, Education, and Welfare are currently administered by *six operating agencies* (the Department is also responsible for *three federally aided corporations:* American Printing House for the Blind, Gallaudet College, and Howard University). As shown in Figure 2-1, three of the operating agencies are components of the Public Health Service, consisting of the Food

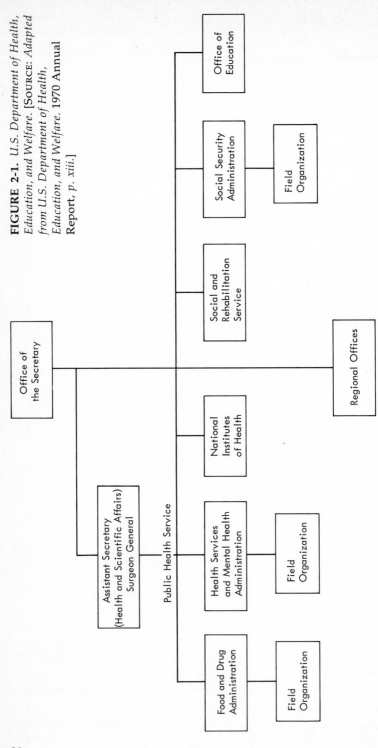

FIGURE 2-1. *U.S. Department of Health, Education, and Welfare.* [SOURCE: *Adapted from U.S. Department of Health, Education, and Welfare. 1970 Annual Report, p. xiii.*]

Office of the Secretary

Assistant Secretary (Health and Scientific Affairs) Surgeon General

Public Health Service

Food and Drug Administration

Field Organization

Health Services and Mental Health Administration

Field Organization

National Institutes of Health

Social and Rehabilitation Service

Social Security Administration

Field Organization

Office of Education

Regional Offices

and Drug Administration (FDA), the Health Services and Mental Health Administration (HSMHA), and the National Institutes of Health (NIH).† The remaining three agencies are the Social and Rehabilitation Service (SRS), the Social Security Administration (SSA), and the Office of Education (OE). The latter agencies, although not primarily concerned with health in the way the Public Health Service is, nevertheless have health-related elements in their programs. For example, the Social and Rehabilitation Service deals with health matters related to the medically indigent (the Medicaid program). The Social Security Administration administers the massive Medicare program. The Office of Education joins with the Public Health Service in the education and training of needed health manpower.

Department regional offices are maintained in each of ten areas in the United States, as shown in Figure 2-2. While regional offices have always had important roles in coordination and general program consultation within their areas, HEW has recently strengthened substantially the regional organization by shifting line authority to regional directors and agency heads.[2]

In the years since 1954, the Department of Health, Education, and Welfare has grown enormously, with vastly increased responsibilities. Federal operating budgets rose tenfold in 17 years, from $1.9 billion in 1954 to $19.9 billion (estimated) in 1971 (Table 2-3). Personnel rose threefold in the same period, from a total of 35,000 to 108,000. Two and a half times as many persons are employed in the regions as in metropolitan Washington.[3]

The Department is thus seen as a large conglomerate superorganization, and there have been many suggestions about

TABLE 2-3. Budget and Personnel in the U.S. Department of Health, Education, and Welfare, Selected Years

	Federal Operating Budget* (in billions)	Personnel	
		Washington, D.C.	All Other Areas
1954	$1.9	10,685	24,757
1960	$3.5	17,803	43,838
1965	$7.1	26,826	60,490
1970 (est.)	$17.4	29,469	77,963
1971 (est.)	$19.9	—	—

* Does not include Social Security Trust Funds, which in 1971 amounted to approximately $46.8 billion.

Source: U.S. Department of Health, Education, and Welfare, Office of the Secretary. *A Common Thread of Service*, 1970, p. 40.

†By January 1974, the Public Health Service had been reorganized into six major operating agencies, as shown in the chart on the front and back covers.

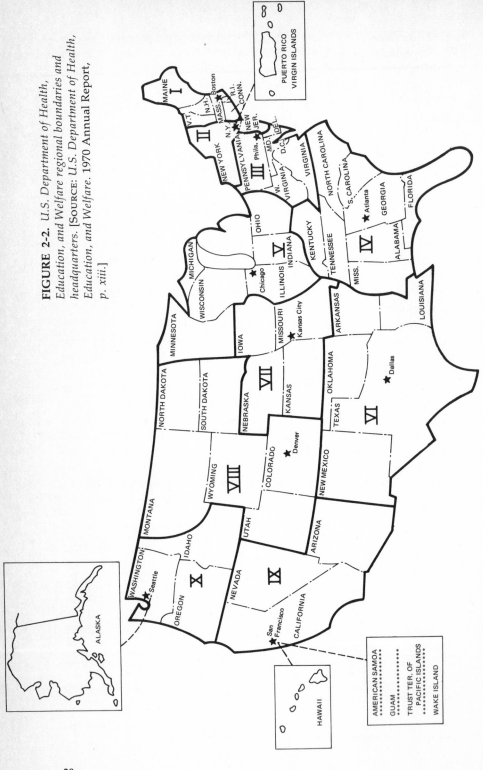

FIGURE 2-2. *U.S. Department of Health, Education, and Welfare regional boundaries and headquarters.* [SOURCE: *U.S. Department of Health, Education, and Welfare. 1970 Annual Report, p. xiii.*]

placing some of the entities in their own separate departments. For example, why should an agency with a health focus be in the same department as one with an education focus? More importantly, can one cabinet officer properly represent all the interests of such a diverse department? Several former secretaries of the Department, in its brief existence of about 20 years, have declared it to be unmanageable. Despite these seeming incongruities, the Department remains the single most potent federal force for health.

The Public Health Service (PHS). As one of the key organizations charged with responsibilities for health protection and health improvement of the nation, the Public Health Service is involved with every imaginable aspect of the health scene. Through its constituent agencies it is concerned with support of direct service programs (not only to states and localities but also directly to federal beneficiary populations such as federal employees and American Indians). It supports scientific and related research. It supports the search for improvement of health services. It is broadly involved in the development of health personnel of all kinds.[4]

These general functions have expanded rapidly in recent years, and countless new specific programs have been added. Annual congressional appropriations have increased in order to keep pace with expanding responsibilities. For example, in 1953 the appropriation to the Service was $222 million; in 1963 it was $1.6 billion; in 1971 it exceeded $3 billion.[5,6]

The extraordinary and rapid growth of the Public Health Service has brought on problems of organization and management of its hundreds of programs and related activities. Since 1946 there has been a dizzying succession of organizational attempts to grapple with the many responsibilities. Figure 2-3 shows the organizational entities *within* the three operating agencies of the Public Health Service that were functional in 1971–1972.*

PHS: Food and Drug Administration. The herculean task of guarding the safety and effectiveness of foods, drugs, medical devices, and cosmetics used in interstate commerce is the responsibility of the Food and Drug Administration (FDA). This embraces most items found on shelves in supermarkets and drugstores as well as prescription drugs and items of manufacture used in health care procedures. Aside from basic concepts of purity, safety, and wholesomeness, examples of concern of the FDA include the honest

---

*By January 1974, the Public Health Service had been further reorganized into six major operating agencies, as shown in the chart on the front and back covers.

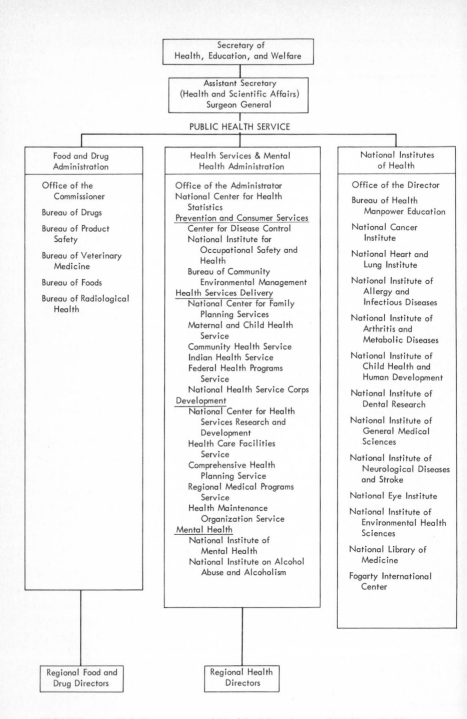

FIGURE 2-3. *U.S. Department of Health, Education, and Welfare, Public Health Service.* [SOURCE: *U.S. Department of Health, Education, and Welfare, Office of the Secretary, January 1972.*]

and informative labeling of contents, adequate warnings for safe use and handling, and the prevention and control of contamination.[2]

Of high concern today is the matter of side-effects of drugs used in medical practice. Few items in the drug, product safety, and food line escape attention by the FDA. Its functions are to establish high standards for manufacture, for product testing and surveillance, and for speedy and corrective action in the event hazards and dangers are detected in products in distribution. While compliance with safety regulations depends on broad voluntary agreement on the part of manufacturers, the FDA is also armed with enforcement powers to back up its findings in specific instances.

PHS: Health Services and Mental Health Administration.   Perhaps the broadest range of activities of any of HEW's operating agencies is found in the Health Services and Mental Health Administration (HSMHA). It comprises no fewer than 17 major components, the unifying threads being the mandate to provide leadership for improvement of health services for physical and mental diseases.[2] In 1972, the HSMHA activities were grouped into four sectors.

First, there is the Prevention and Consumer Services sector, which has organized units concerned with (a) the prevention and control of communicable and other preventable diseases, (b) occupational safety and health, and (c) selected elements of environmental management in communities (e.g., rat control and lead poisoning eradication). In 1972, this group of services had a budget of $145 million, with $79 million earmarked for grant and contract awards.

Second, the Health Services Delivery sector groups together important organized units in the field of maternal and child health, family planning, Indian health, the health of federal employees, and general health of communities. These are a set of programs which involve federal stimulation of state and local services, and frequently also involve substantial research and training support. The newest element is the National Health Service Corps, operational in 1972, designed specifically to attract doctors and nurses to urban ghettos, rural areas, and other settings that ordinarily have a severe shortage of these and other health professionals. The 1972 budget for Health Services Delivery amounted to $857 million, including $586 million for grant and contract awards.

Third, the Development sector, with organized units devoted to broad health planning in the United States, comprises "centers" or "services" for research and development, for health facilities planning and support (hospital construction funds), for comprehensive health planning, and for regional medical programs. Also included

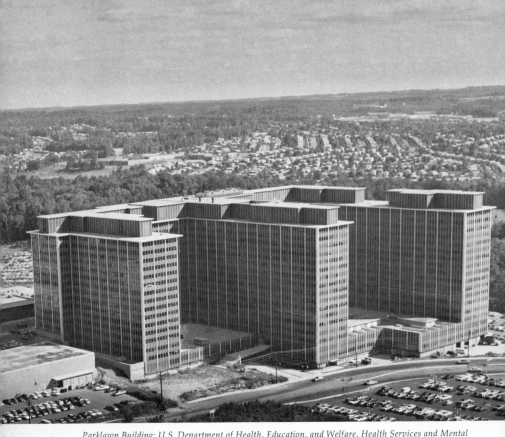

Parklawn Building: U.S. Department of Health, Education, and Welfare, Health Services and Mental Health Administration, and Food and Drug Administration. Courtesy of Parklawn Joint Venture, Bethesda, Maryland.

Courtesy of U.S. Department of Health, Education, and Welfare, National Institutes of Health.

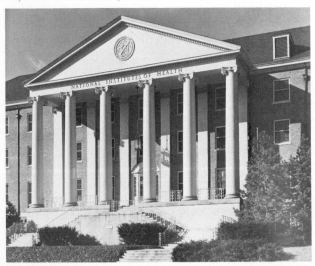

is a new element devoted to the furtherance of the concept of Health Maintenance Organizations, a variety of group medical practice with prepayment features based on known populations served. In 1972, HSMHA provided $418 million in its annual budget for development, including $405 million for grant and contract awards.

Fourth, is a sector devoted to mental health and consisting of the National Institute of Mental Health (NIMH), which addresses itself to the mental health problems of the United States through funding programs of service, training, and research. NIMH funds a broad program of support for construction and staffing of a network of approximately 400 comprehensive community mental health centers across the nation. The 1972 budget for mental health was $639 million, including $556 million for grant and contract awards. Long-range research interests of NIMH include schizophrenia and depression as well as alcoholism and narcotics abuse. NIMH supports training in medical schools and schools of nursing, social work, and public health. A new institute within NIMH is the National Institute on Alcohol Abuse and Alcoholism.

PHS: National Institutes of Health.   Through a system of separate categorical disease institutes designated as the National Institutes of Health (NIH), the federal government supports basic and applied research in the cause, treatment, and prevention of disease. It accomplishes these goals through relevant laboratory activity at the main institute campus and environs in Bethesda, Maryland (just northwest of the city limits of Washington, D.C.) and through a system of grants and contracts to universities, public and private research institutes, hospitals, and health departments.[2]

Manpower development is furthered in two ways by the National Institutes of Health. Each separate institute maintains a training program for the development of scientists and related technical personnel. The Bureau of Health Manpower Education (a component of NIH) has responsibility for the development and training of health personnel generally—doctors, nurses, dentists, and other categories of public health workers. Training of all kinds is supported by grants and contracts for faculty enlargement and improvement, student support in the form of sums (grants and/or loans) for tuition, fees, and personal stipends. The support extends to building and construction of facilities for the enhancement of education in the health sciences.

There are ten categorical institutes, including those devoted to cancer, diseases of heart and lung, eye diseases, child health and human development. There is also an institute devoted to "general medical sciences" (an important catchall). Table 2-4 gives some inkling of the priorities (dollar totals) of grants and awards made by

TABLE 2-4. Grant Awards for Research and Training Made by the National Institutes of Health, Fiscal Year 1970

NIH Component	Total (millions of dollars)
Bureau of Health Manpower Education	485.9
Institutes	
General Medical Sciences	132.3
Heart and Lung	130.3
Cancer	129.3
Arthritis and Metabolic Diseases	102.9
Neurological Diseases and Stroke	73.2
Allergy and Infectious Diseases	69.7
Child Health and Human Development	60.1
Dental Research	20.6
Eye	19.9
Environmental Health Sciences	11.6

SOURCE: U.S. Department of Health, Education, and Welfare. *Public Health Service Grants and Awards,* Part II, 1971, pp. 2 and 3.

the institutes for fiscal 1970. In that year the extramural support programs for all institute and manpower programs exceeded $1.25 billion.

The National Institutes of Health also maintains the National Library of Medicine. The library has the most extensive collection of medical literature in the world, exceeding one million items (books, journal serials, etc.). Bibliographic access to its collections is provided through MEDLARS, a computerized information storage and retrieval system, and through the publication of guides in the form of catalogs, indexes, and bibliographies. The library supports the translation and publication of biomedical literature and administers a program for the support of medical library development.[2]

OTHER FEDERAL AGENCIES WITH HEALTH FUNCTIONS

Significant responsibilities for health aspects of the environment are placed in the Environmental Protection Agency (EPA), which was created in 1970. To it were transferred from other agencies several research, monitoring, standard-setting, and enforcement activities in the environmental health field. The new agency (see Chapter 8) was established to overcome the growing dissatisfaction with the separation and fragmentation that had developed over the years as first one, then another, environmental problem gained public attention and resulted in the creation of a governmental unit to deal with it. In the EPA there are separate offices for air and water quality programs as well as offices concerned with pesticides, radiation, and solid waste management. The hope—not realized in past organizational efforts—is for the development in this new and important agency of a broad policy for the protection of an endangered environment.

Many other federal agencies have health functions which are secondary or supplementary to their main mission. Thus, the Departments of the Army, Navy, and Air Force administer medical services for military personnel and their dependents; the Veterans Administration has a corresponding function for war veterans; the Department of Justice provides medical care for federal prisoners; and the Department of State operates a medical program for Foreign Service personnel on duty outside the United States.

The Department of Labor administers federal laws related to conditions of work, including industrial health, safety standards, and the employment of children. In the administration of these laws, the Department works with the labor departments of the various states in order to coordinate the enforcement of federal and state regulations. Legislation passed in 1971 (the Williams-Steiger Occupational Health and Safety Act) gave the Department of Labor important functions in prevention and control of occupational hazards to life.[7] Training and standard-setting functions of this act reside with the National Institute for Occupational Safety and Health (HSMHA).

The federal government also exercises regulatory powers over certain specific industries which directly affect the public health and safety. Thus, the Bureau of Mines (Department of the Interior) has responsibility for safety and healthful working conditions in the mineral industries. The Atomic Energy Commission has responsibility to protect the health and safety of the public in matters concerning the development, use, and control of atomic energy. The Federal Aviation Agency promulgates a variety of safety regulations with respect to air commerce; the U.S. Coast Guard (Department of Treasury) is responsible for maritime safety; and the Interstate Commerce Commission enforces safety regulations pertaining to common carriers by railroad and highway, including the transportation of explosives and other dangerous items. The Department of Agriculture regulates livestock in an attempt to eradicate animal diseases and inspects domestic and imported meat and meat products. The Office of Economic Opportunity, directed to low-income groups in both urban and rural settings, has health components, particularly in its support of neighborhood health centers.

State and Local Health Services and Organization

BASIC TASKS AND RANGE OF SERVICES

Official state and local health departments customarily perform several basic tasks, including planning of program, organization, and administration in connection with agency operation and the delivery of services, and evaluation of the programs that are in operation. *Planning* generally involves the assessment of health needs and already existing resources, the definition of purposes and objectives of a proposed new program, and the determination of which of several possible needs is most pressing. *Organizational and administrative* tasks consist of policy-making, implementation of program plans, internal management of the agency (e.g., personnel and finances), and coordination of activities both internally and with outside agencies. Through *evaluation,* the agency assesses the quality and effectiveness of its programs, and the results of such activity in turn influence planning and organization. Evaluation, heavily emphasized in recent years, is generally accomplished through the assembly and assessment of various kinds of information which may be accumulated either on an ongoing basis or through special studies.

These basic tasks are performed to some extent by health agencies at both the state and local (county and metropolitan) levels. However, a state agency is more likely to be concerned with policy, planning, legislation, consultation for local agencies, indirect services, financial support, organizational relationships, and research and evaluation. A local agency is more likely to provide direct services to the public such as medical care, preventive services, and environmental control. Many state health departments have provision within their organization for the coordination of planning, policy, and services with the lower-echelon units which implement the programs. In California, for example, this relationship has been recognized by the state legislature, resulting in the formation of a formal operational organization known as the Conference of Local Health Officers. The Conference is concerned with statewide planning, policy, standards, and direct health services.

Wide varieties of services and programs are provided by state and local health departments which are similar at both levels but have different functions. A local agency in connection with its provision of direct services operates clinics, conducts immunization programs, inspects and licenses certain public facilities, monitors air pollution, among its other services. A state agency enforces state health laws and regulations and coordinates and provides overall direction for the programs and services of all local units within its jurisdiction. Typically found in a health department, whether state or local, are the following general kinds of programs, each usually having several specific aspects: preventive medical and personal health care services; environmental health services; patient care facilities and services; and supportive services, including certain professional specialties, research, and laboratory and administrative services.

Preventive Medical and Personal Health Care Services.   Several programs of state and local health departments emphasize prevention (although they may have other functions as well) and are directed essentially toward personal health care. *Communicable disease services* and *chronic disease services* deal with disease entities and are concerned with etiology, prevention, detection, treatment, and rehabilitation. *Maternal and child health services,* in addition to providing programs for maintaining the health and preventing illness of mother and child, are also concerned with maternal and infant mortality, prematurity, school health problems, and the mentally or physically handicapped child (services for crippled children are sometimes in a separate organizational unit). *Occupational health services* exercise surveillance of the work environment in order to prevent illness, injury, and disability and to improve the physical and mental health of various categories of workers. *Dental health services* are involved with public education regarding the need for fluoridation of public water supplies, promotion of individual dental health, local dental health programs, clinics, and increased availability of private and public dental services. *Alcoholism services,* sometimes including narcotic addiction, are concerned with both prevention and rehabilitation.

Environmental Health Services.   Programs and services in this category are responsible for achieving and maintaining a physical and biologic environment for the entire population which will enhance survival, prevent disease and disability, and improve health, safety, and comfort. The environmental health activities of state and local health departments are often subdivided into several programs. *Sanitary engineering services* deal with purity of domestic water supplies, disposal of various kinds of wastes, and prevention of contamination of recreational resources (swimming pools, lakes, streams, and coastal areas). *Food and drug control programs* are concerned with standards of safety and purity in the production and processing of foods and the manufacture and sale of drugs and cosmetics. *Pollution control services* involve the assessment of hazards to human, animal, and plant life that come from a variety of environmental pollutants and contaminants. *Vector control services* deal with the control of insects and rodents when they are sources of the transmission of disease; and more recently, these services have also become concerned with the hazards arising from the overuse or improper use of pesticides. *Radiologic health services* are responsible for monitoring air, water, food, and soil for possible contamination that may result from various practices associated with the use of ionizing radiation. *General sanitation services* include the inspection and sometimes licensing of various establishments such as restaurants, recreational areas, and jails; programs related to the sanitation of milk supplies may also be included. *Housing quality and urban planning services* are concerned with broad programs aimed at improvement of the physical environment through better housing and urban facilities (e.g., medical care, transportation, and recreation) and the elimination of blighted areas.

Patient Care Facilities and Services.   Inspection and licensing of general hospitals, chronic disease facilities, and convalescent and nursing homes are traditional responsibilities of state and local health departments. As the result of federal legislation during the past few years, programs for hospital planning and the allocation of federal-state financial support have been added to the responsibilities of the state agency. These responsibilities were expanded still further as the result of federal legislation providing medical care for the aged and other population subgroups.

Supportive Services.   State and local health departments customarily have supportive programs involving one or more basic *professional specialties,* the most usual being public health nursing, health education, and social services. *Research* is another type of supportive program and may include vital and health statistics, data processing, research planning, statistical consultation, and research training. *Laboratory services* may include specialized units for serology, bacteriology, virology, and parasitology; in general, these services support the other health department programs, engage in research, sometimes provide direct services to physicians and private laboratories, and at the state level are responsible for licensing and certification. *Nutritional services* are concerned with educational programs to improve nutrition and with the provision of consultation on nutritional matters for other programs such as maternal and child health, chronic disease, and occupational health. *Administrative services* comprise basic business and administrative "housekeeping," including fiscal and personnel management, personnel training, management analysis and auditing, and the provision of health information to the public.

HEALTH DEPARTMENT ORGANIZATION

There are 50 state health departments in the United States and several equivalent territorial agencies. Of the approximately 3,100 counties in the nation, more than 1,500 are covered by organized local health departments, and about 700 more are covered by state health departments.[8] There is, as might be expected, great variety in the actual organization of the specific services just described and the way in which they are grouped administratively. Variation may be accounted for (a) through accidental history of organization (a surprisingly potent factor), (b) through local conditions demanding variation in health services (a largely rural prairie state may have different environmental and direct service requirements from a highly industrial state on one of the nation's coasts), or (c) by local organizational practice.

In general, however, most program areas are represented in health departments and occur as divisions or bureaus. Tables 2-5 and 2-6 describe the basic organizational pattern of selected state and local health departments, respectively. Missing elements do not necessarily mean that a service or function is not being performed; other agencies may have those responsibilities.

Both state and local health departments generally have an executive officer or health officer and a board of health; they may also have various advisory committees and consultants. In state health departments, the health officer is usually appointed by the governor on recommendation of the board of health, but in most cases he remains in office indefinitely. As chief administrator, the state health officer has far-reaching responsibilities within the department, and he also has a key role in maintaining relationships with the governor's office, the legislature, other department heads, and nongovernmental organizations that have an interest in health affairs. The state board of health has from five to ten members, appointed by the governor in most states, and may consist of members of the medical profession only, although the trend is to broaden representation to include other professions and the lay public. The board generally serves in an advisory capacity, helps to establish policy, holds hearings, acts as liaison between the health department and the public, and sometimes works with the state legislature and professional organizations. In order better to carry out its various programs and services particularly in a large and populous state, the health department may subdivide the state into regions, placing a departmental representative in each subdivision.

In local health departments, the health officer is appointed by the mayor, the county governing body (commissioners, supervisors, etc.), or the board of health; or he may be selected from a civil service list. The health officer in turn may appoint subordinate per-

TABLE 2-5. Organization of Selected State Health Departments

CALIFORNIA: DIRECTOR'S OFFICE, STATE BOARD OF HEALTH, OFFICE OF COMPREHENSIVE HEALTH PLANNING, REGIONAL OFFICES

Office of Fiscal Management	*Community Health Services and Resources Program*	*Preventive Medical Program*	*Environmental Health and Consumer Protection*
Bureaus:*	Bureaus:*	Bureaus:	Bureaus:
Administration	Planning & Construction	Chronic Disease	Food and Drug
Accounting & Budgeting	Health Education	Mental Retardation	Radiologic Health
Statistics, Registration	Licensing & Certification	Maternal & Child Health	Occupational Health
Office of Special Services	Nursing	Dental Health	Sanitary Engineering
Bureaus:	Social Work	Nutrition	Air Sanitation
Data Processing; Statistics	Contract County Services	Alcoholism	Vector Control & Solid Waste
Evaluation	*Laboratory Services*	Crippled Children Services	
Manpower	Various PH and Environmental Laboratories	Communicable Disease	
Health Intelligence			

ILLINOIS: DIRECTOR'S OFFICE, ADVISORY BOARDS, OFFICE OF HEALTH PLANNING, REGIONAL OFFICES

Bureau of General Administration	*Bureau of Personal and Community Health*	*Bureau of Environmental Health*
Divisions:*	Divisions:	Divisions:
Administration	Family Health	Food and Drug
Personnel	Disease Control	Milk Control
Accounting; Finance	Dental Health	General Sanitation
Data Processing	Nursing	Radiologic Health
Education & Information	Health Facilities	Sanitary Laboratory
PH Laboratories	Chronic Illness	Swimming Pools and Beach Sanitation
Local Health Administration		

NEBRASKA: DIRECTOR'S OFFICE, BOARD OF HEALTH ADVISORY COUNCILS

Bureau of Supporting Services Divisions:*	Bureau of Health Care Services Divisions:	Bureau of Special Health Services Divisions:	Bureau of Environmental Health Services Divisions:
Vital Records & Statistics	Standards	Communicable Disease	Air Pollution
Health Education	Facilities	Chronic Disease	Environmental Sanitation
Laboratories	Emergency Health	Mental Health	Radiologic Health
Administration	Examining Boards	Maternal & Child Health	Environmental Engineering
Personnel	Nursing	Dental Health	Pollution Control
Finance & Budget			

* Titles of bureaus and divisions shown are not exact, but serve to indicate functions.
SOURCE: Annual reports of the selected state health departments (1970–1971).

TABLE 2-6. Organization of Selected Local Health Departments

HOUSTON, TEXAS: DIRECTOR

Personal Health Services	*Supporting Health Services*	*Environmental Health*
Dental Health	Laboratory	Veterinary Services
Maternal & Child Health	Administration (Fiscal & Statistics)	Health Inspection
Model City Planning	Health Education	Health Engineering
Communicable Disease Control	PH Nursing	
Chronic Illness Control		

MILWAUKEE, WISCONSIN: COMMISSIONER

Bureau of Administration	*Bureau of PH Nursing*	*Bureau of Maternal & Child Health*	*Bureau of Preventable Disease*	*Bureau of Laboratories*	*Bureau of Environmental Sanitation*
Divisions:*	Citywide & District Services	Divisions:	Divisions:	Divisions:	Divisions:
Administration		School Health	Acute Contagious Diseases	Chemistry	Housing & Sanitation
Bldgs. & Grounds		Clinics	Venereal Disease	Virology	Technical Services
Statistics		Dentistry	Tuberculosis	Bacteriology	Food and Measures
Health Education		Medical Service Centers	Medical Services		

NEWARK, NEW JERSEY: HEALTH OFFICER, COMMITTEES

General Service	*Medical Services*	*Environmental Sanitation*
Administration	PH Nursing	Food and Drug
PH Laboratories	Dental Health	Veterinary Inspection & Meat Control
Statistics	Child Health	Sanitation
AV Aids to Education	Communicable Disease Control	
Health Education	Venereal Disease Control	
	TB & Chest Disease Control	
	Clinics, Pharmacy, & X-ray	

* Division and bureau titles are not exact, but serve to suggest functions.
SOURCES: Annual reports of indicated local health departments (1967 and 1970).

sonnel or they, too, may be selected through civil service procedures. A large metropolitan or county health department may subdivide its area into health districts in order to facilitate the delivery of services to the public. Each subdivision has a district health officer and appropriate personnel and facilities and is directly responsible to the health officer of the local department.

OTHER OFFICIAL STATE AND LOCAL HEALTH AGENCIES

In recent years, as federal programs have grown, other official and quasi-official agencies have entered the state and local arena, sometimes integrally connected with health departments, and sometimes not. In addition, at state and local levels, certain important health functions—whether federally supported or not—have grown up separate from health departments. Examples of both types include comprehensive health planning agencies, special environmental control programs, and special pollution control districts.

It should also be kept in mind that many of the health department's programs and services are shared by other agencies of government; by medical, dental, and allied professions; by citizens' groups; and by private enterprise. With respect to governmental agencies, efforts are being made in some states and localities to consolidate related programs and offices into a single organization. For example, there is now a Department of Health and Mental Hygiene in Maryland (health, mental hygiene, and juvenile services); a Human Relations Agency in California—to become the *Health and Welfare Agency* (health, welfare, corrections, etc.); a Health Services Administration in New York City (health, mental health and retardation, and hospitals); and a Department of Health Services in Los Angeles County (health, mental health, and hospitals). These consolidations contribute to streamlining of organizations and make easier to some extent the lives of governors, mayors, and county executives because of simpler administrative reporting. It is not yet clear that health protection and health service delivery have been advanced as a consequence.

Voluntary Health Agencies

Voluntary health agencies have, traditionally, come into existence in the United States when a citizen or group of citizens has felt that there is an unmet need for a health service or a need for new knowledge in a particular health field. The resulting organization may be on a local, state, or national basis; a national agency may have state and local units, chapters, or affiliates. Voluntary health agencies are not tax supported and are responsible only to their members and to public opinion, although they are chartered and licensed by appropriate state and local governmental agencies.

In addition to voluntary health agencies, there are also, of course, voluntary organizations that deal with welfare matters, such as the provision of family, youth, and recreation services. One estimate is that there are more than 100,000 health and welfare organizations altogether, a large number of these being concerned with health matters, either exclusively or partly. While exact figures are hard to come by, in 1961 it was estimated that voluntary health and welfare agencies raised approximately $1.5 billion, of which $570 million went to organizations with a *primary* interest in health.[9]

HISTORY OF VOLUNTARY HEALTH AGENCIES

There was scarcely a local voluntary health agency at the turn of the century with the exception of the American Red Cross and a few tuberculosis societies. Late in the nineteenth and early in the twentieth centuries, a combination of several factors initiated a marked and persistent growth of voluntary health agencies.[10] First, new knowledge about, and attitudes toward, physical health emerged as a result of scientific advances of the nineteenth century; second, rapid economic expansion through industrialization provided more financial resources and free time for activities other than mere daily subsistence; and third, government-sponsored health programs were still sporadic, rudimentary, and struggling to emerge as organized public efforts. These scientific, economic, and political realities found a favorable climate in emerging humanitarian impulses to alleviate suffering and privation and in the prevailing American tradition of freedom of enterprise and aggressive individual (rather than governmental) action to solve problems. The result was a gradual acceleration in the number and kinds of organized voluntary health agencies, culminating in particularly rapid growth since 1940.[9]

The voluntary health movement began in the United States with the founding of the Anti-Tuberculosis Society of Philadelphia in 1892, followed by the formation of the National Association for the Study and Prevention of Tuberculosis in 1904. This organization is now known as the National Tuberculosis and Respiratory Disease Association and has 50 state associations and some 3,000 local affiliates. Other problem areas were recognized, stimulating local, and later national, organizations. In New York City, the concern with venereal diseases and prostitution led to the development in 1914 of the American Social Hygiene Association. There was developing interest in mental hygiene, and by 1910 concern arose over excessive illness and deaths of infants and mothers. During the next decade, national movements were initiated for cancer control, for prevention of blindness, for maternal hygiene, for the hard of hearing, and for public health nursing. Subsequently, national organizations were formed which were concerned with child health, crippled children, infantile paralysis, diabetes, and heart disease.

Among the vast number of voluntary health agencies in the United States, the American National Red Cross has a particularly unique history and position, especially since it is the only one that has quasi-official status. It originated during the Civil War through the efforts of Clara Barton, who aroused national and international attention to the need for organized medical care for soldiers on the battlefields. Her activities led to the recognition of the International Red Cross in 1882 and to the granting of a charter to the American Red Cross by the United States Congress in 1900. The President of the United States serves as the president of the organization, and it has diverse peace and wartime functions, including service as the official disaster relief agency of the nation.

CATEGORIES AND ACTIVITIES OF VOLUNTARY HEALTH AGENCIES

The first and most important group of voluntary health agencies which may be singled out consist of those that are essentially categorical and are supported by financial contributions and donations. This group may be subdivided into three classes:[10] (1) those concerned with *specific diseases* such as tuberculosis, venereal diseases, cancer, poliomyelitis, and diabetes (e.g., the National Tuberculosis and Respiratory Disease Association, the American Social Health Association, the American Cancer Society, the American Diabetes Association); (2) those concerned with *special organs and structures of the body* such as diseases of the heart, loss of vision or hearing, and dental, locomotor, or skeletal defects (e.g., the American Heart Association, the National Society for the Prevention of Blindness, the National Easter Seal Society for Crippled Children and Adults); and (3) those concerned with *the health and welfare of special groups or of society as a whole,* including maternal and child hygiene, planned parenthood, mental hygiene, and environmental hazards (e.g., the Maternity Center Association, the Planned Parenthood Federation of America, the National Association for Mental Health, the National Safety Council). Direct service to the public is provided by a few of the categorical voluntary health agencies but is not the major objective of most. Rather, the principal activity is usually the conduct of public and professional educational programs to improve the utilization of health services and to raise the quality of personnel and facilities. Other activities may include assessment of community health needs; support of demonstration and experimental projects as pioneering ventures into new health fields; encouragement of research; cooperation with other agencies, both voluntary and official, in the planning and coordination of health activities; provision of advisory services to official health agencies; and support of beneficial health legislation.

Besides the major group of categorical voluntary health organizations just described, there are also *integrating or coordinating agencies,* organized on national, state, and local levels. They are concerned with community and areawide planning to reduce overlapping interests and objectives of the many specialized voluntary agencies. Examples of such organizations are health councils, community chests, and community councils. The most prominent national organization in this category is the National Health Council, which has the mission of coordinating the activities of all the separate and specialized nongovernmental groups that are in the health field nationally.

ORGANIZATION AND FINANCING OF VOLUNTARY HEALTH AGENCIES

The typical national voluntary health agency has a board of directors frequently composed of prominent persons from industry, business, the arts, professions, and politics. The size of some boards prevents frequent meetings, and much of the day-to-day work is performed by a paid professional staff subject to review by an executive committee. Many of the state and larger metropolitan organizations operate in the same manner.

Principal responsibilities at the national level include development of general policies; creation of a public image; exercise of leadership, coordination, and guidance; and promotion of research and public interest in the specific area of concern. The state level provides broad leadership, stimulation, and guidance to the local affiliates, exerting some influence on program planning and administration, budgets, and fund raising. The local health associations raise money, develop program plans, and determine priorities for activities. Generally, the local organizations are more attuned to immediate community needs, and the state and national levels are more concerned with long-range planning.

The large group of voluntary health agencies that depend on financial contributions and donations obtain such support mainly from individual citizens and to a lesser extent from corporations. Some agencies have other sources of income as well, including payments by clients for services, membership dues, and investment earnings. Contributions and donations are obtained through fund-raising campaigns conducted by local committees as part of a national drive at some designated time of the year. Portions of the funds thus collected on the local level are channeled to the next higher echelons; the actual proportional distribution among local, state, and national levels varies with the organization concerned. The proliferation in recent years of the number of voluntary agencies and hence of the number of individual fund-raising campaigns has led to the formation of community chests and united funds. These are federations of agencies that undertake a single drive or appeal for funds and subsequently distribute the proceeds among the participating organizations. The result in numerous communities has been a considerable lessening of the number of different requests for contributions that are made upon the public in a given year.

CONTRIBUTIONS AND PROBLEMS IN THE VOLUNTARY AGENCY MOVEMENT

As with other sectors of the health scene, voluntary health agencies make some significant contributions, but there are also some problems. Voluntary agencies are promotive of health affairs at national policy levels as well as in connection with research and training support and with local programs. Leverage exercised nationally by voluntary agencies is significant, and they have in the past several decades had important influence on health legislation. Particularly notable have been the efforts of the American Cancer Society, the American Heart Association, and the National Association for Mental Health, in their respective fields. Furthermore, voluntary agencies sometimes can move more freely in advocacy of correctives and preventives, as, for example, the early role of the American Cancer Society in reminding the public on television, radio, and billboards about the health hazards of smoking.[11]

Research advances have been stimulated by voluntary agency support alongside the much greater funding abilities of governmental agencies. A great research triumph of the voluntary agencies has been the assistance rendered in the development of the Salk vaccine for poliomyelitis, although the important accompanying role of the National Institutes of Health in this development is sometimes overlooked.

Voluntary agencies — health and welfare alike, and particularly the large group of categorical health organizations — have been experiencing an increasing number of problems during the past decade or so. Some problems are internal and not unlike those experienced by official health and welfare agencies — for example, issues involving the nature and goals of programs, efficiency of administrative organization and management, shortages of trained personnel. A second group of problems are essentially intra-agency and include the existence of overlap and duplications in programs which still persist in spite of efforts to coordinate activities. A third category of problems pertain to financial matters, and although these might appear to be largely internal concerns, they assume an added dimension because the public, as the source of funds, is involved.

In addition to being the object of criticism for generating a multiplicity of fund-raising campaigns, voluntary agencies have been under scrutiny in connection with the expenditure of funds obtained through public contributions. An analysis in 1961 of 56 national voluntary agencies with a primary interest in health revealed that 52.3 per cent of agency expenditures went for organizational expenses and fund raising, public and professional information, and other expenditures such as cost of goods sold, capital expenditures, and special projects; the remaining 47.7 per cent went for services to patients, professionals, and the public and for professional training and research.[9] A more recent analysis (1969) of 13 major voluntary health agencies showed relatively little change in the situation, 55.5 per cent of expenditures going for patient services and for professional training and research activities, and the remainder for "support" expenditures.[12]

Added to this considerable array of problems is the trend toward increasing governmental participation in health and welfare programs, as described earlier in this chapter. Increased taxes to finance this participation may make inroads on public resources that in the past have supported voluntary agencies. In fact, the rate of increase of support for many agencies is already at or below the rate of population increase. At present, there is pressure for regional and areawide coordinated planning for the advancement of health and welfare services through the most efficient use of total available funds from all sources, whether local, state, or national taxes, or the financial resources of voluntary agencies.

The pressures and forces being exerted on voluntary agencies are leading to reevaluation of programs and are resulting in shifts in emphasis and broadening of activities. Changes may be expected to continue for many years to come, particularly if voluntary agencies are to maintain a role in the organized health-and-welfare effort.

Foundations

Next to governmental and voluntary health agencies in their influence on America's health affairs are the philanthropic foundations. Foundations have grown enormously in number since 1900 and particularly since 1945.

Most of the growth has been in foundations with less than $1 million in assets. One recent tabulation listed 5,454 foundations with assets of $500,000 or more *or* that had made grants of $20,000 or more in the year of record.[13] Of these foundations, 331 had assets of $10 million or more each; 1,841 had assets of $1 million to less than $10 million each; and 3,282 had assets of less than $1 million (Table 2-7). Grants vary with foundation size, the average grant for the very large foundation being in excess of $20,000.

The health field gets its share of foundation support, competing with projects in the areas of "education," international activities, welfare, services, humanities, and religion. Of grants of $10,000 or more made in the period 1961–1970, a total of $814 million was awarded for health projects out of a grand total of $5.7 billion for all projects. This is about 14 per cent of all awards of this size. For 1970 alone, the health figure was in excess of $120 million. "Health" awards are probably higher in actuality since many "educational," "services," and "international" awards involve health matters.[13] Typical foundation support (1970) for health projects includes drug education and therapy, alcoholism, children's health, cancer, biologic study, and health manpower training. Prominent foundations with substantial support for activities in the health field include the Rockefeller Foundation, the Ford Foundation, the W. K. Kellogg Foundation, the Commonwealth Fund, the Milbank Memorial Fund, the Markle Foundation, and the Johnson Foundation. There are many others as well, with endowments, annual income, and disbursements at a far lesser level.

The key to understanding the role of foundations in health is the term *innovation*. Foundations probably have fewer constraints

TABLE 2-7. Foundations: Asset Size and Grants

Asset Category	Number of Foundations	Number of Grants	Total Amount of Grants	Average Grant
$10 million or more	331	42,694	$882 million	$20,655
$1 million to $9.9 million	1,841	102,156	$376 million	$3,680
Less than $1 million	3,282	146,298	$256 million	$1,747
TOTAL	5,454	291,148	$1,514 million	$5,198

SOURCE: The Foundation Center. *The Foundation Directory, Edition 4,* 1971, p.xv (with permission).

than some other sources of support to undertake research, demonstration, and training projects that are untried or even unorthodox. They tend to be less formal about their review procedures and granting operations, although in the last analysis many foundations are as searching and rigorous as governmental agencies in their weighing of the quality and potential impact of the programs they support. As with voluntary agencies, foundations with far smaller funds provide valuable stimulation to the health field in a fashion not always possible in government-operated agencies.

Foundations have in recent years come under closer scrutiny by the Internal Revenue Service and state tax agencies regarding financial matters, method of operation, and to some extent the nature of the projects receiving foundation support. Most foundations are tax-free, and this fact and the very innovativeness of many foundations have given rise to thoughts of closer governmental control of foundation procedures. The result has been national legislation (included in the Tax Reform Act of 1971) that in effect makes it necessary for nonprofit foundations to become self-liquidating over the long run. Foundations are required to spend at least 4.5 per cent of the value of their assets (over and above their income) per annum in grant outlay, with the percentage rising to 5.5 per cent in 1974.[14]

Professional Associations

Professional associations play an important role in the organization of the health affairs of the nation and its states and localities. Every conceivable health-related profession and institution is represented, and such associations frequently are forces for change in the health field. A few of the countless organizations in this category are the American Nurses' Association, the American Medical Association, the American Dental Association, the American Public Health Association, and the American Hospital Association.

These organizations are generally national in character, with state and local affiliates. At every level they function as sources of relevant information for their memberships, often with varied publications regularly available, including journals, magazines, and newsletters of special interest to the respective fields. There are annual meetings that serve as forums for the discussion of current issues and current research, as well as employment exchanges.

By and large these organizations are "professionalizers," the trend being for improved standards of membership (or institutional) performance and for encouragement of research and innovation. On the other hand, these organizations also are motivated by and address themselves to the self-interest of the profession and of the membership. Witness, for instance, the national posture (traditional and conservative) of the American Medical Association and the vast influence this has had in national health affairs.

International Health Agencies

THE NEED FOR INTERNATIONAL HEALTH WORK

By now, every nation in the world has some kind of health program even if minimal or rudimentary. However, local-national health resources frequently are not sufficient to bring twentieth-century scientific technology and disease prevention methodology to bear on health problems. As a consequence a good deal of impetus has been given to the protection of health everywhere by international health work, which transcends national boundaries. Many international health activities are sponsored by the technically more advance and economically more advantaged nations, either on a direct country-to-country basis or through participation in organizations that have developed an administrative apparatus for conducting health programs on a broad scale. Organized international health work is of particular importance in the developing countries of the world, where the greatest lag occurs in the availability of health personnel and application of medical and health technology.

The situation is clearly illustrated in Table 2-8, which shows higher death rates and shorter life expectancy accompanying lower physician and nurse ratios in the countries listed. Thus, in contrast to the more developed countries in Europe and North America, many countries in Asia, Latin America, and Africa have higher death rates per 1,000 population, including far higher infant mortality. At the same time, in the latter countries the number of physicians falls far below 10 per 10,000 population; and the number of nurses falls far below 20 per 10,000. Table 2-8 also illustrates the variations in death rates and professional personnel ratios that can occur within a continent.

While there remain many nations with high death rates, the world as a whole is experiencing a phenomenal increase in population, and this fact has become a major concern in international health work. In many countries, including some developing nations, the control of infectious diseases has reduced the death rate, but the birth rate has not declined proportionally or has even remained stationary. The resulting large net gain in population has produced serious problems in meeting the needs for food, clothing, shelter, and many other necessities of life, and the economic strain is particularly great on nations that already have limited resources.

TABLE 2-8. Death Rate and Life Expectancy, Selected Countries*

	Crude Death Rate (per 1,000)	Infant Mortality (per 1,000 live births)	Life Expectancy† Male	Life Expectancy† Female	Physicians (per 10,000)	Nursing Personnel (per 10,000)
NORTH AMERICA						
United States	9.5	20.8	67.0	74.2	15.3	49.2
Canada	7.3	20.3	68.4	74.2	11.4	56.7
Mexico	10–11	65.7	57.6	60.3	5.5	2.0
SOUTH AMERICA						
Brazil	20–22	77.3‡	49.7	49.7	4.1	3.0
Peru	12–14	61.9‡	52.6	55.5	5.0	3.0
Venezuela	9–10	41.4‡	66.4	66.4	8.5	18.7
EUROPE						
Albania	8.0	86.8	64.9	67.0	5.9	18.4
England & Wales	11.9	18.3	68.7	74.9	11.7	30.4
Italy	10.1	30.3	67.1	72.3	17.5	n/a
Sweden	10.4	12.9	71.8	76.5	11.7	39.2
ASIA						
China (Taiwan)	5.2	19.0	65.8	70.4	3.9	1.4
Israel	6.8	23.0	69.3	72.9	23.6	n/a
Japan	6.7	15.3	68.9	74.2	10.9	24.1
Pakistan	18.0	142.0	53.7	48.8	1.6	0.5
AFRICA						
Congo (Brazzaville)	24.4	180.0	37.0	37.0	1.2	15.5
Morocco	18.7	149.0	47.0	47.0	0.8	2.2
Southern Rhodesia	14.0	122.0	50.0	50.0	1.9	8.0
United Arab Republic	14.4‡	118.5‡	51.6	53.8	4.6	2.3

* Mortality rates and life expectancy are mainly 1968 and 1969 data; some data (South America and Africa) are from the early 1960's. Manpower statistics (physicians and nurses) are mainly 1967 data.
† Average number of years of expectation of life at birth.
‡ Data from civil registers are incomplete or of unknown reliability.
SOURCES: Adapted from United Nations. *1969 Demographic Yearbook*, pp. 129–133. Also, World Health Organization.

A major effort in international health work is directed toward the application of scientific knowledge to control population increase and to find means for sharing world resources.

HISTORY OF INTERNATIONAL HEALTH ORGANIZATION

The devastating and recurring epidemics which began many centuries ago may be considered as marking the advent of international health problems, since the diseases frequently spread from one country to another. However, prior to the mid-nineteenth century, protection and control activities were primarily on a national rather than an international scale. The beginning of serious efforts at organized international health activity occurred between 1851 and 1909 when a series of meetings known as International Sanitary Conferences took place in various parts of the world. The principal topics for these meetings were the control of epidemics through quarantine and the exploration of the origin of infections. The first conference, held in Paris with representation of 12 nations, developed a treaty to limit the spread of epidemic disease through the regulation of international commerce, but it was never ratified by the participating nations. The subsequent conferences had similar limited practical results except for one significant accomplishment, which was the creation of the first permanent, worldwide organization dealing with international health.[15,16] This body was known as the International Office of Public Health (l'Office International d'Hygiène Publique) and came into being in Paris in 1909.

The International Office of Public Health, known as the "Paris Office," had a small full-time staff and responsibilities which were concerned mainly with quarantinable diseases: to gather information, revise international regulations, and arbitrate differences. Over a period of time, the Paris Office broadened the range of international regulations, including, for example, obtaining agreement by 14 countries on measures to control the spread of venereal diseases along the shipping routes. It also began the standardization of serums and the control of drug traffic and created several committees to study a wide range of public health problems.[16]

The establishment of two other international health organizations constituted notable accomplishments of the early twentieth century. These were the Pan-American Sanitary Bureau, created in Washington, D.C., in 1902, and the Health Section of the League of Nations, established in Geneva in 1923.

The Pan-American Sanitary Bureau limited its activities to the Western hemisphere. The Bureau was organized by a Pan-American Sanitary Conference as an agency of the 21 American republics, and its original purpose was merely to serve as an information center for keeping the participating nations informed about outbreaks of epidemic diseases.[15] Subsequently, the Bureau's activities expanded considerably and included the stimulation of all American countries to make greater efforts for the prevention, control, and eradication of disease; the development of a vigorous program in epidemiology; the training of professional personnel; and the encouragement and support of research.

The Health Section of the League of Nations, known as the "Geneva Office," functioned alongside the Paris Office until World War II. Its mandate under the Covenant of the League of Nations was to undertake international activity in the prevention and control of disease. The Geneva Office established a system of epidemic intelligence with a center in Singapore; carried on the work of international standardization and control of drug traffic begun by the Paris Office; established "expert committees" which considered a wide range of subjects including malaria, cancer, housing, and the teaching of medicine; sponsored international conferences which produced well-documented statements about health needs in developing countries; and provided medical services in the field, although these were limited because of meager financial resources.

PRINCIPAL CONTEMPORARY INTERNATIONAL HEALTH AGENCIES

Prior to the establishment of the Health Section of the League of Nations, efforts to develop international cooperation in health matters were directed mainly toward finding an international sanitary code strict enough to prevent transmission of disease from one nation to another, but not so strict that it interfered with commerce. It was not until the mid-twentieth century that significant change occurred in prevailing ideas about the true concerns of international health, the translation of these ideas into programs, and the provision of means to make the programs effective and far-reaching. The turning point was reached in 1948 when the World Health Organization was created as a specialized agency of the United Nations.

The World Health Organization.   The stage was set for the establishment of the World Health Organization as an agent for more effective international health work, first, by the scientific and technical developments which had occurred between the end of World War I and the end of World War II and, second, by the determination of governments and peoples following World War II to rebuild world peace, the means for which, it was felt, would be provided by scientific knowledge.

During the United Nations Conference on International Organization held in San Francisco in 1945, the presentation of a memorandum by the Brazilian delegation led to the inclusion of health as a problem to be considered by the United Nations. As plans for the establishment of a formal international health organization proceeded through a series of conferences and committees, the conception of health became broadened, and the health of all peoples was seen as fundamental to the attainment of peace and security.[17] This philosophy was amplified in the constitution of the World Health Organization, which states that "health is a state of complete physical, mental and social well-being, and not merely the absence of disease or infirmity"; that "enjoyment of the highest attainable standard of health is one of the fundamental rights of every human being without distinction of race, religion, political belief, economic or social condition"; and that "achievement of any state in the promotion and protection of health is of value to all."

The WHO has over 130 member countries which contributed to its 1970 budget of $80 million (U.S. dollars); a nation may be a member of WHO without being a member of the United Nations. It provides epidemic and statistical service; develops international quarantine measures; promotes the international standardization of drugs, vaccines, and other biologics; stimulates health research; and prepares and distributes many publications. Technical and program-planning assistance is available for participating nations and includes (1) strengthening individual national health services; (2) training health workers and developing training programs; (3) aiding the attack on major diseases such as malaria, smallpox, tuberculosis, venereal diseases, and parasitic and viral diseases, especially those that can be controlled environmentally; (4) protecting maternal and child health; (5) improving sanitation and water supplies; (6) promoting mental health; (7) improving nutrition in cooperation with other international agencies; and (8) providing general administrative and technical program assistance. The WHO also is concerned with health education of public and professional groups, exchange of information on dental health, and collaboration with the International Labor Organization to improve occupational health.

The International Office of Public Health (Paris Office) became part of the WHO shortly after the latter was established. The Pan-American Sanitary Bureau (now renamed the Pan-American Health Organization) became a regional office of the WHO in 1949, although it still maintains its own organizational identity. The WHO has an executive board composed of 24 health experts who are designated by, but do not represent, their governments. Proposals and issues are presented to the annual World Health Assembly composed of delegations from all member countries. A sample of

TABLE 2-9. Selected Issues Covered by the 24th World Health Assembly (Geneva, May 1971)

Cholera pandemic in Africa and in Eastern Mediterranean regions—high priority given to long-term preventive programs (sanitation systems) and development and use of improved vaccines

Problems of the human environment—worldwide scale of problems

Drug dependence—role for WHO in scientific aspects as well as in drug abuse control

Smallpox eradication—world smallpox figures show 30,000 cases reported in 1970, smallest incidence of the disease ever reported

Occupational health for miners—worldwide health hazards in mining and WHO role in international information system for mining conditions

Health consequences of smoking—international exchange of information about smoking control programs

Safety and efficacy of drugs—problems of quality, safety and efficacy of drugs imported by nations with little drug-manufacturing capability.

SOURCE: World Health Organization, *24th World Health Assembly*, 1971.

the broad span of issues covered in 1971 at the annual Assembly is shown in Table 2-9. An administrative and technical staff of approximately 3,600 people from more than 98 countries is stationed at the Geneva headquarters, in the regional offices, and with operational field projects in every continent. There are six WHO regional offices, as follows:[18]

African Region: headquarters at Brazzaville—31 member nations and three associate members representing a population of over 229 million

Region of the Americas: headquarters at Washington, D.C., at the Pan-American Health Organization—26 member nations with a population of 488 million

Southeast Asia Region: headquarters at New Delhi—8 member nations representing a population of 721 million

European Region: headquarters at Copenhagen—33 member nations representing 753 million people

Eastern Mediterranean Region: headquarters at Alexandria—21 member nations and a population of 282 million

Western Pacific Region: headquarters at Manila—13 member nations representing a population of 278 million

Other Sponsors of International Health Programs. The United Nations Children's Fund, known as UNICEF at the time it was established, was organized originally as a temporary, emergency agency to assist children in war-torn countries. It later expanded its program to provide food and supplies for child and maternal welfare throughout the world and particularly in developing countries. It has also been concerned with programs of vaccination and the control of yaws, syphilis, and malaria. In 1953, the fund was granted permanent status by the United Nations.

The Agency for International Development emerged in 1961—after a series of reorganizations and name changes since the end of World War II—as the international assistance program of the United States. Organizationally, it is within the State Department, but it is semiindependent inasmuch as its funds are appropriated separately. The agency provides military, economic, and technical assistance to other nations. A significant part of the technical assistance provided involves public health matters through direct services, consultation, and fellowships for training in the United States and in other countries.

There are many nongovernmental agencies which have also made major contributions to international health work. These include foundations such as the Rockefeller Foundation, the Kellogg Foundation, and the Ford Foundation and numerous religious organizations. These international voluntary organizations have provided direct service to population groups throughout the world, contributed to the control of infectious diseases, and supported the training of health workers.

References

1. Hanlon, John J. *Principles of Public Health Administration,* 5th ed. The C. V. Mosby Company, St. Louis, 1969.
2. U.S. Department of Health, Education, and Welfare. *1970 Annual Report.* U.S. Government Printing Office, Washington, D.C., 1971.
3. U.S. Department of Health, Education, and Welfare, Office of the Secretary. *A Common Thread of Service.* U.S. Government Printing Office, Washington, D.C., 1970.
4. Office of the Federal Register, National Archives and Records Service, General Services Administration. *United States Government Organization Manual, 1971–72.* U.S. Government Printing Office, Washington, D.C.
5. U.S. Senate, Committee on Government Operations, Subcommittee on Executive Reorganization and Government Research. *Health Activities: Federal Expenditures and Public Purpose.* U.S. Government Printing Office, Washington, D.C., 1970.
6. U.S. Department of Health, Education, and Welfare, Public Health Service. *The Public Health Service: Background Material Concerning the Mission and Organization of the Public Health Service.* Prepared for the Interstate and Foreign Commerce Committee, United States House of Representatives. U.S. Government Printing Office, Washington, D.C., 1963.

7. U.S. Department of Labor. *Federal Register.* Vol. 36, No. 105, Part II. U.S. Government Printing Office, Washington, D.C., May 29, 1971.

8. U.S. Department of Health, Education, and Welfare, Public Health Service, Health Services and Mental Health Administration, Office of Grants Management. *Directory of Local Health and Mental Health Units,* 1969 revision. Public Health Service Publication Number 118, U.S. Government Printing Office, Washington, D.C., 1970.

9. Hamlin, Robert H. *Voluntary Health and Welfare Agencies in the United States.* The Schoolmasters' Press, New York, 1961.

10. Gunn, Selskar M., and Platt, Philip S. *Voluntary Health Agencies.* The Ronald Press Company, New York, 1945.

11. Carter, Richard. *The Gentle Legions.* Doubleday, New York, 1961.

12. Ducas, Dorothy (ed.). *National Voluntary Health Agencies.* National Health Council, New York, 1969.

13. The Foundation Center. *The Foundation Directory,* 4th ed. Columbia University Press, New York, 1971.

14. Goulden, Joseph C. *The Money Givers.* Random House, New York, 1971.

15. Goodman, Neville M. *International Health Organizations and Their Work.* J. & A. Churchill, Ltd., London, 1952.

16. Brockington, Fraser. *World Health.* The Whitefriars Press, Ltd., London and Tonbridge, 1958.

17. World Health Organization. *The First Ten Years of the World Health Organization.* The Organization, Geneva, 1958.

18. World Health Organization. *The Work of WHO, 1970.* Official Records of the World Health Organization. No. 188, The Organization, Geneva, March 1971.

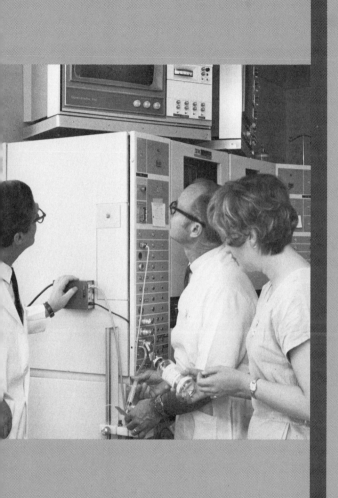

3

HEALTH
PROFESSIONS:
MEDICAL,
NURSING,
AND RELATED
PERSONNEL

CHAPTER OUTLINE

General Status of Health Manpower

Manpower Trends Since 1950
The Health Fields
Manpower Shortages and Opportunities

Some Basic Health Professions

Physician Manpower
Nursing and Related Services
The Dental Profession
Visual Services and Eye Care
The Veterinary Profession
Occupations and Training in Public Health

New Developments in Health Manpower

The Realities of Shortages
New Programs and Enlargement of Training Classes
Physician Expanders
Minority Employment
New Careers

Courtesy of California's Health, *California Department of Public Health.*
Staff photo.

General Status of Health Manpower

The health field provides an extraordinary arena for the employment of men and women in the United States. Most familiar are doubtless those jobs involved in direct service to patients and in the management of institutions and organizations rendering health care. The hospital and private office work settings call to mind nurses, doctors, dentists, practical nurses and aides, technicians in various specialties, nutritionists, and pharmacists. Less visible but equally integral are the personnel in clinical laboratory and radiologic services; these are normally involved in patient assessment and treatment along with health records and social-work staff. Rehabilitation staff are also employed, involving various therapies: physical, occupational, speech, psychologic, occupational, and others. Then there are the health and hospital administrators, the environmental health personnel at all levels, statisticians and data-processing personnel, and others. All these and more constitute the civilian health labor force.

Several aspects of the health field deserve particular mention. First, health careers fit all educational patterns. The extremes are the intensive professional education and training required at present of physicians (10 to 12 years of college and postgraduate work) and the focused training (6 months or less) required of some technical and assistant jobs. In the middle are nursing careers (2 to 5 years of collegiate or diploma training).

Second, health careers are intrinsically interesting. In this regard they are more appealing than many routine jobs, for example, in manufacturing and service industries. Health career jobs often directly serve humanity and are instrumental in reducing pain, relieving illness, and prolonging life. In many instances the focus is scientific, with job settings calling on traits related to imagination, precision, and watchfulness. These added dimensions give personal satisfaction not always found in other jobs.

71

Third, the jobs can be financially rewarding. In other words, the money is good, partly because the skills called upon are intrinsically highly valued in American society and partly because, as will be seen in Chapter 4, the health profession is in a period of high demand.

Finally, since there is the prospect of serious changes in the pattern of health care *delivery*—to consider only one facet of the health industry—there is the likelihood of the development of many new types of jobs. Some of these, like the physician's assistant or health ombudsman, are not yet well-established even in concept.[1,2] Others are bridging jobs, lying between established careers, like the nurse-practitioner, demanding changes in responsibilities, roles, and statuses for some. The upshot is the possibility of careers breaking out of prior fixed molds, and a material opening up of responsibility and reward ceilings.

MANPOWER TRENDS SINCE 1950

As will be seen in other chapters, the health industry of the United States has grown enormously since 1950. Not only have there developed increased demand and utilization of health services, but there has also been a steady expansion of community health programs of every description.

As the health industry has grown, so has the number of professional and technical personnel employed, as well as administrative and supportive staff. The figures for 1970 show approximately 4.2 million persons estimated to be employed in the health field, 5 per cent of the civilian working force in the United States (Table 3-1).

TABLE 3-1. Total Health Personnel, Physicians, Nurses, and Dentists, United States, 1950–1970

	1950	1960	1970
TOTAL HEALTH PERSONNEL	1.7 million	2.6 million	4.2 million
PHYSICIANS			
Number*	232,700	274,800	348,000
Rate per 100,000	149	148	166
PROFESSIONAL NURSES (R.N.)			
Number	335,000	504,000	700,000
Rate per 100,000 population	249	282	345
DENTISTS			
Number*	87,200	102,000	118,200
Rate per 100,000 population	57	56	58

* Includes inactive.

SOURCE: Adapted from U.S. Department of Health, Education, and Welfare, Health Services and Mental Health Administration, National Center for Health Statistics. *Health Resources Statistics, 1971* (and *1965*).

This figure compares with 1.7 million employees in 1950 and 2.6 million in 1960. In other words, the number of persons employed in the health field was more than doubled in the period 1950–1970. By 1960, health services ranked third out of 71 industries in the number of civilian labor force employees, exceeded only by agriculture and construction.

Throughout the period 1950–1970 and continuing today, there is deep concern about the supply and number of qualified health professionals and technicians available to do the jobs called for. There have been, as will be seen later, some imaginative undertakings to provide training for various specialties in the broad *allied health* manpower field. Equally, there are important advances being attempted in the training of new breeds of health personnel to be engaged in direct personal health care service.[3–6]

Symptomatic of the varied picture in health manpower availability are the figures for nurses, physicians, and dentists in the United States. While there has been an increase in numbers of these highly trained health personnel since 1950, the increase has been relatively small when the rise in the American population is taken into account. Table 3-1 shows that the ratio of dentists to population has not risen at all since 1950, and that of doctors has increased only since 1960. Nurses have increased substantially since 1950. Overall, when looked at in the light of the increase of population 55 years and older — persons at high risk of chronic illness (see Chapter 4) — the manpower figures look even less impressive.

THE HEALTH FIELDS

The health industry employs professionals and technicians from more than 30 different health subfields and specialties and in 200 to 300 specific occupations within those fields.[7,8] These numbers include only persons who have had special education or training for work in a health setting; excluded are many other persons who perform the business, clerical, and maintenance services essential to the operation of health facilities and agencies, but whose occupations are not unique to the health field. Table 3-2 shows the principal health fields arrayed in descending order of the estimated number of persons employed and indicates one or more typical occupations within each field. There were almost 2 million persons employed (active status) in the field of nursing and related services in 1970, followed by medicine and osteopathy with 323,000, and dentistry and allied services with almost 245,000. The large number of remaining health fields ranged in magnitude from more than 200,000 persons to several hundred (Table 3-2).

Health workers are employed in many different kinds of set-

TABLE 3-2. Health Fields and Estimated Numbers of Persons Employed, United States, 1970

Estimated Persons Employed	Health Fields and Typical Occupations
1,995,000	Nursing and related services (Registered and practical nurses; aides, orderlies, attendants; home health aides)
323,000	Medicine and osteopathy* (Physicians: doctors of medicine and osteopathy)
275,000–300,000	Secretarial and office services (Medical and dental receptionists, secretaries, assistants, and aides)
245,900	Dentistry and allied services* (Dentists; dental hygienists, assistants, and laboratory technicians)
242,000	Environmental control (Environmental engineers; scientists; sanitarians; technicians; aides)
200,000–300,000	Medical assistants (Office assistants to the physician)
140,000	Clinical laboratory services (Clinical chemists, microbiologists, and other biologic scientists; clinical laboratory technologists, technicians, and assistants)
139,300	Pharmacy* (Pharmacists; pharmacy assistants and aides)
75,000–100,000	Radiologic technology† (Radiologic or x-ray technologists, technicians, and assistants)
55,650	Optometry and opticianry (Optometrists; opticians; optometric technicians and assistants; orthoptists; ophthalmic assistants)
53,000	Medical records (Medical record administrators and technicians)
51,200	Basic sciences in the health field† (Microbiologists, physiologists, biochemists, and other scientists engaged in medical research)
49,000	Administration of health services (Administrators, program representatives, and management officers and their assistants)
47,000	Dietetic and nutritional services‡ (Dietitians; nutritionists; technicians; food service supervisors)

* Estimate indicates active rather than total.
† 1968 estimate.
‡ 1965 estimate.
§ Estimate not available for patients' librarians.
‖ Estimate not available for programmers, operators, and electronic technicians.
Estimate not available for statistical clerks.

SOURCE: Adapted from U.S. Department of Health, Education, and Welfare, Health Services and Mental Health Administration, National Center for Health Statistics. *Health Resources Statistics, 1971,* pp. 8–11.

Estimated Persons Employed	Health Fields and Typical Occupations
29,800	Social work (Medical and psychiatric social workers, assistants, and aides)
29,400	Miscellaneous health services (Ambulance attendants; electrocardiograph and electroencephalograph technicians; inhalation therapy technicians)
26,640	Food and drug protective services (Food and drug technologists, analysts, and inspectors)
25,700	Veterinary medicine*
24,000	Physical therapy (Physical therapists; physical therapy technicians, assistants)
23,400	Surgical and other aides employed in hospitals
23,000	Health education (Public health educators; school educators and coordinators)
19,000	Speech pathology and audiology
13,400	Vocational rehabilitation counseling
13,000	Psychology (Clinical counseling and other health psychologists)
12,800	Occupational therapy (Occupational therapists, technicians and assistants)
12,600	Health information and communication (Biologic photographers; health information specialists and science writers; health technologic writers; medical illustrators)
11,300	Specialized rehabilitation services (Corrective, educational, manual arts, music, recreational therapists; home economists in rehabilitation)
10,900	Biomedical engineering (Biomedical engineers and technicians)
9,500	Library services in the health field§ (Medical librarians, technicians and clerks)
7,000	Podiatry*
3,600	Orthotic and prosthetic technology†
2,500	Automatic data processing‖ (Systems analysts)
1,600	Anthropology and sociology (Cultural and physical anthropologists; medical sociologists)
1,350	Health and vital statistics†# (Health statisticians; vital record registrars; demographers)
500	Economic research in the health field

tings, from private offices to large and complex health organizations where numerous occupations are represented. Hospitals and nursing care facilities are examples of the latter, and nationally they employ the largest number of health personnel. Thus, approximately 7,600 American hospitals employ some 1.9 million health workers, 80 per cent of them (1.5 million) full-time. Approximately 440,000 additional health personnel work in nursing care and personal care homes.[7]

Other big employers of health workers include the federal government (Department of Health, Education, and Welfare; Department of Defense; and the Veterans Administration), state and local health departments, and voluntary agencies, as well as school systems, community health centers, clinics, and laboratories. Business and industry also employ health workers in the conduct of occupational health programs and services.

MANPOWER SHORTAGES AND OPPORTUNITIES

Despite increases in number in health manpower in recent years, shortages remain serious blocks to carrying out health programs that have been launched to meet community needs. There have been documented deficits in a number of fields.[9] For example, even in 1965–1966 there were budgeted vacancies, mainly in hospitals, for at least 75,000 registered nurses and 25,000 licensed vocational nurses.[10]

An inkling of the broad manpower pressures is given in Table 3-3, showing that at least 5.3 million persons could be employed in health occupations in 1980 (compared with 4.2 million in 1970). These estimates include 1.5 million in medicine and allied services; 270,000 in dentistry (a special candidate for expansion) and allied services; 2.7 million in nursing and related services; and 400,000 in environmental health services.

The preceding estimates are conservative and do not take fully into account potential drastic changes in the American health system in the next decade. For example, the impact of Medicare and Medicaid, which are still expanding, has not yet been fully felt. Furthermore, there is the impending adoption of some form of national health insurance that is sure to aggravate further the need for additional direct service personnel. In addition, countless thousands of individuals at all levels, from aides and technicians to health administrators, will be needed to organize, administer, and manage the health organizations of the future. The estimates for environmental health service personnel are also undoubtedly due for expansion as today's environmental consciousness is translated into tangible programs for controlling pollution and other environmental hazards.

TABLE 3-3. Projected Manpower Needs in 1980, United States

Occupation Within Group	1980
TOTAL, ALL HEALTH OCCUPATIONS	5,316,300
Other than "allied health"	3,972,300
"Allied health"—at least baccalaureate	410,000
"Allied health"—less than baccalaureate	934,000
MEDICINE AND ALLIED SERVICES (TOTAL)	1,477,300
Physicians (M.D. and D.O.)	407,300
Selected practitioners	275,000
"Allied health"—at least baccalaureate	320,000
"Allied health"—less than baccalaureate	475,000
DENTISTRY AND ALLIED SERVICES (TOTAL)	271,000
Dentists	120,000
"Allied health"—less than baccalaureate	151,000
NURSING AND RELATED SERVICES (TOTAL)	2,720,000
Registered nurses	895,000
Licensed practical nurses	675,000
Nursing aides, orderlies, and attendants	1,150,000
ENVIRONMENTAL HEALTH SERVICES (TOTAL)	398,000
"Allied health"—at least baccalaureate	90,000
"Allied health"—less than baccalaureate	308,000
ALL OTHER SERVICES (TOTAL)	450,000

SOURCE: U.S. Department of Health, Education, and Welfare, National Institutes of Health. *Health Manpower Source Book,* Section 21 (Allied health manpower, 1950–1980), 1970, p. 33.

While there no doubt *are* shortages of qualified individuals (simply not enough trained people), the situation is worsened by individual geographic preference and mobility of the health personnel. It is no secret that many graduates of health programs prefer serving in the communities or states in which they were trained. There are also the factors of salary level, working conditions, and personal receptivity in different regions and communities. Thus, there are found the severest shortages of health personnel in rural areas and in inner-city ghettos. As a consequence, the federal government and some state governments have initiated programs to encourage dispersal of health manpower more equitably to all areas and sections.[11]

There is broad national recognition of what has been until very recent years a counterproductive lag in training opportunities. The problem originates from many sources: lack of foresight and planning; lack of training imagination; self-protectiveness of professional associations; failure of professional association leadership to apply pressures for training expansion; failure of government to supply funds needed to build or expand teaching facilities and/or to assemble or expand faculties; and failure to make it financially possible for students to obtain health-professions training in competition with other opportunities.[12]

The response by all parties has been a stirring on many fronts—government, professional associations, community leadership, community colleges, and some universities and four-year colleges. Since 1950 there have been increases in the *number of new schools and programs* in various fields: nursing (mainly in associate in arts and baccalaureate programs), approved programs for practical (vocational) nurses, new medical and dental schools, new programs for dental hygienists, and a commensurate increase in schools and programs for every conceivable additional element in the broad allied health field. Of equal importance is the simultaneous *expansion of existing programs,* it being common to observe enlargement of entering classes and, in a few places, the speeding up of existing programs of instruction.

There has also been widespread support for making possible the redirection of individuals in the health fields. For those originally qualified for a health occupation at one level, there is the possibility of expanding horizons sideways or upwards, in response to personal aspirations and/or to community need. Traditional definitions of professional roles are being questioned and some new answers are emerging. Thus, can, or ought, a practical nurse aspire to assume certain responsibilities normally in the province of the registered nurse? Should a practical nurse be encouraged to become a registered nurse (through suitable additional training)? Can the registered nurse assume certain responsibilities of diagnosis and treatment normally jealously guarded by physicians? All these issues are under active consideration in a number of settings in the United States through programs supported by the U.S. Department of Health, Education, and Welfare and other elements of the federal government.[13]

For individuals without prior health employment qualifications, there is the possibility of entry and later upward mobility in what is for such individuals a new field. The range, for example, is from minority training and employment in community health centers and hospitals, to the retraining of unemployed aerospace engineers as health administrators.

Thus, the health field offers countless future opportunities for careers in a wide diversity of specialties, occupations, and settings—careers that can be both challenging and satisfying. The "knowledge explosion" has revolutionized the health fields, and many more skilled persons will continue to be required to develop and apply modern medical science and technology. Moreover, there is an "application explosion," parallel to the expansion of technology, but concerned with organization and delivery of personal and environmental health services. Here, too, many thousands of individuals will be required, combining knowledge about the health field with information about individual and group motivation, the governance of organizations, and the role of health organizations in the community.

Some Basic Health Professions

PHYSICIAN MANPOWER

In the United States, in 1970, there were 348,000 physicians who held the degree of Doctor of Medicine (M.D.) and 14,000 with the degree Doctor of Osteopathy (D.O.) The latter receive training in one of six accredited osteopathic training institutions where the program of study is increasingly similar to that for doctors of medicine.[7] Physicians are in private, solo practice and in group practice (as described in Chapter 4) as well as in hospital service, teaching, public health work, and research activities.

Several characteristics of the medical profession are worthy of attention (Table 3-4). There were approximately 311,000 medical doctors (plus about 12,000 doctors of osteopathy) in actual practice in 1970. Of these, about 192,000 were primarily in office practice (solo or group). Some 86,000 were primarily hospital-based, either in training programs (internship, etc.) or in full-time hospital occupations. The remainder (some 32,000) were in other activities, including teaching, research, and administration. Only one quarter of medical doctors were in general practice, the rest being in some cer-

TABLE 3-4. Type of Practice of Active Physicians, United States, 1970

	Total Active	General Practice	Specialty
M.D.'s			
Total	310,845	77,363	233,482
Office-based	192,439	54,914	137,525
Hospital-based			
Training	51,228	10,400	40,828
Full-time	34,868	5,946	28,922
Other professional*	32,310	6,103	26,207
D.O.'s	11,381	8,651	1,416

* Includes medical teaching, administration, research, and other.
SOURCE: Adapted from U.S. Department of Health, Education, and Welfare, Health Services and Mental Health Administration, National Center for Health Statistics. *Health Resources Statistics, 1971*, p. 155.

tified or accredited specialty (about 80 per cent of doctors of osteopathy were in general practice).

The medical profession recognizes about 30 specialties which may be grouped into four major categories (Table 3-5). There are the *medical* specialties (77,000 physicians), which include cardiovascular diseases, dermatology, internal medicine, pediatrics, etc. There are the *surgical* specialties (97,000 physicians), including anesthesi-

TABLE 3-5. Medical Specialties for Doctors of Medicine, United States, 1970

		Total Active M.D.'s
SPECIALTY PRACTICE		233,482
MEDICAL SPECIALTIES		77,214
Allergy	1,719	
Cardiovascular diseases	6,476	
Dermatology	4,003	
Gastroenterology	2,010	
Internal medicine	41,872	
Pediatrics	18,819	
Pulmonary diseases	2,315	
SURGICAL SPECIALTIES		96,902
Anesthesiology	10,860	
Colon and rectal surgery	667	
General surgery	29,761	
Neurologic surgery	2,578	
Obstetrics and gynecology	18,876	
Ophthalmology	9,927	
Orthopedic surgery	9,620	
Otolaryngology	5,409	
Plastic surgery	1,600	
Thoracic surgery	1,809	
Urology	5,795	
PSYCHIATRY AND NEUROLOGY		26,310
Child psychiatry	2,090	
Neurology	3,074	
Psychiatry	21,146	
OTHER SPECIALTIES		33,056
Aerospace medicine	1,188	
General preventive medicine	804	
Occupational medicine	2,713	
Pathology	10,483	
Physical medicine and rehabilitation	1,479	
Public health	3,029	
Radiology	13,360	

SOURCE: Adapted from U.S. Department of Health, Education, and Welfare, Health Services and Mental Health Administration, National Center for Health Statistics. *Health Resources Statistics, 1971*, p. 155.

ology, general surgery, obstetrics and gynecology, ophthalmology, etc. Specialists in *psychiatry* and *neurology* (including child psychiatry) number 26,000 physicians. *"Other"* specialties (33,000 physicians) include pathology, radiology, public health, etc.

Specialty practice as a proportion of all medical practice has grown enormously since the 1940's and no doubt will remain in ascendancy for some time to come. Reasons for this preference are many, and include the fact that only in recent years has technology been available for individuals to become genuine specialists (to "know a lot about a little"). Specialty incomes range higher than incomes in general practice. Furthermore—and probably an extremely important factor—medical students are taught principally by specialists, whose work, in turn, is supported by impressive research grants in their specialty areas. If ever prestige figures create role models, they no doubt do so in this instance.

Training as a physician normally takes at least 8 years after graduation from high school and, with internship and residencies, may extend to 10 or 12 years. A license to practice is required in all states and the District of Columbia. To qualify for a license, a candidate must have been graduated from an approved school, passed a licensing examination, and, in more than half the states, served a one-year hospital internship.

TABLE 3-6. Selected Health-Professions Students, United States, 1969–1970

	Schools or Programs	Students		
		Total	*Admissions*	Graduates
PHYSICIANS				
Medicine	101	37,669	10,401	8,367
Osteopathy	6	1,997	577	432
NURSES				
Registered nurse	1,328	150,795	*	43,639
Licensed practical (vocational) nurse	1,253	*	55,635	37,128
DENTAL PROFESSION				
Dentists	53	16,008	*	3,749
Dental hygienists	121	6,854	*	2,465
Dental assistants	165	5,074	*	2,955
OPTOMETRISTS	11	2,488	786	445
VETERINARIANS	18	4,875	1,341	1,165

* Data not available.

SOURCE: Adapted from U.S. Department of Health, Education, and Welfare, Health Services and Mental Health Administration, National Center for Health Statistics. *Health Resources Statistics, 1971.*

There were, in 1969–1970, a total of 101 medical schools in the United States and Puerto Rico. Among these, 87 were established and had graduating classes; 8 were recently established and already had first-year or more advanced classes, but as yet no graduates; and 6 were approved schools of "basic medical sciences" from which graduates may transfer to established schools. There were also 6 four-year osteopathic schools. In 1969–1970 there were 8,367 graduates from all medical schools, 37,669 students enrolled, and 10,401 first-year admissions (Table 3-6).

With physician supply short and in high demand, foreign medical graduates (FMG) are found in various apprentice medical roles and actually offering medical services. In 1970, there were in the United States almost 17,000 foreign medical graduates in internship and residency programs, and approximately 50,000 FMG's — not all of them fully licensed — providing patient care.

NURSING AND RELATED SERVICES

Professional Nurses (R.N.). Professional nurses, also known as registered nurses (R.N.) or graduate nurses, are responsible for nursing care received by patients in hospitals, outpatient clinics, medical offices and in new settings in the community. Not only do professional nurses provide direct nursing care, but they also supervise practical nurses and nonprofessional personnel who handle routine care and treatment of patients.

There are a number of clinical specialties in the nursing profession. For example, pediatric nurses specialize in caring for children; obstetric nurses care for mothers and new babies; and medical-surgical nurses care for patients before, during, and after surgery and in most types of illness. Other nursing specialties include the care of patients with particular diseases, such as cardiovascular illnesses, cancer, and pulmonary ailments. Positions in these and other specialties require experience and additional courses of study beyond the basic preparation, sometimes at the master's and even at the doctoral level. For licensure as a registered nurse (required in all states) an applicant must be a graduate of an "approved" nursing school and must pass an examination of the state board of nursing.

In 1971 there were approximately 700,000 active nurses, of whom 515,000 were in full-time practice and the remainder in part-time occupation. As with nonpracticing physicians and dentists, there are additional qualified professional nurses who are not employed in nursing; the figure was estimated in 1966 at 300,000. One recurring theme in the face of nursing shortage is the effort to get these trained individuals back into the nursing field.

TABLE 3-7. Fields of Employment of Registered Nurses, United States, 1970

	Number of Nurses	Per Cent of Total
TOTAL	700,000	100.0
Hospitals and nursing homes	486,000	69.4
Private duty, doctor's office, and other fields	112,000	16.0
Public health and school health	51,000	7.3
Nursing education	31,000	4.4
Occupational health	20,000	2.9

SOURCE: U.S. Department of Health, Education, and Welfare, Health Services and Mental Health Administration, National Center for Health Statistics. *Health Resources Statistics, 1971*, p. 177.

The places of employment of registered nurses in 1970 are shown in Table 3-7. Almost 70 per cent (486,000) worked in hospitals, nursing homes, and related institutions. Sixteen per cent (112,000) worked in doctors' offices or were self-employed. Seven per cent (51,000) were in public health and school health. Four per cent (31,000) had posts in nursing education, and the remaining 3 per cent (20,000) were in occupational or industrial health.

Graduation from high school is a common requirement for admission to schools of nursing that prepare students for licensure as registered nurses. In 1969–1970 there were 1,328 schools of nursing located in every state in the Union as well as in Puerto Rico, Guam, and the Virgin Islands. In that year there were approximately 150,000 students enrolled, and about 44,000 nurses graduated (Table 3-6). More than 50 per cent of the graduates (approximately 23,000) were from hospital-diploma schools; 27 per cent (about 12,000) were from associate degree programs; and 21 per cent (about 9,000) were from four-year baccalaureate programs. Graduate nurses also earned advanced degrees in 1970: 1,988 master's and 27 doctoral degrees.

There has been a quiet revolution in the initial stages of nursing education since 1960. In that year, 78 per cent of nursing graduates came from hospital-diploma (usually three-year) programs. By 1971, 200 of these programs had closed.[14] On the other hand, in 1960, there were about 1,000 graduates of associate degree (two-year) programs, generally in community colleges; baccalaureate program graduates numbered about 4,000. By 1970, graduates of the two-year program had gone up tenfold, and graduates of the baccalaureate programs had more than doubled.

Practical Nurses. Practical nurses, known also as vocational nurses, give nursing care and treatment of patients under supervision of a licensed physician or a registered nurse. Practical nurses must be licensed to practice as L.P.N.'s in each state (or as L.V.N.'s in California and Texas). In 1969–1970, there were approximately 400,000 licensed practical nurses, half of whom worked in hospitals registered with the American Hospital Association; about 50,000 worked in nursing homes and related institutions. Many others are employed in private homes, and some work in doctors' offices, schools, and public health agencies.

Training as a practical nurse usually requires 12 to 18 months and may be obtained in trade, technical, or vocational schools; in other *public* schools; or in *private* schools controlled by hospitals, health agencies, or colleges. A number of proprietary schools have recently gotten into the business of training practical nurses. In 1969–1970, there were more than 1,200 approved (by the states) programs for training practical nurses. In that period, there were 56,000 admissions and 37,000 graduates (Table 3-6). Approved programs, admissions, and graduates doubled in the 10-year period following 1959–1960.

Related Nursing Services. There are several kinds of workers who provide auxiliary nursing services in hospitals, clinics, and nursing homes. *Nursing aides,* who are usually women, assist professional and practical nurses by performing less skilled tasks in the care of patients. *Orderlies* and *attendants,* who are usually men, perform routine duties in caring for male patients and certain heavy duties in the care of the physically ill, mentally ill, and mentally retarded. There were an estimated 850,000 of these auxiliary workers in the United States in 1971. Such occupations are not licensed (except for psychiatric aides, who are licensed in Arkansas, California, and Michigan), but hospitals generally have their own standards of service and their own training programs. *Ward clerks,* sometimes also known as floor clerks or ward or unit secretaries, act as receptionists and relieve the nurse of much of the paperwork in the patient care units of an institution. They receive on-the-job training for duties such as preparing patients' charts, distributing the records needed by physicians on their rounds, and similar clerical tasks.

Workers who provide auxiliary nursing services in the home rather than in an institutional setting are *home health aides* (also known as home aides or visiting health aides) and *homemakers.* In general, the duties of the home health aide include a large element of personal care for persons who are ill or disabled, while those of the homemaker are more likely to be associated with various problems of household management that have arisen because of illness or disability in a family. Home health aide—homemaker services are organized and administered under various auspices, including more than 500 public or voluntary agencies which provide such programs. The number of home health aides and homemakers was estimated to be in excess of 17,000 in 1971 in the United States. Such workers receive on-the-job training, are not licensed, and work under professional supervision.

THE DENTAL PROFESSION

Dentists. Dental care in the United States is provided primarily in private dental offices and in private and public clinics. Increasingly, group dental practices are emerging, a few of which have prepayment features. Some dentists also serve in hospitals and military installations. Others are involved in teaching, research, or administration of dental programs. A number of dentists are found in part-time community work, for example, examining the teeth of schoolchildren and offering dental services to ghetto dwellers and migrant worker groups.

In 1970, there were 118,000 dentists in the United States, of whom 102,000 were professionally active in dental work. Of these, about 7,500 were in federal employ (Veterans Administration, Public Health Service, and Armed Forces). Although most dentists are general practitioners, about 10 per cent (more than 10,000 dentists) are in specialty practice, the number having tripled since 1958 (Table 3-8). There are eight recognized dental specialties; not quite

TABLE 3-8. Dental Specialists, United States, 1970

	Number
TOTAL	10,315
Endodontists	497
Oral pathologists	97
Oral surgeons	2,406
Orthodontists	4,335
Pedodontists	1,159
Periodontists	1,003
Prosthodontists	715
Public health dentists	103

SOURCE: U.S. Department of Health, Education, and Welfare, Health Services and Mental Health Administration, National Center for Health Statistics. *Health Resources Statistics, 1971*, p. 77.

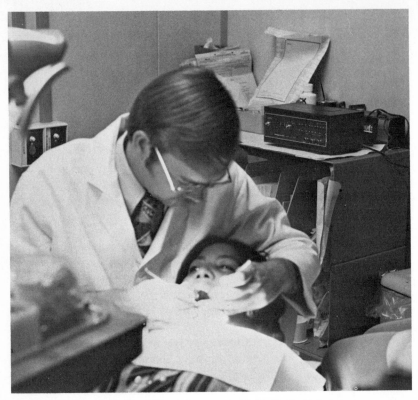

Courtesy of California's Health, *California Department of Public Health. Staff photo.*

half the specialists engage exclusively in orthodontics (straightening of teeth) and a quarter are oral surgeons.

Dentists receive four years of professional education in an accredited dental school, and must pass licensing examinations (written and clinical) in all states in order to practice. Dental specialties normally require at least two years of advanced study. In 1969–1970, there were 53 dental schools in the United States and Puerto Rico (12 more than in 1949–1950), and there were almost 3,800 graduates and 16,000 students enrolled, as shown in Table 3-6.

Various factors have enhanced the pressures on dental manpower. One is the Medicaid provision of the Social Security Act that provides for dental treatment for a wide group of eligible recipients. Another is the increasing pressure from labor-management negotiations to include dental care in employee fringe benefits.

Allied Occupational Groups in Dentistry.   There are three principal allied occupational groups in dentistry: dental hygienists, dental assistants, and dental laboratory technicians. *Dental hygienists* are the only dental auxiliaries who provide service directly to the patient and who, like the dentist, are required in each state to obtain a license to practice. The hygienist, working under the direction of the dentist, performs prophylaxes (scaling and polishing of the teeth), exposes and processes dental x-ray films, applies fluoride solution to the teeth of children, instructs individual patients in toothbrushing techniques and proper diet as related to teeth, among other services. In 1970, an estimated 16,000 dental hygienists were in practice, but there are still only 16 active hygienists per 100 practicing dentists, and a number of these are employed part time. The number of schools offering training in the dental hygiene program has increased significantly in recent years, from 37 in 1960 to 121 in 1970. Almost 2,500 dental hygienists graduated in 1970, and there were more than 6,800 students enrolled (Table 3-6). Dental hygiene training can be obtained in community colleges (two-year associate degree) or in baccalaureate programs (four-year college).

Dental assistants, who numbered about 90,000 to 95,000 in 1970, assist the dentist at the chairside by preparing the patient for treatment, keeping the operating field clear, mixing filling materials, passing instruments, and so on. Other duties involve exposing and processing x-rays, sterilizing instruments, assisting with laboratory work, ordering supplies, and handling the office records and accounts. More than 85 per cent of the dentists in private practice now employ one or more dental assistants. Traditionally, dental assistants have been trained on the job by their dentist employers. However, the number of institutions offering accredited training programs (one-year certificate and two-year associate) for assistants increased from 26 to 165 within the period 1961–1970. In 1969–1970 there were almost 3,000 graduates from the nation's accredited dental assistant program and more than 5,000 students enrolled.

The *dental laboratory technician* is a highly skilled craftsman who performs many tasks involved in the construction of complete and partial dentures, fixed bridgework, crowns, and other similar dental restorations and appliances. The technician does not have direct contact with the patient but performs his work in accordance with instructions received from the dentist. There were an estimated 32,000 technicians in 1970, approximately 25,000 of whom worked in commercial dental laboratories; the remainder were employed by dentists in private practice.

VISUAL SERVICES AND EYE CARE

The responsibility for visual services and eye care is divided among three categories of health personnel: ophthalmologists, optometrists, and opticians. *Ophthalmologists,* constituting one of the surgical specialties mentioned earlier in this chapter, are physicians who specialize in the medical and surgical care of the eyes and who may prescribe drugs or other treatment as well as lenses.

Optometrists specialize in vision analysis by examining the eyes, and they prescribe lenses and other vision aids, visual training and orthoptics, or other forms of treatment. They do not treat eye diseases or perform surgery. In 1969, there were about 18,000 active optometrists in the United States, the number having been relatively constant for many years. Almost 90 per cent are self-employed. Nearly three quarters are in private practice, either solo practice, in partnership, or in group practice. All states and the District of Columbia require a license for the practice of optometry. To qualify for a license, the applicant must be a graduate of an accredited school of optometry and pass a state board examination. In 1969–1970, there were 11 accredited colleges of optometry in the United States, requiring a six-year curriculum leading to the degree of Doctor of Optometry (O.D.). There were 445 graduates in 1969–1970, and about 2,500 students enrolled in all schools (Table 3-6).

Opticians fit and adjust eyeglasses according to prescriptions written by ophthalmologists or optometrists; they do not examine eyes or prescribe treatment. The actual grinding and polishing of lenses and assembly in a frame are done by an *optical technician,* who is also known as an optical laboratory mechanic, lens grinder, or polisher. The dispensing optician then fits and adjusts the eyeglasses to the individual's requirements. There were an estimated 11,000 opticians and contact lens technicians employed in the United States in 1970. Opticians are required to be licensed in 17 states; some of these states also require licenses for optical technicians in retail optical shops or for the retail optical establishment itself.

THE VETERINARY PROFESSION

Veterinary medicine deals with the prevention and treatment of disease and injury in animals. Veterinarians, in addition to providing treatment, also give advice regarding the care and breeding of animals and help prevent the outbreak and spread of disease among them, by physical examinations, tests, and vaccinations. One of the newest developments in the health field is the veterinarian's role in disease prevention among human beings by protecting them from the various diseases that can spread from animals to man, including tuberculosis, rabies, brucellosis, and salmonellosis.

The number of veterinarians in the United States increased from 15,800 in 1950 to 27,000 by the end of 1970. Ninety-five per cent are actively practicing. All states and the District of Columbia require that veterinarians have a license to practice. To obtain a license, an applicant must be a graduate of an approved veterinary school and pass a state board examination. A few states also require some practical experience under the supervision of a licensed veterinarian. Graduates of a veterinary school earn the degree of Doctor of Veterinary Medicine (D.V.M.), which requires a minimum of six years beyond high school. In 1969–1970, there were 18 approved schools of veterinary medicine in the United States, with 1,200 graduates and approximately 5,000 students enrolled (Table 3-6).

About three quarters of the veterinarians go into private practice, and most handle all kinds of domestic animals. An additional number work directly in regulatory and public health aspects of veterinary medicine for federal, state, or local governments or are engaged in teaching, research, and other types of practice. For positions in public health, research, or teaching, the master's or doctoral degree in a field such as pathology, epidemiology, public health, or bacteriology may be required, in addition to the D.V.M. degree.

OCCUPATIONS AND TRAINING IN PUBLIC HEALTH

The health personnel described thus far, as well as in subsequent chapters, sometimes find employment directly in governmental *public health* work—that is, in federal, state, and local official health agencies. It has already been mentioned (Chapter 2), for example, that the U.S. Department of Health, Education, and Welfare has approximately 100,000 employees, many of whom are formally trained physicians, nurses, dentists, engineers, health educators, social workers, biostatisticians, environmental sanitarians, laboratory personnel, and others. There are also a like number of health personnel employed in state and local health departments.

Physicians with a specialty in public health are certified by the American Board of Preventive Medicine. In addition to a medical degree and training as a general practitioner or a specialist, the career public health physician usually has a graduate degree in public health. Such physicians are employed by federal, state, and local health departments and by voluntary health agencies. Their activities range from clinical practice to consultative and administrative positions. They work closely with other public health personnel, such as nurses, sanitarians, health educators, and social workers. Many public health physicians specialize in particular areas, including maternal and child health, chronic disease, communicable disease, mental health, alcoholism, and others.

Public health nursing is a specialty within both professional nursing and the broad area of organized public health practice. It is responsible for the provision of nursing service on a family-centered basis in the home and for individuals and groups at work, at school, and in public health centers. The public health nurse works to prevent disease and promote health through case finding, by encouraging individuals to seek medical care, and by providing facts about health to the individual, the family, and the community. Local health departments constitute the typical settings in which public health nurses are employed. Public health nurses also work in voluntary agencies, notably visiting nurse associations. In addition, school nurses and occupational health, or industrial, nurses are often considered a part of public health nursing. Areas of particular concern in public health nursing include maternal and child health, communicable disease control, chronic illness and rehabilitation, psychiatric care, and nutritional education. The public health nurse may also provide instruction in public health matters to community groups, volunteer personnel, and professional nursing groups.

Public health dentists assess the dental health needs of a community and assist in the planning and development of programs of education, prevention, and care on a communitywide basis. Direct services on the local level are primarily for the treatment of indigent children. A few large cities have fairly extensive programs, employing dentists in local clinics. Dental public health programs on the state level provide dental consultation to local communities. Such programs also offer diagnostic laboratory services to practicing dentists; conduct screening examinations, postgraduate training, research, and demonstration projects; and provide dental treatment for patients in state institutions. On the national level, Public Health Service dentists provide direct care for Service personnel and for the special population groups for which the Service is responsible. The National Institute of Dental Research of the National Institutes of Health carries on research in the basic sciences of dentistry and the epidemiology of dental diseases. The Armed Forces and the Veterans Administration employ dentists who render direct care to military personnel and in Veterans Administration hospitals, respectively.

The *public health aspects of visual problems and eye care* are becoming increasingly recognized. Public education regarding eye care and the desirability of early diagnosis and optimum treatment to forestall visual impairment is an important part of public health programs. Glaucoma and cataracts, which are major eye disorders, are particularly important public health problems because the blindness to which they may otherwise lead is preventable if the diseases are discovered in early stages. Early detection of these and other eye conditions depends on the provision of broad programs for examining apparently healthy eyes—by specialists in their own offices and by comprehensive screening and testing programs.

Veterinary public health is a specialty within the broad field of veterinary medicine. Veterinarians in public health conduct research, develop diagnostic and laboratory methods, provide special training and advisory services, and conduct epidemiologic investigations and preventive medical programs concerned with diseases transmissible from animals to man. Veterinarians are employed by the U.S. Department of Agriculture and by the Food and Drug Administration (HEW). Veterinarians in the Public Health Service develop programs for controlling animal diseases that affect public health, help the states establish veterinary public health programs, and serve as consultants in other Public Health Service activities. This nationwide service provides a broad base for tackling widespread problems and has proved effective in reducing the spread of many diseases from area to area. Veterinarians employed by state and local health departments cooperate with private practitioners and federal field workers to control disease among animals and also to protect human health.

The *training* of the various specialized categories of community health workers has for some time been recognized as the particular responsibility of schools of public health, although many other educational forces are getting in on the act. Professional schools of public health were established in the United States early in the present century. In 1912, a formal program of instruction in biologic sciences and public health was organized by William Sedgwick at the Massachusetts Institute of Technology in cooperation with Harvard University. Subsequently, a conference of leaders of public health, medicine, and education set the pattern for schools of public health by recommending that they be established as separate entities but affiliated with universities and their schools of medicine. In 1918, the Johns Hopkins University established a School of Hygiene and Public Health based on this principle. Professionalization of the field continued to develop thereafter, and in 1945, a system of accreditation of schools of public health was begun by the American Public Health Association.

In 1971–1972, there were 19 accredited schools of public health in the United States and Canada. Of the schools in continental United States, four offered bachelors' degrees (the University of California at Berkeley and at Los Angeles, the University of Michigan, and the University of North Carolina), and all offered master's and doctor's degrees. Some students undertake master's or doctoral programs directly after they obtain a bachelor's degree with, perhaps, a major in public health. Many other students in the graduate-degree programs are already practitioners in various health fields, for example, in medicine, dentistry, nursing, veterinary medicine, engineering, environmental health, and numerous additional fields.[15]

Several broad areas have been delineated in the curricula of schools of public health.[16] One of these has to do with the *health problems of the general population,* including the provision of comprehensive health care services and several special considerations such as environmental hazards, infectious diseases, mental illness and retardation, and chronic diseases. A second broad area is concerned with the *health problems of special population groups,* such as mothers and children, occupational groups, and the aged. A third area consists of *special services for the general population or for special groups* and includes medical and hospital care, family planning, health education, nursing, nutrition, occupational health services, and rehabilitation. A fourth area pertains to *health resources and health economics,* and a fifth includes *technical and background subjects* such as epidemiology, biostatistics, demography, behavioral sciences, and research methodology.

New Developments in Health Manpower

THE REALITIES OF SHORTAGES

In all health specialty fields there is the cry of manpower shortages, and the problem has been subjected to detailed and sophisticated analysis, resulting in countless articles, books, and position papers. There have been major conferences on health manpower, sponsored by and involving the federal government (e.g., Department of Labor; Department of Health, Education, and Welfare) as well as the major professional associations. Manpower estimation is a notoriously difficult field, and few agree on the extent of shortages.[17] In some respects, failure to reach agreement on exact figures matters little, since even the more modest manpower aims are likely to be hard to achieve in some fields.

One important observation is that manpower shortages are linked to the nature of the nation's health system. According to this view, some of the shortages are really a consequence of fragmentation and duplication of health service delivery as well as other administrative and logistical deficits.[2,3,18] It is, however, unlikely that even a considerably more streamlined health care system than now exists in the United States would solve the manpower problem completely or even substantially in the short run.

NEW PROGRAMS AND ENLARGEMENT OF TRAINING CLASSES

Manpower growth in the health field has been the result of several developments. One has already been commented on in this chapter, and consists of the expansion of existing training. Thus, in many traditional fields there have been added new schools and programs in the decades since 1950. Table 3-9 summarizes this development for instruction in several health fields. These schools and programs have sometimes been established at great financial cost (particularly medicine and dentistry and, to a lesser extent, nursing) and depend on support principally from federal and state funds.

Corollary to inauguration of new training sites is expansion of the training capabilities of existing ones. Until 1971 this sort of expansion was accomplished essentially by the institutions themselves at their own cost. However, late in 1971, federal legislation—the Comprehensive Health Manpower Training Act and the Nurse Training Act—provided new methods of assistance. The aim of these acts is to increase the number of practicing physicians to 436,000 by 1978 and the number of nurses to about 1.1 million by 1980. In an effort to accomplish these goals, some ingenious approaches are used in the legislation. For example, schools of medicine, osteopathy, and dentistry are awarded special funds if they pledge to increase student enrollment. The new legislation also provides direct loans of up to $3,500 and $2,500 a year for medical and nursing students, respectively. In addition, there is provision for loan forgiveness of up to 85 per cent for medical students who agree to work for two years in an area that has a doctor shortage. Similar provisions exist for nurses, and there are already lists of public or

TABLE 3-9. Increase of Programs and Schools, 1960–1970

	1961–1962	1969–1970
Medicine	87	101
Osteopathy	5	6
Registered nurse	1,123	1,328
Licensed practical (vocational) nurse	739	1,253
Dentistry	47	53
Dental hygienists	37	121
Dental assistants	26	165
Optometry	10*	11
Veterinary medicine	18	18

* 1964–1965 data.

SOURCE: Adapted from U.S. Department of Health, Education, and Welfare, Health Services and Mental Health Administration, National Center for Health Statistics. *Health Resources Statistics, 1971.*

nonprofit hospitals in scarcity areas where employment for a stated period results in 100 per cent loan cancellation.

PHYSICIAN EXPANDERS

Another important manpower thrust relates to the establishment of new programs which, in effect, expand the range of talent and skill of highly trained (and expensive) physician manpower. The objective is to identify elements in diagnosis and treatment of patients that may properly be delegated to individuals with less preparation than is needed to train physicians. Such delegation would thus have the direct result, presumably, of making physicians' time available to supervise more patients. In addition, there would be added to many health careers a new dimension of high technical and social value. The objective presumably is not alone to reduce costs, but also to expand expert medical care.

One major set of physician expander programs involves *extension of the roles of nurses*. In 1971, there were at least 47 programs under way in 16 states, which were designed to extend duties and responsibilities beyond those normally within the nurse's province.[19] Included among new duties are the taking of medical histories, initiation of certain diagnostic procedures and, under supervision, the prescribing of some medication. Table 3-10 gives the titles of 25 of these programs. As can be seen, most are in the pediatrics field, although some branch out into other health care areas.

The nurse extender programs bring to the surface viewpoints that express the fears and hopes involved in any serious innovation. On the one hand are the many nurses who by virtue of training, experience, and other personal qualifications are genuinely ready to alter the basic framework of their present responsibilities. Many have already been performing as nurse practitioners, but without formal training or recognition. Many nurses, on the other hand, probably are not ready to accept such responsibilities, and no doubt would not wish to do so. It is not surprising that some physicians are wary of these potential new nurse-associates, and are made uneasy by the proposed new relationships. However, many physicians welcome the new developments; most nurse-practitioner training programs have physician directors or co-directors. A recent report by a committee appointed by the Secretary of the Department of Health, Education, and Welfare (including many physician members) endorses the nurse extender idea as basically sound.[20]

The other type of physician expander is the *physician's assistant*. In 1971, there were 78 programs that accepted students with various qualifications (generally not nursing) for training as physician's assistants. Table 3-11 gives the titles of a number of operational pro-

TABLE 3-10. Programs for Extending Nursing Roles

State	University or Agency	Title
Arizona	University of Arizona	Family nurse practitioner
California	University of California, Berkeley	Family health practitioner
	Loma Linda University	Pediatric nurse associate
	UCLA School of Medicine	Nursing pediatrist
Colorado	University of Colorado	Pediatric nurse practitioner
	University of Colorado	School nurse practitioner
Connecticut	University of Connecticut	Pediatric nurse associate
	Yale University	Pediatric nurse practitioner
Illinois	Rush Presbyterian—St. Luke's Hospital	Pediatric nurse associate
Kentucky	Frontier Nursing Service	Family nursing program
Maine	University of Maine	Pediatric nurse associate
Massachusetts	Bunker Hill Health Center	Pediatric nurse practitioner
Michigan	Wayne State University	Pediatric nurse practitioner
Missouri	Washington University	Pediatric nurse practitioner
New York	Albert Einstein College of Medicine	Nurse physician surrogate
	Albert Einstein College of Medicine	Triage or screening professional
	Dr. Martin Luther King, Jr., Health Center and Montefiore Hospital	Public health nurse practitioner
	University of Rochester	Pediatric nurse practitioner
Ohio	University of Cincinnati	Pediatric nurse associate
Pennsylvania	St. Christopher's Hospital for Children	In-service education for ambulatory pediatric nurse
	Allegheny County Health Dept.	Pediatric specialist program for public health nurses
Tennessee	University of Tennessee	Pediatric nurse clinician
Texas	Baylor University	Ophthalmic nursing
	U.S. Air Force Medical Center	Pediatric nurse practitioner
Virginia	University of Virginia	Nurse clinician

SOURCE: U.S. Department of Health, Education, and Welfare, National Institutes of Health. *Selected Training Programs for Physician Support Personnel,* Pub. No. 72-183, 1971, pp. viii–ix.

TABLE 3-11. Listing of Selected Physician's Assistant Programs

State	University or Agency	Title
Alabama	University of Alabama	MEDEX
	University of Alabama	Pathology assistant
	University of Alabama	Surgeon's assistant
California	De Anza Junior College	Pediatric assisting
	Foothill Junior College	Orthopedic assistant
Colorado	University of Colorado	Child health associate
District of Columbia	Washington Hospital Center	Cardiovascular technician
Georgia	Emory University	Medical specialty assistant
	Georgia State University	Pediatric assistants
Kentucky	University of Kentucky	Clinical associate
Michigan	Western Michigan University	Physician's associate
	Veteran's Administration Hospital	Urological assistant
New York	Brooklyn Cumberland Medical Center	Medical services associate
	Columbia-Presbyterian Medical Center	Orthoptics and ophthalmic assistant
	Manhattan Community College	Medical emergency technician
	U.S. Public Health Service Hospital	Marine physician assistant
North Carolina	Duke University	Pathology assistant
	Bowman-Gray School of Medicine	Physician's assistant
Ohio	Cincinnati Technical Institute	Surgical assistant
	University of Cincinnati	Urological assistant
	Cleveland Clinic Hospital	The corpsman
	Ohio State University	Circulation technology
Pennsylvania	Hahnemann Medical College	Graduate art therapist
	Hahnemann Medical College	Mental health technology
Texas	University of Texas	Clinical associate
	Baylor College of Medicine	Ophthalmic assistant
Washington	University of Washington	MEDEX
West Virginia	Alderson-Broaddus College	Physician's assistant
Wisconsin	Marshfield Clinic	Physician's assistant

SOURCE: U.S. Department of Health, Education, and Welfare, National Institutes of Health. *Selected Training Pro-*

grams in various states. Some, like *Medex* programs, give preference to ex-military or ex-navy medical corpsmen, or persons with other health experience. These programs appeal at present principally to male students, although there is no reason why women would not be equally appropriate. The *generalist* programs train graduates to keep records, perform emergency care, take histories, and do routine diagnostic tests. In the training, there are studies in basic sciences, laboratory procedures, medical instrumentation, and clinical experience. Most *specialist* programs train graduates to perform specialty physical examinations, to do routine diagnostic tests, and to take histories. Almost all specialist programs require basic sciences, the rest of the curriculum being geared to specialty needs. Although physician's assistant training is relatively new, some programs have graduated their first classes, with graduates now in employment, and most seem to be enjoying a measure of success.[21]

For both the nurse extender and the physician's assistant programs, several concerns about career outcome are worthy of mention. First, for the newly prepared health professional, there is concern about the definition of the role to be played in the actual medical care situation. There needs to be common agreement by the parties involved, about the nature of day-to-day authority and responsibility in the new role. Second, an extremely important consideration is the effect of the new jobs upon the patient. From meager studies undertaken thus far, there is full acceptance of the new roles only in connection with certain routine tasks,[22] although there may well be increased acceptance as patients gain more experience with the new personnel. Third, it is clear that, as in all education for skilled jobs, selection of particular candidates for instruction is of high importance. Finally, there is the matter of licensure and legal responsibility. Not all states in which there are the programs listed in Tables 3-10 and 3-11 have yet licensed the careers in question.

MINORITY EMPLOYMENT

Cutting across these efforts at expansion and extension of health delivery skills are simultaneous efforts to introduce into the health labor force several groups previously underrepresented in such employment. One such group consists of America's racial minorities—Black, Chicano, Puerto Rican, American Indian, and American Oriental. There are relatively few physicians and dentists in the United States who have a minority-group background, although the nursing field has long held some opportunities for minority women. The situation is changing slowly. For example, the 1971–1972 entering classes in medical schools had 1,275 minority students, compared with 998 in the entering class of 1970–1971, an increase of more than 25 per cent. There is a corollary interest in the medical school enrollment of women. A total of 1,673 women enrolled in America's medical schools in 1971–1972 compared with 1,256 in 1970–1971, an increase of one third.

The situation is more serious concerning preparation for entry-level health jobs requiring less education than that which qualifies for medicine, nursing, or dentistry. Minority students (particularly Negroes, Mexican Americans, Puerto Ricans, and American Indians) have educational deficits that often hinder ready admission to colleges and universities where training programs for a broad variety of health careers are available. This situation also is slowly changing, with many institutions making special allowances for admission (e.g., accepting experience as educational equivalent in some instances) and providing special tutoring after admission.

One important new force in education for all races, but of great meaning for racial minorities in particular, is the emergence of the community college (two-year program) in training for health careers. A recent query of the 1,000 colleges listed in the 1970 junior college directory revealed that of 708 colleges responding, 620 were offering at least one program in the health instruction field and more than half were offering two or more such programs.[23] The array of programs is very broad and includes "basic" programs, short programs, continuing education, and refresher courses. The basic health occupation programs include assistant and/or technician categories in several broad fields, as shown in Table 3-12.

NEW CAREERS

Still another and extremely important subvariety of health manpower is the "new careerist." New health careers are part of a broad movement to employ indigenous poor people in health and welfare settings where educational requirements are normally much higher.[24,25] The jobs are variously titled: health aide; family aide; community health aide; environmental health aide. There are even "community health research aides," and one of the newest titles is "service guide." There are at least 150 different job titles of individuals found employed in neighborhood comprehensive health centers, migrant health programs, community mental health centers, maternal and infant care projects, Indian health centers, and elsewhere.

Typical tasks performed by new careerists include collecting data about agency clients; explaining agency or institution services to clients and preparing them for interaction with professionals; seeing that appointments are kept; acting on behalf of clients and

TABLE 3-12. Basic Health Occupations Education Programs Offered in Junior Colleges, United States, 1971

ADMINISTRATIVE SERVICES	12		MEDICAL CARE ASSISTANTS	
Health administrative assistant	7		(continued)	
Nursing home administrator	5		Inhalation therapist	87
BIOMEDICAL ENGINEERING AND			Intravenous technician	—
INSTRUMENTATION SERVICES	6		Orthopedic assistant	5
Biomedical engineering			Physician's assistant	—
technician	5		Podiatric assistant	—
EEG technician	1		MISCELLANEOUS SERVICES	14
EEG-EKG technician	—		Dietary technician	9
DENTAL SERVICES	210		Geriatric assistant	—
Dental assistant	125		Medical photographer	2
Dental hygienist	63		Pharmacy technician	—
Dental laboratory technician	22		Veterinary technician	3
ENVIRONMENTAL CONTROL			NURSING SERVICES	661
SERVICES	24		Home health aide	1
Environmental science aide	4		Licensed practical nurse	281
Environmental science			Nursing aide	—
technician	19		Registered nurse	340
Radiological health technician	1		Surgical technician	39
EMERGENCY SERVICES	1		OPTICAL AND VISUAL CARE	
Medical emergency aide	—		SERVICES	10
Medical emergency technician	1		Optician	5
LABORATORY SERVICES	123		Vision care technician	5
Cytotechnologist	1		RADIOLOGICAL SERVICES	105
Histology/cytology technician	1		Nuclear medicine	
Medical laboratory assistant	22		technician	6
Medical laboratory technician	97		Radiation therapy	
Medical technologist	2		technician	2
MEDICAL RECORDS AND OFFICE			Radiologic technician	97
SERVICES	247		REHABILITATION SERVICES	46
Medical office assistant	104		Occupational therapy	
Medical records technician	44		assistant	21
Medical secretary	99		Physical/occupational	
MENTAL HEALTH AND			therapy assistant	2
PSYCHIATRIC SERVICES	64		Physical therapy assistant	19
Mental health assistant	50		Prosthetic/orthotic	
Mental retardation specialist	6		technician	3
Psychiatric aide	8		Recreational therapy	
MEDICAL CARE ASSISTANTS	92		technician	1
Cardiovascular technician	—		Speech and hearing	
Dialysis technician	—		technician	—

SOURCE: American Association of Junior Colleges. *Allied Health Education Programs in Junior Colleges/1970.* U.S. Department of Health, Education, and Welfare (NIH) Pub. No. 72-163, pp. 6–7.

cutting red tape for them; taking initiative in organizing neighborhoods and communities; and so on.[26] Sometimes new careerists are trained to offer emergency health care.

While new careerists are not prepared to carry out complex technical or medical procedures, intelligent application of their skills can make or break a health program in inner-city ghettos and kindred settings. Employment of new careerists also has other important consequences. It adds to the economic base of a poverty area. If the job is permanent, is integral to the health system, and has opportunities for higher career development, an invaluable element of credibility of the agency or institution is created. Not only are useful role models created in this way, but also the new careerist can bridge the gap between client (the poor) and the professional (not poor, often white). Most important, the presence of the new careers employee communicates that someone in the health system cares and is protective of indigenous interests.

Although no reliable count is available of new careerists, they number in the thousands. Their ages range from very young to middle age. Education varies, but often is less than high school graduation. All are poor, and nearly all are from racial minorities. Commonly sought attributes are relationship abilities, capacity to handle crises and emergencies thoughtfully and without panic, willingness to follow instructions of professional staff, among other qualities.

An employer of new careerists in a rural mental health program in North Carolina is convinced that one such new career—the "service guide"—more than warrants the stipulated $5,500 annual salary. There is evidence that rehospitalization rates began to drop when "service guides" who were assigned to follow up ex-patients began identifying their relapses early and getting them into the aftercare clinic without delay.[27]

References

1. American Medical Association, Division of Medical Practice, Department of Health Manpower. *Current Status of the "Physician's Assistant" Concept.* American Medical Association, Chicago, Illinois, September 1971.
2. Kroepsch, Robert H., Bunnell, Kevin P., Elliott, Jo Eleanor, Feldman, Raymond, and Palmer, Paula. Health manpower: adapting in the 70's, education and training. In: *Health Manpower Adapting in the Seventies.* Report of the 1971 National Health Forum. National Health Council, New York, 1971.
3. Doster, Daphine D. Utilization of available "nurse power" in public health. *Am J Public Health,* **60**:25–37, January 1970.

4. Cowin, Ruth. Some new dimensions of social work practice in a health setting. *Am J Public Health,* **60:**860–69, May 1970.

5. Fisher, Morton A. New directions for dentistry. *Am J Public Health,* **60:**848–59, May 1970.

6. Applewhite, Harold L. A new design for recruitment of blacks into health careers. *Am J Public Health,* **61:**1965–71, October 1971.

7. U.S. Department of Health, Education, and Welfare, Public Health Service, Health Services and Mental Health Administration, National Center for Health Statistics. *Health Resources Statistics, 1971.* U.S. Government Printing Office, Washington, D.C., 1972.

8. U.S. Department of Labor, Bureau of Employment Security. *Health Careers Guidebook.* U.S. Government Printing Office, Washington, D.C., 1965.

9. U.S. Department of Health, Education, and Welfare, Public Health Service, National Institutes of Health, Bureau of Health Professions Education and Manpower Training. *Health Manpower Source Book,* Section 21. U.S. Government Printing Office, Washington, D.C., 1970.

10. Bonnet, Philip D. Health manpower needs and requirements. In: U.S. Department of Labor-U.S. Department of Health, Education, and Welfare. *Training Health Services Workers: The Critical Challenge.* (Proceedings of the Conference on Job Development and Training for Workers in Health Services.) U.S. Government Printing Office, Washington, D.C., 1966.

11. U.S. Department of Health, Education, and Welfare, Public Health Service, National Institutes of Health, Bureau of Health Manpower Education, Division of Nursing. *Handbook for Loan Cancellation Benefit.* HEW Publication No. (NIH) 72-220. U.S. Government Printing Office, Washington, D.C., January 1972.

12. American Medical Association, the Council on Health Manpower. *Expanding the Supply of Health Services in the 1970's.* Report of the National Congress on Health Manpower. American Medical Association, Chicago, Illinois, 1970.

13. Points, Thomas C. Guidelines for development of new health occupations. *JAMA,* **213:**1169–71, August 17, 1970.

14. Altman, Stuart H. *Present and Future Supply of Registered Nurses.* HEW Publication No. (NIH) 72-134. U.S. Government Printing Office, Washington, D.C., November 1971.

15. American Public Health Association, Committee on Professional Education. Educational qualifications of management personnel in health agencies. *Am J Public Health,* **60:**345–50, February 1970.

16. American Public Health Association, Committee on Professional Education. Criteria and guidelines for accrediting schools of public health. *Am J Public Health,* **56:**1308–18, August 1966.

17. Lynch, Michael. The physician "shortage": the economists' mirror. *Ann Am Acad Pol Sci,* **399:**82–88, January 1972.

18. Roemer, Ruth. Legal regulation of health manpower in the 1970's. In: *Health Manpower: Adapting in the Seventies.* Report of the 1971 National Health Forum. National Health Council, New York, 1971.

19. U.S. Department of Health, Education, and Welfare, Public Health

Service, National Institutes of Health, Bureau of Health Manpower Education, Division of Manpower Intelligence, Professional Requirements Branch. *Selected Training Programs for Physician Support Personnel.* HEW Publication No. (NIH) 72-183. U.S. Government Printing Office, Washington, D.C., March 1971.

20. U.S. Department of Health, Education, and Welfare, Secretary's Committee to Study Extended Roles for Nurses. Extending the scope of nursing practice. *JAMA,* **220:**1231–36, May 29, 1972.

21. Hughbanks, Janet, and Freeborn, Donald K. Review of 22 training programs for physician's assistants. *HSMHA Health Rep,* **86:**857–62, October 1971.

22. Litman, Theodor J. Public perceptions of the physicians' assistant—a survey of the attitudes and opinions of rural Iowa and Minnesota residents. *Am J Public Health,* **62:**343–46, March 1972.

23. American Association of Junior Colleges. *Allied Health Education Programs in Junior Colleges/1970.* HEW Publication No. (NIH) 72-163. U.S. Government Printing Office, Washington, D.C., 1970.

24. Pearl, Arthur, and Reissman, Frank. *New Careers for the Poor.* Free Press, New York, 1965.

25. Gartner, Alan. *Paraprofessionals and Their Performance.* Praeger Publishers, New York, 1971.

26. Lenzer, Anthony. New health careers for the poor. *Am J Public Health,* **60:**45–50, January 1970.

27. Hollister, William G. The service guide. *Am J Public Health,* **60:**428–29, 1970.

SECTION

II

MEDICAL CARE,
MENTAL HEALTH,
AND
ENVIRONMENTAL
HEALTH

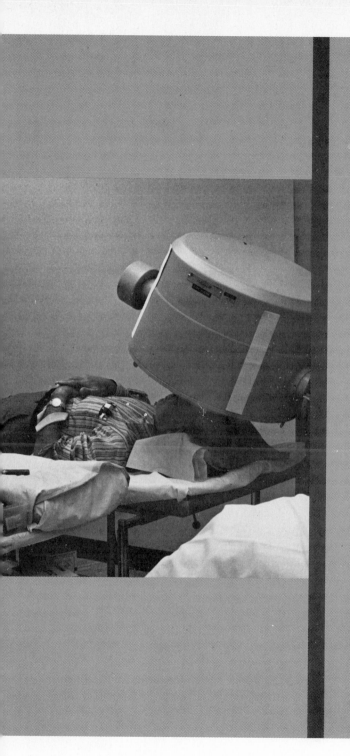

4

PUBLIC HEALTH
ASPECTS OF
MEDICAL CARE

CHAPTER OUTLINE

The Scope and Nature of Medical Care

Medical Care Dilemmas of the 1970's

Shifts in Population
Increased Consumer Demands and Expectations
Lags in Training Health Care Personnel
Rising Costs of Medical Care
Failure to Organize the Delivery of Health Services

Basic Organizational Modes for Providing Medical Care

Private (Solo) Practice
Group Practice
Outpatient Clinics
Hospitals
Nursing Homes
Home Health Services

Maintaining the Quality of Medical Care

Financing and Delivery of Health Services in the United States

Paying for Health Care
Present Privately Sponsored Health Insurance Plans
Present Government-Sponsored Financing Plans
Proposed Private-Government Plans
Workmen's Compensation

Direct Medical Care Provided by the Federal Government

Courtesy of California's Health, *California Department of Public Health.*
Staff photo.

The Scope and Nature of Medical Care

The aim of a rational system of medical care is to provide health service when it is needed, with use of the best health technology available and with efficiency, warmth, and compassion. The system should provide services to individuals with the intention of preventing illness or of mitigating the course of illness once it has begun.

From a community vantage point, medical care services are all the personal health services, including the care of sick and disabled persons, which are rendered by individual physicians, nurses, and related personnel and by private and public agencies. Thus, it is generally recognized that to be effective, medical care extends well beyond the provision of treatment to the sick and covers the entire range of services: preventive, curative, and rehabilitative.

Sometimes this service can be best and most expeditiously provided as ambulatory care, that is, in visits to a physician and nurse for diagnosis and treatment, often involving some combination of change in health behavior and prescription of drugs. Sometimes referral is necessary for review of the case from specialty viewpoints. Sometimes hospital stay is indicated, for further observations and tests, for controlling the patient's environment, or for surgery. Sometimes there is the need for hospital aftercare in a nursing home or in a home care program.

Organizing the delivery of medical care is far from a simple matter. The parties to a system of medical care include trained *health manpower* or providers, in proper numbers, with the appropriate skills and specialties, and with an outlook broad enough to be mindful of various sociomedical responsibilities. The parties include, also, *health consumers* — young and old alike — of different racial, economic, and educational backgrounds, and with an astonishing variety of health habits and practices. Linking health provider and consumer requires an organizational scheme that ensures medical care of high quality and concern. Public policy dictates that care be rendered with an eye to the benefit of the health consumer rather than mainly at the convenience and for the gain of the health provider. Needless to say, the system should provide geographic matching up of populations needing care, on the one hand, and professionals and technical personnel, institutions and other agencies ready to offer it.

The system should take into account and make provision for consumers who are unsophisticated in dealing effectively with organized bureaucracies, let alone with medical organizations that are too easily perceived as intimidating. The system must forecast its manpower requirements and plan for changes in need and demand. And finally, an effective medical care organization must provide service at prices individuals can afford. Financing—as well as technical skill, geographic placement, and sheer management—becomes critical to medical care organizations.[1]

Quality of medical care begins with availability, and is further concerned with diagnostic acumen, treatment regimen, hospital bed provisions, and aftercare procedures. It includes the concept of *continuity of care* and, last but not least, some concern for the sensibilities of the patient. Some problems of quality of care are really not related to the technical excellence of the physician. Even the best physician is hampered when a case comes too late to cope with optimally, or when gaps in continuity of care interfere with proper patient management. However, serious erosions in quality take place when doctors for various reasons—including overly busy practices—fail to keep up with advances in medicine and surgery.

Medical Care Dilemmas of the 1970's

Much has been said about how health care differs in the 1970's from the health care of the early 1900's, with some idealization of the devotion and quality of service rendered in the earlier time. In those days, for persons who could afford a family doctor, there was one who made house calls when necessary, who was cordial and friendly, and who knew the family history. He was, in short, a source of comfort, regardless of whether or not he was able to do much for a particular ailment.

Whatever the true state of medical care in the United States in earlier times, the present reality is far different from the idealized past. There is no doubt that, individually, today's physicians, nurses, and dentists are technically far better trained than their earlier counterparts. Today's diagnostic procedures are extraordinarily sophisticated. There is also today a far more impressive armamentarium of treatment modalities, including pharmaceuticals and surgical procedures. And hospitals are governed by exacting licensing and accreditation procedures unknown in an earlier period.

Yet there appears today substantial discontent in many quarters with the American medical care scheme.[2] There is discontent with availability of care when needed, discontent with quality of care when rendered, and universal discontent with its costliness. Many persons, in fact, consider the United States to be in the midst of a medical care crisis. The situation, having developed over a long period of time, results from the convergence of several circumstances, including shifts in population, increased consumer demands and expectations, lags in the training of health care personnel, rising costs of medical care, and failure to organize the delivery of health services.

SHIFTS IN POPULATION

Certain demographic facts of recent decades have affected supply and demand for medical care services. For example, there has been since the 1900's, a steady migration of individuals from farms to cities and, in the 1960's and 1970's, from the central cities to the suburbs. Doctors, dentists, and to some extent hospitals have tended to follow population migrations, with consequent loss of professional manpower, first, from the rural and farm communities and later from the inner cities. The consequence has been millions of Americans without ready access to health care personnel when needed. Since central cities are increasingly occupied by Blacks and Spanish-speaking and other minorities, there has been the additional factor of racial estrangement.

A direct press on demand for health care services derives from the steady rise of the population of older persons in the United States. Table 4-1 shows that there were 20 million persons 55 years

TABLE 4-1. Population of the United States, 55 Years and Older, Selected Years

Age in Years	Population in Millions			
	1940	*1950*	*1960*	*1970*
55–64	10.7	13.3	15.5	18.6
65–74	6.4	8.4	11.0	12.4
75 and older	2.6	3.9	5.6	7.6
Total 55 years and older	19.7	25.6	32.1	38.6

Sources: Adapted from U.S. Department of Health, Education, and Welfare, National Center for Health Statistics. *Facts of Life and Death,* 1970, p. 3. Also, U.S. Bureau of the Census. *General Population Characteristics, United States Summary,* 1970 Census of Population. Also, U.S. Bureau of the Census. *Statistical Abstract of the United States, 1971,* p. 23.

and older in 1940; by 1970 this number had almost doubled to 38.6 million. Older persons, of course, tend to suffer from chronic illness at a far greater rate than do younger adults or children. Chronic diseases are long-lasting and require more medical attention, and the individual often requires protracted care and institutionalization. The doubling of this drain on medical care resources is bound to present significant additional strain on the system.

INCREASED CONSUMER DEMANDS
AND EXPECTATIONS

Added to the preceding set of pressures is the "revolution of rising expectation in consumer demand," brought about in part by World War II, when many Americans experienced for the first time in their lives the benefits of comprehensive medical care for themselves and their dependents as a by-product of military service. This demand was underwritten by the advance in medical technology, which affected a host of techniques, from blood banking to surgery, and gave medicine capabilities that were undreamed of only a few years before. The revolutionary advances in communication which paralleled these gains created an expanded awareness of the new developments in medical care. Many population groups previously unaffected by medical care advances soon emerged with kindred medical care demands. All these forces have led to a recognition of the existence of great pockets of unmet medical needs within a generally affluent society. The benefits to be derived from the advances of medical technology have been particularly unattainable for the segments of the population who are in impoverished circumstances. These segments include minority groups, the elderly, migrant workers, and numerous others who are at or near the poverty level. In such groups are found the most urgent medical needs, often compounded by a complex of health and social problems.

LAGS IN TRAINING HEALTH CARE PERSONNEL

Another source of the present medical care problem is the lags that have occurred in training and preparation of health care personnel. As reviewed in Chapter 3, while there have been rising demand indicators, the supply of critical professional health manpower has either remained stationary (dentists) or has risen only slightly (physicians). Only nurse training has to some extent kept pace with population trends.

TABLE 4-2. Index of Medical Care Prices, United States, Selected Years

	1950	1960	1970
TOTAL MEDICAL CARE	57.7	79.1	120.6
SELECTED COMPONENTS			
Physicians' fees	55.2	77.0	121.4
Dentists' fees	63.9	82.1	119.4
Hospital daily service charges	28.9	56.3	143.9
Drugs and prescriptions	88.5	104.5	103.6

SOURCE: U.S. Bureau of the Census. *Statistical Abstract of the United States, 1971,* p. 62.

RISING COSTS OF MEDICAL CARE

Costs of physician, nursing, and dental care have been rising steadily since 1950 and have been accompanied by soaring increases in costs of hospital and nursing-home stay. Cost increases have been due in part to the demand and supply factors already mentioned. Advances in medical technology are also extremely expensive. For example, improved diagnostic procedures and complex treatment programs require increased time from health providers per patient served as well as longer stays in hospitals and nursing homes.

Inflation, of course, is a significant factor in mounting medical costs. From 1950 to 1965, the cost of physicians' services, dentists' fees, optometric examinations, and particularly hospital charges rose ahead of the rising cost of living. In 1965, the introduction of Medicare and Medicaid, largely because of the method of financing, made doctors' fees rise more than twice as fast as before and hospital daily costs rise even more steeply.

The index of medical care prices reveals how steeply prices have risen in the period 1950–1970 (Table 4-2). Physicians' fees have more than doubled in the 20-year period (increasing from 55.2 in 1950 to 121.4 in 1970). Dentists' fees have gone up nearly 90 per cent (from 63.9 to 119.4). Hospital daily charges in 1970 were more than four times their price in 1950. The costs of drugs and prescriptions have gone up since 1950, but have stabilized from 1960 to 1970. The consequences of the medical care cost-crunch are felt everywhere in society, among the poor to be sure, but also pressing hard on the broad range of middle-income families.

FAILURE TO ORGANIZE THE DELIVERY OF HEALTH SERVICES

There has been notable failure to organize the medical care effort in the United States to make up for the deficits noted in the foregoing. While many observers have called attention to various faults in the system in the decades from 1930 to 1960, the 1960's saw the emergence of serious national debate about solutions to the medical care problem. The critical issues in this debate center around the method of payment for medical care (including preventive care)—how and by whom payment is to be made—and around the method of arranging for care—how and by whom it is to be rendered.[2]

Elements in the debate touch some deep and sensitive nerves that cause conflict between major themes in American life. One theme suggests that individuals should pay for what they get and be responsible for debts so incurred. Another important theme is the growing national consciousness that, while material things fit that model, health has the quality of a *right*.

Thus, although health care is a purchasable commodity, it defies the normal rules of the free-enterprise marketplace. There ought to be only one standard of health care, not a flimsy one for those who can only afford that, and a better one for those who can afford better.[3] Moreover, there are too few normal marketplace forces that reward good quality of care, availability of health care, and efficiency of service, thus reducing the cost. In fact, at present the normal market mechanisms probably work in unison *against* a fair and equitable distribution of health care services to all Americans. Such broad planning and reorganization efforts as have actually been instituted have been substantially ineffectual in altering the main difficulties, since they tended to avoid coming to grips with the prerogatives of the private practice of medicine and dentistry. Two exceptions are the enactment in 1965 of Medicare and Medicaid legislation (substantial relief for the payment of medical care for persons 65 and older as well as for certain other classes of impoverished patients) and the rise of prepayment group practices.

Basic Organizational Modes for Providing Medical Care

The direct provision of medical care normally begins with contact between the health consumer (the patient) and a health professional—either a licensed physician or someone under the direction and supervision of a physician. A vast array of different kinds of health professionals may be involved in the rendering of this care (see Chapter 3). There are several organizational modes of medical practice today and a variety of settings and institutions in which health services are provided. One need hardly be reminded that, however slowly, the American health service system has been evolving over many years and that changes, experiments, and other innovations in organization are increasingly being undertaken.

PRIVATE (SOLO) PRACTICE

The private practice of medicine has for decades been a primary entry point for the rendering of medical care. Under private practice the patient employs whatever physician he wishes or is able to afford. "Free choice" of physicians has been for decades a hallmark of private practice. The physician attends the patient for as long as the arrangement is mutually satisfactory and has responsibility to the patient alone. The physician must, of course, be licensed to practice medicine in the state in which he practices and must observe the laws of the state regarding medical practice. Should he exhibit what the patient regards as carelessness, neglect, or incompetence the patient may bring suit for malpractice through the courts.

Private practice depends for high-quality medical care on familiarity with the patient's history, good record keeping, competency of referrals, and a deep concern by the physician regarding continuity of care. It depends, moreover, on the physician's personal competence and ability to keep up to date on current developments in the art and science of medical practice.

In private solo practice, the physician is a businessman as well as a provider of care. Particularly when medical costs are high it would be surprising if the relationship between patient and physician did not suffer as a consequence of the finances of care, and if medical judgments were not sometimes affected. The situation has, in fact, been aggravated by the introduction of third-party payments in which someone other than the patient participates in compensating the physician for the services rendered. As a consequence, there are few inhibitions to charging what the traffic will bear, since "someone else" is paying the bill. In the last analysis, the patient pays through higher premiums and fees.[4]

GROUP PRACTICE

A principal alternative to solo practice of medicine is group practice, which seeks in several ways to improve medical care rendered to patients. In the most advanced group practice situations there are assembled in one organization physicians of different specialties, often in a location where they have joint use of personnel and equipment, all organized to aid in the diagnosis and treatment of the patient's illness. Until recent years, group practice was opposed by the American Medical Association, and there remains today substantial opposition from many elements of organized medicine particularly against group practices that depart from fee-for-service principles.

A survey conducted in 1969 by the American Medical Association revealed that there were in the United States approximately 6,400 medical groups involving 40,000 physicians.[5] Most of the groups could be properly referred to as "combined practice" groups, with only limited advantage generally taken of the group concept. Two thirds of the groups were small—consisting of at most three to four physicians—and almost half were *single-specialty groups* (e.g., radiologists, surgeons, etc.). The vast majority of all medical groups operated on a fee-for-service basis, maintaining at least this characteristic in common with solo practice. Of special interest are the approximately 2,400 *multispecialty groups* involving 24,000 physicians. These hold the promise of offering organizationally based comprehensive care to their patients. More than 1,000 of these are small (fewer than 5 affiliated physicians), and the vast majority operate on a fee-for-service basis, charging by item for services rendered.

Group practice is in a state of flux, and it is possible to forecast rapid growth of the idea as a significant factor in the delivery of medical care in the United States in the future.[6] Of high interest are some 400 to 500 group plans in operation in 1971 that in varying degrees applied the concepts of *organization for health care delivery*.[5,7] These plans are variously sponsored, some by private medical (or dental) groups, by medical (or dental) societies, by health consumers, by union and/or employer welfare funds or associations, and by others. There is endless variation in the plans in the precise health benefits available and in the manner and setting in which health care is obtained by the subscriber or patient. To be noted particularly are the group practices that operate on a prepayment plan, that is, provide contract services on a per capita basis to a defined population for major health care coverage. In such plans, capitation payments are calculated actuarially, that is, on illness and medical care utilization experience of members in the plan. Coverage is generally broad and some plans operate their own hospitals and laboratories as well as providing doctors' offices, examining rooms, and other facilities. Most of the larger plans operate on a nonprofit basis. Pioneering and eminently successful examples of this type are the Kaiser Foundation Health Plans (California, Oregon, Hawaii, Ohio, Colorado), Group Health Cooperative of Puget Sound (Seattle, Washington), Community Health Association (Detroit, Michigan), and Group Health Association (Washington, D.C.).

From the standpoint of quality of medical care rendered, groups offer several distinct advantages over solo practice. First, the close collaboration among several physicians tends to establish an atmosphere of peer review of each person's professional activity. Second, each physician has easy access to consultation when he is in an area of uncertainty and has no fear of losing his patient to the consultant. Third, many groups have sufficient income and volume of patients to permit the purchase of superior, expensive equipment and to justify a laboratory on the premises. Both these measures aid the physician in improving the quality of care he delivers. Fourth, many group practice agreements specify that the physicians may take time each year to attend medical conferences and refresher courses, thus again increasing the potential for betterment of quality of care.

For the consumer likewise there are many benefits from receiving care through a group practice. First, in a well-developed group, he is offered the benefits of an entire array of specialists, each ready to consult as his case may require. Second, many groups offer patients preventive care of a kind that is not readily available from solo practitioners. Some groups effect a cost saving to patients by stressing the use of out-of-hospital treatment wherever possible. Finally, groups offer the patient continuity of care and coverage that is available every hour of every day.

Existing nonprofit group practices have found a large measure of favor with subscribers who express general satisfaction both with medical care received and with financial arrangements. Chief dissatisfactions are cliniclike atmosphere for certain procedures (waiting rooms), lengthy waiting times, and bureaucratic impersonality.

OUTPATIENT CLINICS

Health Department and Hospital Clinics. Outpatient clinics are at present a significant element in the initiation of medical care for hundreds of thousands of individuals in the United States. One segment is the outpatient clinics of the 1,800 city and county health departments throughout the nation. Services typically include prenatal clinics, child health conferences, tuberculosis clinics, venereal disease clinics, and immunization clinics. More advanced health departments also may conduct alcoholic rehabilitation clinics, dental clinics, and clinics for glaucoma testing and diabetes screening. Most recently some health departments (still very few) conduct clinics for adolescent and youth groups, pregnancy testing, drug treatment, family planning, and other programs.

Hospital outpatient activities constitute the other significant segment of the outpatient scene. In 1970, there were in all hospitals in the United States almost 200 million outpatient visits, double the approximately 100 million visits in 1962. Analysis of about 130 million outpatient visits to community hospitals alone (nonfederal, nonchronic disease, and nonpsychiatric) reveals that about a third are emergency visits, a third are as regular clinic patients, and a third are referrals from physicians. Visits to emergency departments and referrals have sharply increased since 1962 and reflect the extent to which the outpatient clinic (health department or hospital) has evolved as the source of medical care for ambulatory patients who are poor, although there are some private outpatient clinics that charge substantial fees.

The rise in use of hospital emergency rooms is of particular interest, and a number of reasons other than poverty have been advanced for their popularity, including 24-hour service and the fact that hospital emergency visits are often covered by health insurance, but doctor visits are not. Moreover, population mobility is such that families new to a town may not yet have found a physician. In any event, many office practices are crowded and do not encourage unscheduled visits.

Neighborhood Health Centers and Projects.   Practical and psychologic impediments to the search for good ambulatory medical care have given rise in recent years to several new varieties of outpatient clinics for low-income families and individuals. These include neighborhood health centers supported largely or wholly by the federal Office of Economic Opportunity (OEO) or by the Public Health Service (Community Health Service). They also include projects supported by the Children's Health Service (the Maternal and Infant Care Projects and the Children and Youth Projects) as well as centers supported by federal migrant health funds.

All the centers and projects aim not merely to provide direct categorical health service, but also to search out actively those who might benefit from care. The latter intention is helped materially by location of the facility in the immediate neighborhood of greatest utilization, with evening and weekend hours, minimum eligibility screening procedures, and so on.

A recent review of neighborhood centers in 24 large American cities (populations of about 500,000 or more) revealed a varied picture, with a number already established and a number in the process of development. While most centers are organized independently, a few are run by local health departments in a fashion representing radical departure from traditional clinics. Thus, for example, by 1970, New York City had 8 comprehensive health centers (6 supported by OEO and 2 by the Public Health Service) plus a number organized by the city health department which were already operative or in planning. Chicago had 3 OEO centers and 3 children and youth centers. Philadelphia had 3 OEO centers, 1 Public Health Service center, and several run by the health department.

Significant problems in connection with neighborhood centers are funding, staffing, and community participation in clinic affairs. In addition to OEO, Public Health Service, and Children's Health Service sources, there is some support from the Model Cities Program of the Department of Housing and Urban Development and from special project grants (e.g., for drug control programs). Some centers have combined support from several agencies. Support from granting agencies has been shrinking since the beginning of the programs, and local support is also increasingly difficult to come by. Staff problems are sizable, since a hallmark of such operations is to employ personnel not only technically qualified but culturally sensitive as well. Such operations are also seen as opportunities for employment of persons from the neighborhood, usually ethnic minorities. The matter of community voice in the running of the clinic is another issue in connection with neighborhood centers. It sometimes can be resolved with few problems, but often there is wrangling among various factions who desire to be spokesmen for the community regarding clinic affairs. The medical effectiveness of the neighborhood centers is now under study, and it remains to be seen to what extent community health is advanced in this way.[8]

Free Clinics. The free clinic is another new phenomenon, about as old as the neighborhood health center. A survey in 1971 showed at least 135 volunteer clinics in the United States, including about 80 that started up during 1970–1971. While free clinics are located in all parts of the United States (and in Canada), the largest state-concentration appeared to be in California, where there were 42 clinics.[9]

Staffed mainly by volunteers (physicians, nurses, and others) the free clinics are open mainly evenings and cater to youth and young adults under 25 years of age. Many clinics serve principally white youth of the counterculture. Others (neighborhood free clinics) serve principally minority group members in the surrounding area, or specially designated ethnic groups (e.g., in Los Angeles, the Barrio Free Clinic and the American Indian Free Clinic).

Free clinics mainly treat emergencies, venereal disease, problems of pregnancy, and drug problems as well as providing a scattering of services including infant care, dental care, and psychiatric or psychologic counseling. One of the attractions of free clinics for their clients is freedom from red tape, hassle, and constraints of "the Establishment." As with other new modalities, contributions of these clinics to the medical care scene is as yet unclear.

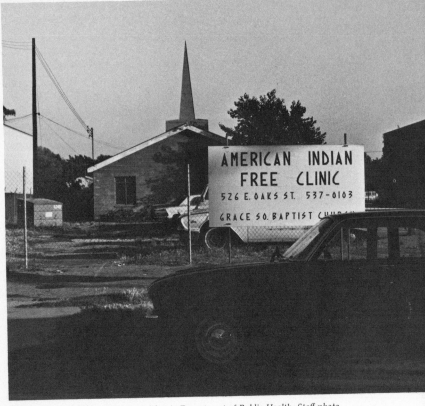

Courtesy of California's Health, *California Department of Public Health. Staff photo.*

HOSPITALS

Changing Role of the Hospital.   The place of the hospital in American medical care has undergone dramatic change in recent years. Not long ago, the hospital was a place where the very poor and the terminally ill languished in their misery. Today the situation has changed for several reasons. First, the hospital is the logical site of delivery of many of the advances in medical technology that have provided previously undreamed of potential for altering the course of disease. This technology involves complex and often expensive equipment as well as large numbers of personnel whose jobs may require special training. The hospital, properly organized, is also an unparalleled place to conduct surgical procedures and to maintain careful surveillance and monitoring of patient progress, functions not possible to carry out in a doctor's office. Hospitals, as has been noted, are also the site of emergency rooms and outpatient departments which provide valuable adjuncts to the practice of medicine.

In 1970, there were approximately 7,600 hospitals in the United States. This figure is up from 1946, but stable since about 1965, particularly among general medical and surgical hospitals. About 6,600 are general hospitals, and there are 501 psychiatric, 108 tuberculosis, and 126 geriatric and chronic disease hospitals; there are in addition more than 300 highly specialized hospitals (maternity, orthopedic, alcoholic, etc.). Included among the 7,600 hospitals are about 400 federal and almost 2,500 state-local governmental hospitals.[10] As shown in Table 4-3, all hospitals taken together provided 1.54 million beds in 1970, with a daily census of 1.23 million patients, representing a 79.9 per cent occupancy rate. Total admissions in 1970 were 31.6 million patients (double the total admissions in 1946, and up 6 million patients from 1960).

Recent trends in types of hospitals available reflect new treatment modalities and policies. There was closing (without attendant replacement) of some federal hospitals, some tuberculosis and other long-term care hospitals, and some large psychiatric hospitals (replaced by smaller ones). There has been a sizable increase in smaller community hospitals: in 1970, there were 5,900 of them, with 848,000 beds, 29.3 million admissions, an average daily census of 662,000 patients, and an occupancy rate of 78 per cent. A new thrust is the increase in the number of proprietary (for profit) hospitals, one estimate being that 50 to 100 of these hospitals are built per annum in the United States.

Rising costs of hospitalization are found generally, of course, but are particularly apparent in community hospitals (nonfederal, nonspecialty). In these hospitals, there has been an 8.6 per cent average annual increase in expense per day, and the daily rate has reached $80 to $110 (plus extras) in some localities. Factors in this rise have already been alluded to, including increased utilization and the costs of specialty equipment and other nonpayroll items. Of particular note are the increases in salaries of hospital personnel. In

TABLE 4-3. Basic Hospital Data, United States, 1970

Number of hospitals	7,638
Number of beds	1.54 million
Average daily patient census	1.23 million
Occupancy rate (daily)	79.9 percent
Admissions (annually)	31.6 million
Average hospital size	202 beds
Outpatient visits	197.5 million

SOURCE: Adapted from U.S. Department of Health, Education, and Welfare, Health Services and Mental Health Administration, National Center for Health Statistics. *Health Resources Statistics, 1971.*

the period 1960–1970, average annual salaries of all employees rose from $3,239 to $5,921, an increase of 83 per cent in the ten-year period. An additional factor in mounting costs is the sizable proportion of unpaid patients' bills. The percentage of these is greater among outpatients and emergency clinic patients than among inpatients. The expansion of the former services results in an enlarged deficit which must be added to the inpatients' bills if the hospital is to remain solvent.

Quality of Hospital Care.   Hospitals in the United States operate with a fair degree of autonomy in regard to quality of care delivered. The major effort to achieve quality care is through the mechanism of accreditation, which is granted by the Joint Commission on Accreditation of Hospitals, sponsored by the American Hospital Association, the American Medical Association, the American College of Physicians, and the American College of Surgeons. Only hospitals having approved intern and residency training are required to be accredited; for other hospitals, accreditation is voluntary. Eleven per cent of hospitals are approved for intern training, and 17 per cent are approved for residency training (only 9 per cent are affiliated with a medical school). Altogether, 71 per cent of hospitals are currently accredited, and they contain over 80 per cent of the nation's hospital beds.[11]

The standards set for accreditation are not excessive. Many of the regulations refer to proper record keeping. In addition, an accredited hospital must have at least 25 beds, a proper system for dispensing of drugs, clinical and pathology laboratories, and an x-ray department. The hospital staff must be organized into committees, including a tissue committee to review surgical practices at the institution. Since the passage of Medicare legislation, accredited hospitals are also required to have utilization review committees to examine bed occupancy in terms of admitting diagnosis, length of stay, and treatment prescribed. Many of the better hospitals have long maintained standards far in excess of these rather minimal requirements, but the existence of the accreditation process has helped motivate institutions to achieve at least minimal quality standards.

Construction and Planning of Hospitals.   Prior to World War II most hospitals in the United States were built under private or voluntary financial auspices. In 1946, under the provisions of the Hospital Survey and Construction Act (Hill-Burton), federal matching funds were made available to the states for hospital construction. The purpose of the act was to improve the distribution of hospitals, particularly in the many rural areas which were far removed from adequate facilities. In order to qualify under the program, the states had to develop a statewide priority list for hospital construction, so that the majority of construction under the joint program would take place in areas of greatest need. Rural facilities were of necessity stressed, because population-to-bed ratios were the basis for setting statewide priorities. In the 25 years that the Hill-Burton program has been in operation, the states, with federal participation, have invested over $6 billion for hospital construction, providing over 450,000 beds and almost 3,000 laboratories, diagnostic and treatment centers, and other health facilities.[12]

The net effect of the Hill-Burton program has been perhaps an overbuilding of rural facilities, since in the same 25 years the population of the United States has shifted markedly into urban centers. The plight of urban hospitals, many of them old and overcrowded, was not alleviated by the Hill-Burton Act. Recent amendments to the act, however, now make it possible to modernize urban hospitals. In 1970, there were 316 projects initiated nationwide with Hill-Burton assistance, 95 per cent being earmarked for additions, alterations, and replacements rather than for new construction.

In spite of these advances, systematic planning for the construction of hospitals in a given geographic area still remains a knotty problem. In the absence of consistent areawide planning, hospitals have tended to grow in an unplanned manner. More often than not, the final decision to add costly equipment or beds has been based on local pride rather than demonstrated need. This has resulted in much duplication of effort, waste of funds, and construction of facilities that were not subsequently fully utilized. This is the picture by and large across the nation today, despite the fact that state governments were empowered by Hill-Burton regulations to set bed quotas for geographic regions. Some of these bed-allocation functions have been absorbed by Comprehensive Health Planning (CHP) agencies, particularly at state levels. These agencies can conduct studies to identify health needs and are required to inventory health resources and to consider alternative courses of action as well as evaluating the results of priorities recommended. Such activities provide an informed background for decisions regarding hospital need and approval for hospital construction.[13]

NURSING HOMES

Unlike American hospitals, which are still principally nonprofit or governmental, the network of American institutions for long-term care has grown up largely within the proprietary arena. The cause of this lies mainly with the reasoning of the framers of the Social Security Act of 1935. The original act, which has often been amended in the intervening years, contained not only sections setting up old-age and unemployment insurance programs, but also provisions for federal matching funds to be given to states in order to provide public assistance to the aged and to needy children. Mindful of the existence of public poorhouses, however, and anxious to empty these out, the federal legislators specified that recipients of public assistance under this program could not be residents in public institutions. Residents in private institutions were not similarly excluded, however. The net result was that nursing homes, privately owned and catering primarily to old people eligible for public assistance money, sprang up all over the country (the act subsequently was amended to allow payment for medical care in public institutions).

Nursing home costs for the individual patient are met to a large degree by federal Medicare and Medicaid provisions, with many patients augmenting nursing home fees from public assistance payments. Charges for nursing home stay in many localities range from $12 to $25 per day ($16 per day, is "average" in California), with far higher ceilings for patients who can afford more luxurious accommodations.

Nursing homes are of three types, geared to some extent to the requirements of the elderly resident. In 1969, there were a total of 18,910 homes in the United States, of which 11,484 offered nursing care; 3,514 offered personal care with some nursing; and 3,792 offered personal care without nursing. There were almost 1 million persons residing in these institutions, three quarters in homes with nursing care.[10]

Today 77 per cent of nursing homes are proprietary, about 7 per cent are government-sponsored, and 16 per cent are private nonprofit. The high proportion of for-profit homes raises a question as to whether or not the profit motive is consistent with the goal of rendering satisfactory, humane care to the elderly at reasonable prices. Advocates of the entrepreneurial nursing home say that, with proper organization and modern management methods, they can effect sufficient economies of purchasing to provide a laudable service for the money. The truth is that no one has a monopoly on problems of quality of nursing home care, with nonprofit homes also coming in for their share of criticism.

Nursing homes tend to be depressing places and, in contrast to the majority of American hospitals, are no credit to the general system of medical care. The patients in these institutions, average age around 80, offer little challenge to the medical and nursing professions and have been ignored as much as possible by the medical care system of the average American community. In older nursing homes the physical plant is outmoded and often hazardous. Newer nursing home construction, of course, offers better standards of hygiene and nursing staff convenience. With exceptions, quality of care within nursing homes has in the past been largely inadequate, with absence of even such minimal measures as a nurse in attendance around the clock, a physician on call at all times, and acceptable maintenance of patient records.

Federal Medicare legislation, in its provision for extended care, has brought improvements in the quality of care provided by nursing homes. The Medicare law specifies that, in order to qualify for treating Medicare beneficiaries, a nursing home must have an arrangement with a hospital for an orderly transfer back and forth of both patients and records. In addition, to qualify, a nursing home must have round-the-clock nursing services, with at least one registered nurse employed full time; a physician available to handle emergencies; appropriate medical policies governing the facility's skilled nursing care and related services; specified methods and procedures for the handling of drugs; and utilization review procedures similar to those required of hospitals participating in the Medicare program.[14] At the time of the passage of the Medicare legislation, only a small percentage of American nursing homes met even these minimal standards, and therefore, the beginning of the extended care benefits under the law was delayed six months beyond the start of the rest of the program in order to allow a reasonable number of nursing home beds to come into compliance. The Medicare legislation has also stimulated the formation of a Joint Committee on Accreditation of Nursing Homes, similar in sponsorship and purpose to the body that has for years been successfully handling the hospital accreditation program.

There still remains the problem of redefining the function of nursing homes, so that they may be organized to suit more closely the needs of the patients themselves. Within the nursing home population there are those whose primary needs are for nursing care and those whose primary needs are for custodial care. These two groups would benefit from widely differing institutions, and ultimately one would hope that nursing homes, in their architecture and staffing, would reflect a recognition of this divergence in patient needs. Certain countries in Europe have recognized this difference and are far ahead of the United States in almost every aspect of nursing home care today.

HOME HEALTH SERVICES

When a seriously ill patient no longer needs the 24-hour care and supervision provided in a hospital or nursing home, it is possible that promotive care may be rendered in the patient's home. The cost is estimated to be one tenth that of hospital care. Furthermore, for the patient with a satisfactory home environment, many comforts are available that no institution can provide. It is important, however, to emphasize that home care is a desirable alternative to hospitalization only when the home itself is adequate. There are many patients whose home situation precludes rest or proper attention, and for these, care in an institution is preferable even though more expensive.

Medicare legislation stimulated progress in this area. The law provides funds for home care, in addition to care in institutions, and it is widely recognized as being to the taxpayer's ultimate advantage to develop this alternative maximally. The federal law requires that Medicare patients on home care be under a treatment plan established by a physician within 14 days of discharge from a hospital or extended care facility. In addition, home health agencies, in order to qualify, must be either publicly owned or nonprofit; or, if they are proprietary, they must meet specified staffing and quality regulations. Under Medicare, a patient may receive as many as 100 home health visits a year following a most recent hospitalization.

In 1971, there were about 2,300 home health programs in the 50 states and territories approved for Medicare participation and reimbursement. An additional 500 programs were in existence but were not so approved. Of the 2,300 approved programs, 57 per cent were based in official health agencies (e.g., health departments), 24 per cent in visiting nurse associations, and only 9 per cent in hospitals.[10] Some local health departments have viewed the development of comprehensive home care programs as one of the chief roles that they can fulfill under the Medicare program, and their multidisciplinary staffing would appear particularly well suited for this. Various ancillary programs devoted primarily to other than the medical aspects of home care, such as meals-on-wheels and the homemaker programs, need to be expanded and integrated with the developing programs of home medical care.

Maintaining the Quality of Medical Care

Quality, in the context of medical care, has at least two connotations, one dealing with its community character ("coverage"), and the other involving the care rendered an individual patient. On a communitywide basis, quality of care is related to the range of services available; the range of medical need in the population; the extent of coverage of the population by the services available (including the appropriateness of the services to the needs of the patients); the cost of care in both money and personnel; and the relation between cost and benefits. These issues already have been discussed in connection with solo and group practice of medicine, hospitals, nursing homes and related services.

Quality of care in the case of the individual patient is particularly complex. Probably the best of the indirect measures of quality is peer judgment, that is, an assessment of competence by acknowledged experts in the field of specialization of a professional person or in the area of operation of an institution. Licensure, accreditation, and specialty certification are all variants of peer judgment, and have come into increasing use as mass means for trying to assure quality of care. It is still common enough, however, to see an unaccredited hospital or extended care facility in operation, and many professional services requiring the skill of a specialist are still rendered by physicians who lack specialty certification. In many instances, licensing requirements for facilities and personnel are likewise not sufficiently stringent to ensure high-quality care.

Tissue committees and bed occupancy committees have long been features of the staff organization of better hospitals. The tissue committees have focused on the elimination of unnecessary surgery and have had a high degree of success in many institutions. Bed occupancy committees have so far focused largely on the fiscal aspects of underutilization or overutilization of hospital beds. However, with the advent of the Medicare program, these committees, renamed utilization review committees, are focusing on the appropriateness of bed use in relation to admitting diagnosis, length of stay, and treatment prescribed.

The technique of medical audit provides procedures in which an institution's practices are continuously assessed against standards derived from comparable institutions. It involves an evaluation of total performance from the audit of various individual operations within the particular institution being examined. Medical audit is still in its infancy, but gives promise of developing into a most useful measure of quality.

Continuing postgraduate education for all levels of professional personnel involved in medical care also predisposes to improved quality. The advance of medical knowledge and technology today is so rapid that it is difficult to avoid obsolescence after leaving school. Professional associations, the universities, and government and private organizations are all developing programs to provide continuing education opportunities on a broad scale.

One important program designed to influence quality of care is the federal Regional Medical Program (RMP). As originally conceived, Regional Medical Programs were to provide a mechanism to bring the benefits of up-to-date medicine from the large medical centers to medically underdeveloped health providers in both urban and rural areas. Thus, the plan was to transmit scientific knowledge, particularly about heart disease, cancer, and stroke as well as "related diseases." By 1971, there was developed a network of 56 Regional Medical Programs covering every state in the union. As the general programs unfolded, operating experience and more recent legislation broadened the original "centers of excellence" idea considerably.[15]

Each Regional Medical Program operates through a series of planning and operational grants. Personnel include RMP staff, advisory committees, and a variety of task forces responsible for categorical diseases, continuing education and training, planning, and so forth. Local involvement of health providers is very broad. For example, throughout the nation in 1971 there were hundreds of task forces, committees, and advisory groups involving in excess of 12,000 health professionals (physicians, nurses, dentists, and others) as well as health consumer representatives.

A principal thrust of this important program is the upgrading of individual medical care by development of diverse activities. Program and planning aspects of RMP's engage with an area's hospitals (including Veterans Administration), professional societies (medical, nursing, dental, etc.), voluntary agencies, and Comprehensive Health Planning agencies.

Government, while constituting a large and increasingly dominant force in the provision of medical services, traditionally has been loath to assert itself in questions regarding quality of care. Too often attempts by government to enforce quality controls have been fearfully rejected as steps leading toward "socialized medicine," a system in which it was asserted doctors and patients alike would lose freedom of action, with consequent disastrous effects on quality of medical care. As has been seen in Medicare legislation, the federal government has moved into the area of quality control by insisting that utilization review be carried out regularly at participating institutions. Some state governments also have attempted to establish quality controls by various measures, including strengthening the functions of regional hospital planning councils with the added force of comprehensive health planning legislation. It is likely that, among health professionals, auditing the quality of care rendered by health providers will be viewed increasingly as simply good practice.

Financing and Delivery of Health Services in the United States

PAYING FOR HEALTH CARE

As has been suggested earlier, the great health debate of the 1970's and 1980's can be expected to center on provisions for financ-

TABLE 4-4. National Health Expenditures by Object of Expenditure, United States, Fiscal Year 1970–1971

Object of Expenditure	Amount in Billions
HEALTH SERVICES AND SUPPLIES: TOTAL	$69.5
Hospital care	29.6
Physicians' services	14.2
Dentists' services	4.7
Other professional services	1.5
Drugs and drug sundries	7.5
Eyeglasses and appliances	1.9
Nursing home care	3.4
Expenses for prepayment and administration	2.3
Government public health activities	1.6
Other health services	2.8
RESEARCH AND MEDICAL FACILITIES CONSTRUCTION: TOTAL	5.5
Research	2.1
Construction	3.5
TOTAL	$75.0

SOURCE: *Social Security Bulletin*, Vol. 35, No. 1, January 1972, p. 7.

ing health care. A first step in understanding the complexities of the problem is to grasp the amounts of money at stake. They are formidable. In fiscal year 1970–1971, national health expenditures came to $75 billion, with government spending amounting to $28.5 billion (38 per cent) and private spending totaling $46.6 billion (62 per cent). Public expenditure (government) has increased markedly since the advent of Medicare and Medicaid in 1965.

How was the $75 billion spent? Table 4-4 shows that the vast bulk (93 per cent) went for consumer health services and supplies—that is, hospital stay ($29.6 billion), doctors' and dentists' services ($19 billion), etc. Approximately 6 per cent went for research or facilities construction.

Trends in national expenditures for health purposes are shown in Table 4-5. The rise since 1950 has been extraordinary. In that year, total health expenditures were $12.9 billion, an average of almost $84 for every man, woman, and child in the United States. In 1970–1971, the per capita expenditure had increased to $358. This is more than a fourfold rise in per capita costs.

Costs and methods of paying for health care are of high interest to United States legislators. Furthermore, with so much money at stake, the issue has excited the interest of insurance companies and other business entrepreneurs. With so many parties involved, one can be certain of continual high political interest. One can also be sure that organized lobbies will be busy trying to get their view-

TABLE 4-5. Total and Per Capita National Health Expenditures, United States, Selected Years

Calendar Year	Total in Billions	Per Capita*	
		Actual	Adjusted†
1950	$12.9	$ 83.19	$162.62
1955	18.0	107.11	177.61
1960	27.0	147.20	197.69
1965	40.6	205.55	238.74
1970	67.8	324.00	—
1971	75.0	358.00	—

* Based on total population, including Armed Forces and federal civilian employees aboard as of July 1.
† Adjusted to 1964 prices in order to take into account changes in the purchasing power of the dollar as shown by the Bureau of Labor Statistics Consumer Price Index for all items.
SOURCE: Adapted from *Social Security Bulletin*, Vol. 35, No. 1, January 1972, p. 5. Also, House of Representatives, Committee on Ways and Means. *Basic Facts on the Health Industry*, 1971, p. 11.

points built into any legislation that is likely to have far-reaching effects.

The personal cost of and expenditure for health care are of extreme concern to every American citizen. Illness may strike at any time—and sometimes more than once in a given family. Everyone has heard of cases of catastrophic illness, the treatment of which—in the acute phase and its aftermath, or because it is chronic and lengthy—is extraordinarily expensive, and can bring financial ruin on a family. Particularly vulnerable groups in the medical cost squeeze are the elderly and the poor.

The elderly are generally no longer employed and are usually found in the nation's lowest income brackets. They are also the primary sufferers from three of the major killers—heart disease, cancer, and stroke. Compared with younger persons, the elderly (65 and older) have twice as many days of disability per annum and see physicians for their ills far more often. The paradox is that at the point in life when health care is most needed, the elderly are least able to pay for it.

The poor are in the same general fix as the elderly, but with some important differences. Health status of the poor is inferior to that of better-off persons. On almost every index of sickness and health and on various indicators of medical care sought for and received, the poor are at a serious disadvantage. The disadvantage occurs at every age, including, most tragically, mothers-to-be, infants, and young children. For nonwhites, the vast majority of whom are poor, the issue is reflected in such basic health indicators as infant mortality (higher for blacks than for whites) and life expectancy (lower for blacks than for whites).

PRESENT PRIVATELY SPONSORED HEALTH INSURANCE PLANS

The idea of purchasing insurance to cover the costs of illness is not new and has historic roots in some European national health schemes of the nineteenth century. In the United States, health insurance emerged parallel to workmen's compensation, which provided some coverage for injuries and sickness incurred on the job. Health aspects of one sort or another have for some time been built into various insurance policies such as life insurance ("disability"), automobile insurance, and others.

Health insurance, per se, emerged as a basic solution to the problem of providing for the rising and possibly catastrophic costs of medical care. Several types of voluntary health insurance plans, including Blue Cross and Blue Shield, have been in operation since about 1930, but growth was slow until after World War II. The immediate postwar period saw the simultaneous emergence of entrepreneurial interest of the big insurance companies in the health insurance field and the development of interest in government-sponsored health insurance.[16] Government health insurance (for the elderly)

FIGURE 4-1. *Per cent of health expenditures paid by health insurance, United States, selected years.* [SOURCE: *House of Representatives, Committee on Ways and Means. Basic Facts on the Health Industry, 1971, p. 103.*]

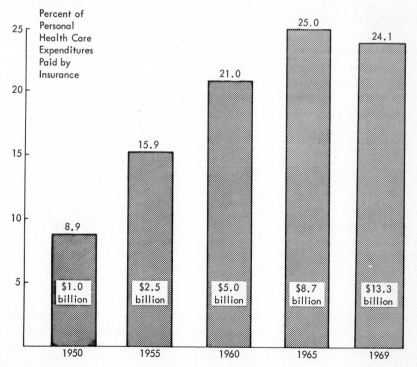

had to wait until 1965 (passage of Medicare legislation), but private health insurance grew dramatically. In 1950, as shown in Figure 4-1, health insurance covered almost 9 per cent (or $1 billion worth) of all health expenditures. By 1969, the proportion had risen to about 24 per cent ($13.3 billion). By that same year, approximately 80 per cent of the population under age 65 had hospital and/or surgical insurance.[17]

Types and Provisions of Privately Sponsored Health Insurance. There are three principal types of privately sponsored health insurance: provider-sponsored hospital insurance (Blue Cross); provider-sponsored physician's care insurance (Blue Shield); and commercial health care insurance issued by a variety of commercial insurance companies. A fourth type is the "independent" health insurance plans, which account for about 5 per cent of the total health insurance coverage in force.

In Europe, where government has long operated most of the hospitals, there was no need for hospital insurance, and the advocates of health insurance concentrated on providing coverage for the cost of out-of-hospital physician services. By contrast, in the United States, general hospitals are mostly nongovernment owned, and the first effort, of necessity, was an attempt to underwrite hospital costs.

"Major medical" insurance plans were pioneered by the commercial insurance companies, and cover many items, including hospitalization, physician services, drugs, and nursing care in the event of expensive illness. "Major medical" insurance may be supplementary to basic health insurance or may represent the only coverage that the patient has. In either case, it is typically characterized by a *deductible* amount of expense which the patient must pay before the policy begins to reimburse his expenses. Furthermore, there is usually a *coinsurance* feature whereby the patient pays about 20 per cent of all expenses beyond the deductible, and there is a large but definite maximum sum beyond which the insurance policy will not be liable. "Major medical" plans have by now become a feature of Blue Cross and Blue Shield policies.

Blue Cross Plans. Blue Cross was generated by the American Hospital Association, and the Association's Blue Cross Commission must approve any plan that wishes to use the Blue Cross symbol. There are currently 80 plans in the United States (and in several Canadian provinces). The plans operate with a great deal of autonomy. Almost all are enabled, by special state legislation, to operate outside of the confines of state insurance laws. The Blue Cross Commission originally required of each approved plan that it be nonprofit, be organized as a public service, be financially sound, have an advisory board containing hospital trustees and physicians, allow all recognized hospitals to participate in benefits, grant the subscriber free choice of hospital, and allow responsibility for services to rest with the hospitals. These criteria were widely interpreted as endorsing the *community rating system of premiums,* which involves uniform premium rates for all persons regardless of differing risks of illness. The criteria were also interpreted as endorsing *service benefits* (such as coverage for a stated number of days in hospital) rather than *indemnity benefits* (such as a fixed dollar sum per day in hospital regardless of charges incurred).

The Blue Cross principle, while laudable in theory, proved very difficult in practice, partly owing to rapidly rising hospital costs and partly owing to competition from the commercial insurance companies. Younger, healthier workers were offered "package deals" by the commercial insurance companies, which included life insurance, disability insurance, and various other benefits in addition to low-cost health insurance. In these "packages," the profitable policies, such as life insurance, covered losses incurred through the health benefit being offered at low premium rates. Blue Cross suffered under this competition and was left with a progressively larger percentage of poor-risk clients attracted by the community rating system of premiums. In 1950, Blue Cross plans paid out in benefits, or put into reserves for future payments, about 88 cents on the dollar, leaving 12 cents to cover administration costs. By 1958, about 97 cents on the dollar were being paid out in benefits, leaving only 3 cents for administration.[17]

In recent years, Blue Cross has kept up with the commercial companies in expanded benefits and more flexible contracts for groups, so that today it is common to find major medical protection included in group Blue Cross contracts. This has been possible through rate increases which, as might be expected, have often been opposed by rate-setting bodies, bringing Blue Cross premiums in line with those set by commercial companies.

Commercial Health Care Plans. The commercial companies, arriving on the health insurance scene after the Blue Cross plans and the "independent" plans, soon acquired the dominant position. The "package deals," including health insurance which the commercial companies offered labor groups, as already described, were one reason for their ascendancy. Another reason stemmed from the fact that the commercial companies had no commitment to the ideals of the community rating system of premiums or to service benefits. Using the *experience rating system of premiums* — where the premiums are determined by the actual loss experience in past years of the group at risk — the commercial companies could offer broad health insurance coverage to the better health risks at reduced rates.

By paying indemnity benefits rather than service benefits, the companies limited their risk even further.

By 1969, commercial health care plans generally had come to the point where they compared favorably with Blue Cross plans. Recent experience is that commercial *group* health insurance (which most commercial policies are) pays out 94 per cent of income in benefits, retaining 6 per cent for expenses and profit. *Individual* policies purchased from commercial carriers are another matter; only half the premium costs are returned as benefits.[17]

Blue Shield Plans. Blue Shield, while often working closely with Blue Cross plans, and identified with them in the minds of many people, has had a different history from Blue Cross. The origin of the Blue Shield idea was in the "medical bureaus" set up by local medical societies in the states of Washington and Oregon as an alternative to the closed-panel medical plans provided by the lumber companies. Only gradually were statewide plans formed, and not until 1948 did the American Medical Association consolidate the idea nationally. Blue Shield plans were then required to operate with approval and under responsibility of the state and local medical society; to provide free choice of physician to subscribers; to be nonprofit; and, if possible, to provide service benefits rather than indemnity benefits.

There are today 72 Blue Shield plans in the country. In 30 states they operate outside of the insurance laws, under special enabling legislation which differs, however, from the Blue Cross enabling legislation in the same states. In the remaining 20 states, regular insurance laws cover the Blue Shield plans as well.

Unlike Blue Cross, which has had fairly smooth relations with the hospitals that gave it origin, the relations between Blue Shield and its parent—the medical profession—have been more troubled. There has been much debate about whether physicians should be allowed to charge patients with higher incomes a surcharge beyond the established Blue Shield schedule of fees, thus in effect converting the service benefit of Blue Shield policies into an indemnity benefit for one category of patients. The general rule adopted has been to surcharge patients earning more than a specified amount, or at least to allow the physician freedom to do so. Blue Shield has been more expensive to administer than Blue Cross but still has managed to pay out benefits of around 90 cents on the premium dollar.

"Independent" Health Insurance Plans. The "independent" health insurance plans, although providing only a very small percentage of the coverage nationally, have pioneered the principle of combining prepayment for medical care with group practice and have shown the combination to be workable. The "independents" cover a broad spectrum, from small fraternal programs and consumer cooperatives to giant operations such as the Kaiser Foundation Health Plans and the Health Insurance Plan of Greater New York.[7] Some plans own their own hospitals, some are closely affiliated with one hospital although they do not own it, and some use a variety of totally unaffiliated community hospitals. The "independents," unlike the Blue Cross and Blue Shield plans or the commercial insurance plans, have always kept close watch on the type of medical care rendered to purchasers of their insurance and have found that, as a result, they are often able to counter the trend toward increased use of hospitalization which has helped to inflate the costs of other types of insurance plans.

Coverage and Problems in Private Health Insurance.   While most health insurance policies originate as group fringe benefits in employment situations, the actual contract is an individual one between the insurer and the policyholder. Terms of health insurance policies vary widely. Most policies offer hospital stay coverage for 70 to 100 days per "confinement," with varying coinsurance arrangements after the initial coverage period. Most policies also cover "usual, customary and reasonable charges" in hospital either in full or up to a fixed limit. Psychiatric care is covered only spottily. Maternity cases are generally covered by flat fee.

Figure 4-2 shows the percentages of persons under age 65 who had insurance coverage for various kinds of health services in 1969. While about 80 per cent were covered by hospital and/or surgical insurance, as stated earlier, other benefits were available to far fewer individuals. For example, about 70 per cent were insured for in-hospital doctor visits and 65 per cent for x-ray and laboratory examinations, but less than 50 per cent were covered for prescribed drugs and for office and home visits. Only about 5 per cent were insured for dental care. Thus, there is considerable unevenness of coverage for the general public holding health insurance.

Another inequity occurs in the fact that some segments of the population are less likely than others to hold health insurance. For those under age 65, private health insurance is held by 90 per cent of persons with income exceeding $10,000; but only about one third of individuals earning less than $3,000 have policies. The situation is even worse for the children of the poor: less than a quarter of these children (in families with incomes under $3,000) are covered by health insurance. Rural families have far less health insurance coverage than do urban families, largely because rural people are less likely to work in a setting where group enrollment is possible. In 1963, the National Health Survey found that only 51 per cent of the rural population in the United States had some kind of insurance for hospitalization.

Health insurers—the commercial carriers and the Blue Cross

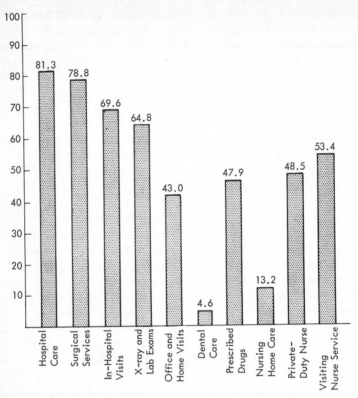

FIGURE 4-2. *Per cent of population under age 65 with health insurance, United States, 1969.* [SOURCE: *House of Representatives, Committee on Ways and Means.* Basic Facts on the Health Industry, *1971, p. 97.*]

plans alike—have tended to see themselves more as fiscal agents than as monitors of the quality of the product their money is buying. They have been inclined to steer clear of using the enormous fiscal power at their command to effect improvements in the health care delivery system. The opportunity is recognized for change in this situation, and some insurers and some Blue Cross Plans are beginning to show more concern for the quality of care rendered to the insured.

PRESENT GOVERNMENT-SPONSORED FINANCING PLANS

Health Insurance: Medicare. Some national means was sought to rectify the serious health care deficit for the elderly, and in 1965, after much debate, Congress passed Title XVIII, amending the Social Security Act. This measure became known, popularly, as Medicare. Title XVIII established a federal program of health insurance for almost all Americans age 65 and over, regardless of means and, currently, regardless of whether or not they are eligible for the Social Security old-age pensions. The Medicare program is divided into two parts: *Part A* is financed largely from the Social Security tax and *Part B,* which is voluntary, required at the outset a monthly payment of $3 from the beneficiary (since gone up to $5.80) and, as far as the government's portion is concerned, is financed from general revenues.[18–20]

Medicare, Part A, provides hospitalization up to 90 days per spell of illness; posthospitalization care in an extended care facility for up to 100 days; posthospitalization home health care services; and outpatient hospital diagnostic services. Part B provides physician's and surgeon's services; home health visits even with no prior hospitalization; many diagnostic tests; dressings, splints, casts, rental of certain medical equipment, and many other ancillary services; and limited out-of-hospital treatment for psychiatric disorders. In line with private health insurance practice, many of the services in Part A and all services in Part B require the payment of deductibles and coinsurance charges by the beneficiaries.

Hospital benefits (Part A) provide the first 60 days of hospitalization except for $72 which the patient pays. For the next 30 days, the coinsurance goes up to $18 per day paid by the patient. The first 20 days of posthospitalization (extended care) are provided fully by Medicare; the patient pays $9.00 per day for the next 80 days. For home health care, there is provision for up to 100 visits for part-time nursing, various specified therapies, and certain medical supplies. The patient pays 20 per cent of costs of outpatient diagnostic service, after a $20 deductible feature. Lifetime psychiatric benefits are limited to 190 days. Part B of the Medicare legislation provides for 80 per cent (the patient pays 20 per cent) of the cost of "reasonable charges" for covered services after a $60 deductible.

Medicare—Parts A and B—is clearly a "best buy," and has gone a long way toward alleviating the financial catastrophe of illness for the aged. The costs of out-of-hospital pharmaceuticals, private-duty nurses, eyeglasses, and so on are not covered under either Part A or Part B. No doubt changes over the years may bracket these items in, probably with some deductible and coinsurance features. In the meantime, additional financial help is afforded the elderly through assistance to the medically indigent (Medicaid) and through various private health insurance policies, now with more modestly priced premiums since the major risk has been absorbed through Medicare.

In fiscal 1970, 20.4 million persons 65 and older were enrolled in the Medicare program. In this group were almost 8 million people 75 years and older. Costs for the program are enormous and in fiscal year 1971 came to $7.9 billion ($5.6 billion for Part A—Hospital

Insurance, and \$2.3 billion for Part B—Medical Insurance). The total is more than double the expenditures of 1967, the first year of the program. Per capita expenditure was \$380 per elderly person in 1971. In that same year, there were an estimated 6.3 million "Medicare" admissions to short-term hospitals, with average length of stay of 12.4 days.[19]

Medical Assistance Program: Medicaid.   Title XIX of the Social Security Act (as amended in 1965) became known as Medicaid. This potentially far-reaching program (costing \$5.5 billion in 1970) has replaced the medical components of most federal-state assistance programs. Medicaid provides grants to the individual states of from 50 to 83 per cent of the costs of the program. The richer states pay more of the share (based on state per capita income) and the poorer states pay less.[20,21] There are five basic health services mandated by the legislation: inpatient *and* outpatient hospital services, diagnostic (laboratory) tests, physicians' services, and nursing home services. At least ten other services—including home health care services, private duty nursing, and dental services, among others—may be provided by individual states, costs for which may be shared by the federal government.

The Medicaid law gives the states financial incentives to participate. Persons on public assistance (welfare) are automatically covered. Equally important is the recognition and establishment of the category of "medical indigency" that is determined by amount of family income and not by welfare status. Most states have kept Medicaid eligibility requirements very close to welfare levels. In some states permissible annual income for Medicaid eligibility at one point reached \$6,000 (e.g., New York). But the financial drain on the state became so great that there resulted amendments to the Social Security Act that put a lower ceiling on eligibility.

While there is enormous variability in benefits among the states, Medicaid seeks to establish, at least within each state, uniformity of medical care benefits available to public assistance recipients in all categories. Furthermore, medical indigency is recognized by Medicaid to exist not only among the aged but also among every other group for whom categorical welfare assistance is provided. However, any medical benefit offered to one category or subgroup of public assistance recipients must be offered in identical amount, duration, and scope to every other person or group receiving public assistance support.

PROPOSED PRIVATE-GOVERNMENT PLANS

Health Maintenance Organizations.   The successful experience of health plans combining prepayment with group practice (as described earlier) has led to their espousal as elements of major health policy by the United States government. Called Health Maintenance Organizations (HMO's), the provisions entail four basic elements.[22,23] First, an HMO must be an organized health care delivery system, including health manpower and facilities capable of providing, or at least arranging for, all the health services a population might require. Second, it must have an enrolled population, consisting of individuals and groups who contract for a range of health services to be made available. Third, an HMO must have a financial plan which incorporates underwriting the costs of the agreed upon set of services on a prenegotiated and prepaid basis. Fourth, it must have a managing organization which assures legal, fiscal, public, and professional accountability.

All four elements must be present in an HMO, although any one element may undertake the responsibility for organization and management. For example, a physician group, a medical society, or a hospital may initiate HMO development, as may a group of consumers, an insurance company, or an industrial or management corporation. Any one of these may take the initiative to organize the other three elements and constitute an HMO.

While Health Maintenance Organizations, as national policy, represent a break from the past, their success depends on the two familiar, critical and interrelated factors: what are the benefits (quality and extent of care), and who will pay the bill? Present successful "independents"—Kaiser Foundation Health Plans and others—which are models for the HMO concept have a broad set of inpatient and outpatient benefits, but do not provide dental and general psychiatric service. Furthermore, Kaiser's success, in part, depends on the fact that subscribers constitute employed groups (not particularly high-risk) in certain industries, guaranteeing ability to meet substantial monthly premium payments (Kaiser's monthly payments in Los Angeles, 1972, for one subscriber group were: subscriber only, $21; subscriber and spouse, $42; family, $59). High-risk groups (e.g., ghetto dwellers, the elderly, migrant workers) will undoubtedly need financial assistance in meeting premiums.[24] It remains to be seen whether the comprehensive services rendered and the economies encountered in existing plans can be duplicated in HMO's across the nation in proprietary (profit) as well as nonprofit circumstances.

One important problem for nonprofit as well as profit-making HMO's has to do with potential corner-cutting in medical care rendered in order to make the HMO finances come out right. It is easy to see how a patient might have attention to important medical problems deferred or needed hospital stay shortened because they are "expensive" to the organization. HMO's, having the quality of a public utility, will require regular monitoring and evaluation to ensure that the consumer is getting high-quality medical care, as needed, for the premiums paid.

National Health Insurance. In the welter of discussions for modifying or "correcting" the American health system, one recurrent theme is the search for a satisfactory national health care *financing* plan, also known as national health insurance. National health *insurance* is not to be confused with a national health *system* such as those found in the Scandinavian countries, England, and Canada. Such a system normally involves not only a method of financing health care and compulsory membership in the system, but also a regulated plan for *delivering* health care. Groundswell has developed in the United States for adoption of some national health measures — aside from Medicare and Medicaid — that would extend benefits more widely in a rational manner. None of the proposals combines a comprehensive national *insurance* (financing) plan with a comprehensive *delivery* plan, although some schemes come closer to this goal than do others.

The details of any national health insurance scheme must answer some searching questions about coverage, organization and quality of care, provisions of premium payments, and so forth. Some significant points needing attention are as follows:[25]

1. *Target population, extent of coverage, and utilization.* What populations are covered? What deductibles and coinsurance features for what individuals, for what conditions, and for what services?
2. *Quality controls.* What quality measures are specified or implied?
3. *Provider payment.* How will doctors (and other health workers) and hospitals be paid ("usual and customary charges"; "reasonable charges")? Will organized health entities be paid differently from solo practitioners?
4. *Financing mechanisms.* How will payments originate: by payroll tax (part or whole, either by employer and/or employee); by credit against income tax; by general federal revenues?
5. *Administrative mechanism.* By whom will the plan be administered: by private insurance carriers; through Medicare; through specially created mechanisms, councils, etc.?
6. *Incentive mechanism.* Are there special incentives for efficient operation or for group practices (as against solo practice), or to discourage overutilization?
7. *Organizational modality.* Is there an attempt to change the medical care organization scheme, for example, to encourage

or to mandate schemes like Health Maintenance Organizations? Or is there no change, or prohibition against change, in the system?

There are no doubt other important dimensions which need to be considered in connection with the national health insurance proposals of the next few years.[26] But measuring a plan against the foregoing yardsticks quickly reveals the degree to which the proposal wishes seriously to alter the contours of the American health delivery system.

WORKMEN'S COMPENSATION

Just as industrial accidents are the inevitable companion of industrialization, so programs for treating and rehabilitating workers injured on the job have been generated in almost every country with any degree of industrialization. In some developing countries which have a minimum of industrialization and a severe general scarcity of medical care resources, the care available under workmen's compensation is actually superior to that available for the remainder of the population's health needs.

Workmen's compensation is based on an understanding by both the worker and his employer that work injuries are predominantly related to the intrinsic nature of work itself rather than to negligence on anyone's part. In line with this understanding, all work-related injuries are considered to be compensable, and the amount of the award, covering both loss of wages and necessary medical care, is related to the degree of injury, the age of the worker, his occupation, and the number of his dependents. The award is determined without having reference to the courts, and this results in substantial savings to the worker, who is spared the cost of legal fees. In the early years of this century, prior to the enactment of workmen's compensation laws, it was estimated that only one in eight industrial accidents resulted in compensation to the injured workers. In cases where compensation was awarded, legal costs ran as high as 50 per cent of recovery. In New York, Pennsylvania, and Minnesota, fully one third of on-the-job fatalities received no compensation, while another 24 per cent received less than $100. By 1970, workmen's compensation expenditures in the United States as a whole stood at almost $3 billion, and included hospital and medical benefits of almost $1 billion.[27]

Another problem which workmen's compensation tries to solve is that of lapsed time between injury and compensation. When the worker must resort to the courts, the time interval is likely to be long. Meanwhile the injured worker's bills, medical and otherwise, continue to pile up. Under workmen's compensation, this time lapse is reduced to a minimum so that the worker can begin, soon after injury, to receive payments which help meet his household expenses and enable him to pay his medical care bills as they arise.

In the United States, workmen's compensation is administered through autonomous programs set up by the individual states, with the insurance carried mainly by commercial insurance companies. Injured workers are treated by private physicians in the community and are hospitalized in community hospitals. This contrasts with many other countries, where injured workers receive care in government-sponsored hospitals and health centers.

A great advantage inherent in the American system of workmen's compensation is that it provides incentive to employers to reduce any hazardous working conditions that may exist. Since, as in most insurance, the premium under workmen's compensation varies with the loss experience, employers benefit when the number of work accidents is reduced.

One major task of the workmen's compensation program is to arouse interest in the rehabilitation aspect of medical care in all parties concerned. Employers and insurance companies have found it less troublesome to make a cash settlement than to get involved in the intricacies of a rehabilitation program. The worker, dazzled by the temporary windfall of a sizable sum of cash, has also often missed the point that, in the long run, the cash offered has little value in comparison to what a full rehabilitation effort would offer. Workmen's compensation represents a major step forward in extending health benefits, but until the program is focused on restoring the worker to maximal productivity, it has not yet met the full challenge of its mission.

Direct Medical Care Provided by the Federal Government

As has already been described, the federal government of the United States has many essential stimulative, supportive, and financial roles in the health field. One significant role is in the direct medical care it provides to specified populations. The earliest beginnings of this activity were in the assumption of responsibility for the care of merchant seamen in special marine hospitals which were operative in 1798. This program was in fact the origin of the U.S. Public Health Service.

Today, the Public Health Service's direct medical care programs are conducted through the Federal Health Programs Service and provide care for American seamen, Coast Guard personnel and dependents, military personnel and dependents, and federal employees injured on the job or who became ill as a result of their work.[12] Medical care for these individuals is offered in eight Public Health Service general hospitals (e.g., Baltimore, Boston, Seattle). There is also a hospital for leprosy patients (in Carville, Louisiana). There are also 30 outpatient clinics and several hundred contract physicians' offices throughout the country. All told, in 1969, there were 37,000 admissions to Public Health Service hospitals and almost 2 million visits to clinics and to contract physicians.

Another long-standing responsibility of the national government has been the rendering of medical care to American Indians. This obligation began informally when U.S. Army doctors sought to control smallpox and other contagious diseases among the Indians living near military posts. Subsequently, as the tribes were pushed back onto reservations, the federal government entered into numerous treaties with the tribes, a number containing government promises to render medical and hospital care. Health care responsibility for American Indians remained with the War Department for some time, was later shifted to the Department of the Interior, and since 1955 has resided in the Department of Health, Education, and Welfare.

The health of American Indians has been one of America's "pockets of neglect" and in many respects is analogous to the situation found in inner cities and among the rural poor. For example, compared to the nation as a whole, Indian infant mortality is 50 per cent higher and the tuberculosis rate is 3.5 times greater.[28]

Today, the Indian Health Service (Health Services and Mental Health Administration) provides medical care to more than 415,000 Indians, Eskimos, and Aleuts through a system of 51 hospitals, 71 health centers, and more than 300 field clinics. Strong national efforts are under way to provide training opportunities for Indians in health careers. Largely through these programs, the health standards of the American Indian population have begun to improve since 1960.

A very large category of individuals for whom the federal government assumes responsibility in health care consists of military personnel, military dependents, and service veterans. *Military personnel* are served by a system of general and field hospitals and medical stations wherever U.S. troops are found. Since the military is at a serious disadvantage in competing for career medical and dental officers, it must depend on the draft to carry out its health care function. Nevertheless, the military has been able to introduce throughout its facilities such well-accepted guarantees of high-quality care as the requirement that all surgery be done by specialists. Furthermore, there are such renowned institutions as the Walter Reed Army Hospital and the Bethesda Naval Medical Hospital that have the highest medical standards.

Military dependents, who are eligible for medical care in the health programs of the federal government, exceed 4.7 million persons. Finally, there are 28.2 million *service veterans* in the United States, including those who have served in Vietnam. There are veterans with service-connected disabilities and those with acute and chronic nonservice-connected conditions, some of which are compensable.

To accommodate the possible health needs of these millions of service veterans, the Veterans Administration (VA) operates 166 general hospitals located in approximately 140 communities across the nation. There are about 107,000 beds, including those reserved for psychiatric conditions. There are also tuberculosis hospitals, domiciliaries for chronically ill veterans, and more than 70 outpatient clinics. The Veterans Administration Hometown Medical Care Program allows eligible veterans who are distant from VA facilities to receive care at civilian hospitals and clinics.

The Veterans Administration employs more than 5,000 full-time salaried physicians, approximately 15,000 full-time nurses, and about 750 full-time dentists as well as personnel in countless other health specialties. In former years, the VA had much difficulty in recruiting the professional personnel to assure high quality of care at its facilities. In recent times, however, the veterans' facilities have become affiliated with medical schools wherever possible and have become involved in the teaching program of the schools. As a result, many Veterans Administration physicians are now full-time members on the teaching faculties of the nation's medical schools. As a consequence, medical care in affiliated veterans' hospitals is equivalent in quality to the care given at other hospitals affiliated with these schools.

References

1. U.S. Department of Health, Education, and Welfare. *Towards a Comprehensive Health Policy for the 1970's.* A White Paper. U.S. Government Printing Office, Washington, D.C., May 1971.
2. Greenberg, Selig. *The Quality of Mercy.* Atheneum, New York, 1971.
3. Fein, Rashi. The case for national health insurance. *Sat Rev*, pp. 27–29, August 22, 1970.
4. Cray, Ed. *In Failing Health, The Medical Crisis and the A.M.A.* The Bobbs-Merrill Company, Inc., Indianapolis, 1970.
5. Balfe, B. E., Lorant, J. E., and Todd, C. (eds.). *Reference Data on The Profile of Medical Practice.* American Medical Association, Center for Health Services Research and Development, 1971.
6. Roemer, Milton I. Group practice: a medical care spectrum. *J Med Educ*, 12:1154–58, December 1965.
7. Reed, Louis S., and Dwyer, Maureen. *Health Insurance Plans Other Than*

Blue Cross or Blue Shield Plans or Insurance Companies, 1970 Survey. Research Report No. 35. U.S. Department of Health, Education, and Welfare, Social Security Administration, Office of Research and Statistics. U.S. Government Printing Office, Washington, D.C., 1971.

8. Sparer, G., and Johnson, J. Evaluation of OEO neighborhood health centers. *Am J Public Health,* **61:**31–42, January 1971.

9. Schwartz, Jerome L. First national survey of free medical clinics. *HSMHA Health Rep,* **86:**775–87, 1971.

10. U.S. Department of Health, Education, and Welfare, Public Health Service, Health Services and Mental Health Administration. *Health Resources Statistics, 1971.* Public Health Service Publication No. 1509. U.S. Government Printing Office, Washington, D.C., February 1972.

11. American Hospital Association. *Hospitals, Journal of the American Hospital Association Guide Issue,* Part II. Vol. 45, No. 15, August 1, 1971.

12. U.S. Department of Health, Education, and Welfare. *1970 Annual Report.* U.S. Government Printing Office, Washington, D.C., 1971.

13. Colt, Avery M. Elements of comprehensive health planning. *Am J Public Health,* **60:**1194–1204, July 1970.

14. U.S. Department of Health, Education, and Welfare, Social Security Administration. *Conditions of Participation; Extended Care Facilities.* U.S. Government Printing Office, Washington, D.C., February 1968.

15. U.S. Department of Health, Education, and Welfare, Public Health Service, Health Services and Mental Health Administration, Regional Medical Programs Service. *Fact Book on Regional Medical Programs.* U.S. Government Printing Office, Washington, D.C., August 1971.

16. House of Representatives, Committee on Ways and Means. *Basic Facts on the Health Industry.* U.S. Government Printing Office, Washington, D.C., 1971.

17. Mueller, Marjorie Smith. Private health insurance in 1969: a review. *Soc Sec Bull,* **34:**3–18, February 1971.

18. U.S. Department of Health, Education, and Welfare, Social Security Administration. *Your Medicare Handbook.* U.S. Government Printing Office, Washington, D.C., May 1968.

19. West, Howard. Five years of Medicare—a statistical review. *Soc Sec Bull,* **34:**17–27, December 1971.

20. Newman, Howard N. Medicare and Medicaid. *Ann Am Acad Pol Sci,* **399:**114–24, January 1972.

21. Alexander, Raymond S., and Podair, Simon. *Medicaid: the People's Health Plan.* Public Affairs Pamphlet No. 422. Public Affairs Committee, New York, August 1968.

22. Ellwood, Paul M. Health maintenance organizations—concept and strategy. *Hospitals,* **45:**53–81, March 16, 1971.

23. Myers, Beverlee A. Health maintenance organizations: objectives and issues. *HSMHA Health Rep,* **86:**585–91, July 1971.

24. Williams, Greer. *Kaiser-Permanente Health Plan—Why It Works.* The Henry Kaiser Foundation, Oakland, California, February 1971.

25. Berki, Sylvester E. National health insurance: an idea whose time has come? *Ann Am Acad Pol Sci,* **399:**125–44, January 1972.

26. Somers, Anne R. The nation's health: issues for the future. *Ann Am Acad Pol Sci,* **399:**160–74, January 1972.

27. U.S. Department of Commerce, Bureau of the Census. *Statistical Abstract of the United States, 1971.* U.S. Government Printing Office, Washington, D.C.

28. U.S. Department of Health, Education, and Welfare, Public Health Service, Health Services and Mental Health Administration, Indian Health Service, Office of Program Planning and Evaluation, Program Analysis and Statistics Branch. *Indian Health Trends and Services.* Public Health Service Publication No. 2092. U.S. Government Printing Office, Washington, D.C., January 1971.

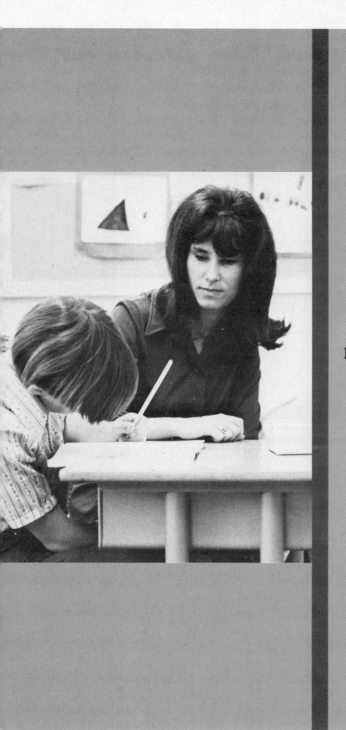

5

COMMUNITY MENTAL HEALTH CONCEPTS AND ORGANIZATION OF SERVICES

CHAPTER OUTLINE

The Basis of Community Mental Health

Mental illnesses range in intensity and nature from mild to severe, and from episodic emotional disturbances to persistent mental disorders. Years ago attention was paid mainly to severe mental disorders. More recently concern has developed for the milder forms along with growing recognition of the personal suffering they cause as well as the serious social and economic toll they take. Aside from the milder emotional disturbances which are considered to be in the "normal" range, the more severe categories share characteristics with many chronic physical illnesses. Chronic *mental* and chronic *physical* conditions both are likely to be due to a number of factors; to be long term, with acute episodes or flare-ups; and to be difficult to manage and treat.

Mental health problems have existed throughout history; they may, today, be the most pressing and complex of all health disorders. Community mental health concepts and practices are very recent developments in the effort to cope with these burgeoning problems. The concepts of community mental health involve the recognition that mental health and illness are community responsibilities and that attention must be directed not only toward overt and severe manifestations of mental illness but also toward prevention, treatment of incipient conditions, and rehabilitation. Community mental health practices involve the translation of these concepts into a variety of programs and services which ultimately are of sufficient magnitude to meet the needs of all segments of the population.[1]

Community mental health activity is based on concepts of *what constitutes mental health and illness,* on knowledge of *the types and causes* of mental disorders, and on measurements of *the extent* of mental illness. At present, there is a considerable deficit of information in all these areas, but the number and variety of scientific investigations under way provide hope for reducing the gap in the future.

Concepts of Mental Health and Illness

Concepts of mental health and illness have changed appreciably throughout history. At one time, the mentally ill were considered to be "possessed," and witch-hunting and exorcism of demons were integral parts of a community's approach to mental health problems. A book entitled *Malleus Maleficarum* (*Hammer Against Witches*), which was published in 1489, contained instructions for the recognition of a witch. Many of the listed criteria are those now associated with mental illness. This book was used for nearly 300 years as the standard guide for handling the "mentally afflicted," and "handling" frequently resulted in violence and death to the handled.

The early organicists maintained that disease could not exist without some organic defect or injury. Therefore, if no lesion could be found, "insanity" (which in modern usage is a legal rather than a scientific term) could not be regarded as disease, nor the patient as sick; rather, he was simply immoral or criminal.

In recent times, many attempts have been made to define mental good health and distinguish it from mental ill health. Anthropologists have found that what constitutes mental illness varies from one culture to another.[2,3] Behavior that in one culture may be considered as symptomatic of mental disorder may in another culture be considered as relatively normal. For example, the Navajos may perceive senility as neither illness nor deviance, but merely as behavior to be expected of old people.[4]

In contemporary Western societies, as in other cultures, concepts of mental health reflect dominant cultural norms. Thus, good mental health has been conceptualized in general terms as characterizing the individual who is emotionally stable, intellectually efficient, and effective in relationships with others. A further element is the ability to accept the need for delayed rewards and to have enough self-control to lessen dependency on the support of external authority. At first glance, these concepts seem sound enough. But as with other definitions, their generalness requires further specification, and attempts at refinement soon run into difficulty. The fact that the definition is rooted in *dominant* social norms also poses problems when applied to the individual who does not conform to the norm.

Is the person who conforms to the norms of a subgroup rather than to the norms of the larger group to be categorized as mentally ill solely on that basis? Bizarre behavior is usually considered as evidence of emotional disturbance or mental disorder.[5] However, there are extensive differences among cultural subgroups in acceptable and unacceptable behavioral patterns, and it is often difficult to

decide whether behavior is actually bizarre or is merely characteristic of the group with which the individual identifies.

General conformity and adaptation are not themselves sufficient evidence of good mental health. Adapting to or accepting
degrading, dehumanizing, or humiliating experiences may be an
index of poor, rather than good, mental health. Conforming to an
unstable social world, accepting impersonal relationships, and feeling powerless to participate in determining one's own destiny may
be indicative of an unhealthy passivity.

Profound personal suffering that is not explained by the individual's circumstances is another generally accepted signal of
mental illness. However, even this concept cannot be taken completely at face value.[5] A certain amount of psychologic stress is built
into daily living and is contributed to by numerous well-established social institutions. Stress, in fact, is viewed as providing
incentives and facilitating the development of desirable goals. The
objective of mental health workers usually is to reduce distress that
has no social function. Functional stress is not easy to distinguish
from nonfunctional stress.

The preceding discussion highlights the idea that concep-
tualizing good and poor mental health has come a long way since
the early days of witch- and demon-hunting. It also makes clear that
as yet there is no simple, unambiguous, all-inclusive definition by
which to distinguish the mentally healthy from the mentally ill.

Types and Causes of Mental Illness

A significant problem in considering the types and causes of
mental illness has to do with the breadth or narrowness of range of
mental conditions to be included. Some mental health workers
include only limited sets of clear-cut psychiatric disorders, while
others take a broader view, including feeling states such as "un-
happiness" or "nervousness," as well as problems of social relationships, family conflict, and deviant behavior such as delinquency, criminality, and a wide array of other social pathologies.

Psychologic impairment may affect any person, at any age, at
any time. It is usually long-standing, and can range along a
continuum from feelings of inferiority or guilt, through psychosomatic disorders and psychoneuroses, to the organic and functional
psychoses.

Personality disorders include *neuroses,* which may be relatively
mild conditions. The neurotic or psychoneurotic suffers from
unreasonable fears, obsessions, compulsions, and unwarranted exhaustion and is frequently very depressed. Although able to interpret his environment, he has reduced personal satisfactions.

Psychoses are more serious disturbances, the most common of which is *schizophrenia*. The psychotic is considered suffering from a major mental illness and has great difficulty interpreting the world around him. Occasionally, he is dangerous to himself or others and usually requires some hospitalization.

Mental health is not just a function of the mind (psyche). Rather, the body (soma) interacts with the mind, thus giving rise to the term *psychosomatic*. Stress on either may be reflected in the functioning of the other. Many individuals seek the services of physicians because of what are basically psychosomatic problems.

CLASSIFICATION OF MENTAL ILLNESS

A corollary to the difficulties in defining mental health is the equally difficult task of categorizing mental disorders. The present trend in treatment and in attempting to understand mental illness is away from pigeonholing mental diseases; but for diagnostic and statistical purposes some system of categorization is needed. In addition, a certain amount of confusion arose over the years in connection with the use of psychiatric terms, and it became apparent that some standardization of usage was in order. To serve these various purposes, the American Psychiatric Association developed a system of classification of mental disorders, the details of which are embodied in a manual.[6]

The classification system of the American Psychiatric Association makes a basic distinction among three categories of conditions: those mental disturbances that result from, or are precipitated by, lesions of the brain; those in which brain damage is secondary, absent, or not demonstrated; and mental deficiency. Briefly, the classification covers:

1. Disorders caused by or associated with impairment of brain tissue function. This general category includes acute versus chronic brain disorders associated with infection; intoxication; trauma; circulatory disturbances; convulsive disorders; disturbance of metabolism, growth, or nutrition; neoplasms; and uncertain causes.
2. Mental deficiency of a familial (hereditary) or idiopathic nature.
3. Disorders of psychogenic origin, or without clearly defined physical cause or structural change in the brain. This general category includes the following:
   a. Psychotic disorders such as *schizophrenia*, which may be manifested by delusions, hallucinations, and inappropriate reactions including showing unsuitable emotion in

a given cultural context (e.g., laughing when sadness is more appropriate); and *paranoid states,* which may express themselves in delusions of persecution and/or grandeur, hostility toward others, and depressive and manic states.

  b. Psychophysiologic disorders such as peptic ulcer, colitis, asthma, hypertension, or skin eruptions.

  c. Psychoneurotic disorders such as anxiety reactions, depression, dissociative reactions including amnesia, phobias about objects or situations, and obsessive-compulsive reactions.

  d. Personality disorders such as general emotional instability (e.g., a tendency to go to pieces under ordinary conditions), passivity, hostility, aggression, dissocial functioning represented by amoral disregard for the norms of society, antisocial behavior, and addiction to chemicals or drugs.

CAUSES OF MENTAL ILLNESS

Since one essential in understanding and treating or controlling any disease is a knowledge of its cause, establishing the etiology of mental disease is a major concern in the field of mental health. It is a complex matter partly because of the number of diverse conditions involved, and partly because of the difficulties of conducting scientific investigations of the kind that, for example, have been successful in pinpointing the specific cause of infectious diseases.

Physical causes of certain mental disturbances have been established slowly, and over time some conditions believed to have no physical cause have been shown, in part, to have such bases. An example is paresis, a mental disorder in which the individual is disturbed, irresponsible, and perhaps even violent. At one time there was no known cause of this condition, but it is now recognized as being due to syphilis. Similarly, it has been established that certain mental disturbances are caused by pellagra, a nutritional disease. It is possible that, as new scientific knowledge is accumulated, certain other biochemical or physiologic deficits or pathologies may be found to cause or at least to predispose individuals to the development of particular mental illnesses.

The vast, remaining array of mental disorders — those that have no known physical cause and thus are considered psychogenic in origin — constitute the principal problem with regard to establishing etiology. Theories as to the causes of psychogenic disorders have existed for many years and serve as hypotheses in research and as guides in treating the sick. However, there are as yet only meager scientific demonstrations of causal relationships between specific factors in the individual's history and/or environment and the development of a particular mental disorder.

The concept of multiple factors in the cause of psychogenic disorders has become generally accepted; the factors are considered to involve the individual, his family, and the community. The role of heredity is open to question. It may play some part in schizophrenia although the evidence to date is not too persuasive. It is possible that a disturbing pattern of behavior in a family may be conducive to the development of psychotic behavior in other family members.[7]

It is also possible that certain mental disorders may be associated with socioeconomic factors, environmental stress, deprivation,[8,9] and other phenomena which characterize modern life. Thus, the mass migration from simple, rural or small-town social systems to large, impersonal, automated, urban environments has contributed to individual conflict, group conflict, and frustration, which often lead to psychologic disturbances and feelings of alienation and isolation.[10] Rapid social change has caused tension and conflict among adults, and this creates disturbed and problem children. Some children, deprived of normal affectional ties and stable families, go through a passive childhood only to break down later when confronted by the responsibilities of adult life.

The Extent and Cost of Mental Illness

MENTAL ILLNESS IN THE GENERAL POPULATION

In the past two or three decades, more than 40 community studies have attempted to determine the number of people with mental disorders.[11-13] That the results varied widely is a considerable understatement.

Estimates of the number of persons with mental problems have varied from 1 or 2 per cent of the population to 81.5 per cent. The latter finding was from a study[13] in which, of the population sampled, 2.7 per cent were considered incapacitated because of extreme mental disturbance, another 7.5 were considered to have severe disturbances, 13.2 had marked symptoms, 21.8 moderate, and 36.3 mild symptoms. Thus, in this particular study only 18.5 per cent were found to be without some degree of mental disturbance.

The wide range in estimates of mental illness has obviously resulted from different criteria used and varying kinds of mental conditions included. If only clearly disabling conditions are counted, the estimate of mental illness in the general population will be relatively low. If milder emotional disturbances, psychosomatic complaints, and any of the vast array of "problems of living" are included, a much larger proportion of the population will be found to have some form of mental illness. As with physical conditions, it is difficult to enumerate mental and emotional conditions until diagnoses have been made, and even then the problem of uncounted psychiatric cases looms large (e.g., noninstitutionalized private patients). The situation is made more complicated by the fact that the very criteria for diagnoses remain controversial.

MENTALLY ILL PATIENTS IN TREATMENT FACILITIES

Counts of the number of persons receiving care in various types of organized psychiatric or mental treatment facilities are easier to make and are more accurate than attempts to count cases of mental illness in the general population. There is some lag in data reporting, however, and consequently the most recent data available at a given time are likely to be estimates which only gradually become replaced by "final" figures. It should also be kept in mind, of course, that resulting numbers, percentages, or rates cannot be construed as representing the amount or kinds of mental illness in the general population.

In 1970, as shown in Table 5-1, there were 501 mental hospitals in the United States consisting of 312 state and county, 150 private, and 39 Veterans Administration neuropsychiatric facilities. In addition, there were an estimated 1,316 general hospitals that reported psychiatric treatment facilities. In these various categories of *inpatient* facilities, about 1,603,000 patients were served in 1968 in connection with psychiatric disorder. In that same year an estimated 1,507,000 patients were served in 2,282 *outpatient* clinics (Table 5-1) in connection with psychiatric, behavioral, or emotional complaints.

Prior to 1956 the number of resident patients in state and county mental hospitals (which constitute a majority of the facilities in that category) had been increasing annually. Since then the resident patient population has been decreasing steadily. On the other hand, the number of total admissions has been increasing, continuing another trend that began in the mid-1940's. These figures would indicate that, in recent years, more patients are being admitted to state and county mental hospitals but they are staying for shorter periods.

Reports from 263 (out of 312) of the state and county mental hospitals revealed that, among first-admission patients in 1968, there were more males than females (60 per cent and 40 per cent, respectively), and almost three fourths were young adults and middle-aged persons. Thus, nearly half (47 per cent) of the first-ad-

TABLE 5-1. Mentally Ill Inpatient and Outpatient Care: Facilities and Patients

	Number of Facilities	Number of Patients Served* (in thousands)§		
	1970‡	1955	1965	1968
INPATIENT				
Mental hospitals	(501)			
State and county	312	819	805	792
Private	150	123	125	118
Veterans Administration	39	88	116	134
General hospitals with psychiatric facilities	1,316	266	519	559
Total inpatient	1,817	1,296	1,565	1,603
OUTPATIENT CLINICS	2,282†	379	1,071	1,507

* Includes resident patients at beginning of year, or those on active rolls of outpatient clinics, plus those admitted during year.
† 1968 data.
‡ SOURCE: Adapted from National Institute of Mental Health. *Mental Illness and its Treatment,* Public Health Service Publication No. 1345, revised 1970.
§ SOURCE: Adapted from U.S. Bureau of the Census. *Statistical Abstract of the United States, 1971,* p. 73.

mission patients were in the age group 20–44, and a quarter were 45–64 years old; relatively fewer were younger than 20 (12 per cent) or older than 64 (16 per cent). As to diagnosis, three fourths of the first-admission patients were divided almost equally among three categories of mental disorders: acute and chronic brain syndromes; personality disorders; and psychotic disorders, most of which were subclassified as schizophrenic reactions.[14]

COSTS OF MENTAL ILLNESS AND PSYCHIATRIC CARE

Since the early 1950's, various attempts have been made to estimate the total "cost" of mental illness to society as a whole. The "cost" was placed at almost $21 billion in 1968.[15] This figure represents the total of two basic components of the estimate: treatment and prevention cost, and loss in productive capacity.

Estimate of the cost of treatment and prevention included expenses of therapeutic, medical, and nursing care provided to the mentally ill as well as expenditures for research, training, and construction. The cost of reduction in productive capacity consisted principally (although not exclusively) of estimates of the loss of earnings caused by mental illness.

Biometricians consider that whatever the figure arrived at through estimation of these two components, the "cost" would be even higher if dollar values were assigned to additional appropriate components. These would include the cost of illegal and antisocial behavior as well as several kinds of intangible costs such as the cost for maintenance of the dependents of the mentally ill. The process of arriving at total "cost" is exceedingly complex and many of the elements unavoidably are speculative. However, from the standpoint of determining social policy, a speculative estimate of the *total* "cost" may be preferable to a firm estimate of *part of the total* "cost."

Although reflecting only a fraction of the total "cost" to society, some indication of the economics of mental illness may be obtained from considering the cost of psychiatric inpatient care (for which relatively firm data are available). Similar to cost of inpatient care in the health service field generally, the cost of psychiatric inpatient care has been rising steadily in recent years. The experience of state and county mental hospitals illustrates this development strikingly.

Even though the number of resident patients in state and county mental hospitals has been declining, maintenance expenditures have been increasing, as shown in Table 5-2. The cost of care in these institutions rose from about $620 million in 1955 to $1.2 billion in 1965 and almost $1.6 billion in 1968. The costs per resident patient per day increased from $3.06 in 1955 to $10.47 in 1968.

These increasing costs have been due not only to factors contributing to the general cost spiral in the United States but also to the increasingly greater numbers of personnel employed in mental hospitals. The upward trend in personnel is also illustrated by Table 5-2, which shows that in 1968 there were approximately 217,000 full-time employees in state and county mental hospitals, compared with about 146,000 in 1955.

TABLE 5-2. Number of Resident Patients, Number of Personnel, and Maintenance Expenditures, State and County Mental Hospitals, Selected Years

	1955	1965	1968
Resident patients, at end of year	558,922	475,202	400,681
Personnel (full time), at end of year	146,392	204,879	217,128
Maintenance expenditures	$618,087,247	$1,204,345,256	$1,577,631,758
Per resident patient			
Per year	1,116.59	2,503.99	3,831.49
Per day	3.06	6.86	10.47
Per patient under treatment			
Per year	849.31	1,499.75	1,996.11
Per day	2.33	4.11	5.45

SOURCE: Adapted from National Institute of Mental Health. *Mental Health Statistics—Current Facility Reports,* Series MHB-H, January 1965, p. 6 and January 1969, p. 3.

SOLUTIONS TO COST OF CARE

Mounting costs (for a variety of reasons) that are associated with psychiatric care (in a variety of settings) have led to concerted searches for solutions. Indications are that at least part of the solution to the problem of mounting costs may lie in the further development of community-based psychiatric facilities of the kind described earlier. For example, in psychiatric units of general hospitals, although the *daily cost per patient* is much greater than in state and county mental hospitals, the *total cost per patient* is much less because the treatment period in the community hospital is much shorter. Also, there is evidence that the cost of psychiatric care in modified residential service facilities is even less than in general hospitals. In one community, the cost of care in a 24-hour psychiatric unit of a general hospital was compared with that of a day/night care unit. The fee per unit of time in the day/night unit was found to be considerably lower mainly because approximately twice as many patients could be treated in a day or night unit as in a 24-hour unit of similar size and staffing.

In state and county and other public mental hospitals and clinics, the taxpayer—and not the individual patient—pays most of the cost of care. In private settings, the patient pays the cost and, depending on circumstances, the financial burden to the individual is likely to be considerable. For public and private arrangements alike, there is as yet no widespread systematic provision for keeping costs down and for making it easier to meet expenses when psychiatric care is needed.

Insurance plans providing coverage for mental illnesses offer a promising avenue of attack on these problems. Such plans, by spreading the cost among a large group of subscribers, more readily permit the individual who needs psychiatric care to obtain it. An additional gain is that there may be prompting to seek help sooner, thus possibly forestalling a prolonged period of costly inpatient care.

Insurance carriers have been reluctant to provide coverage for mental illness for several reasons. One of the most important is their concern with the problem of distinguishing between "real illness" and "the ordinary strains of living" for the purpose of paying benefits for treatment. Another concern has to do with the chronic nature of mental illness and the possibility of the need for protracted treatment. Finally, insurance carriers are concerned with the problem of how to engage with an area of service in which there are public funds already available to pay for care—as in state and county mental hospitals and, more recently, community mental health centers.

In spite of serious obstacles, there have been expansion and improvement in insurance coverage for psychiatric care during the past decade.[16] The first major experiment in providing large-scale psychiatric outpatient care began in 1959 under the auspices of Group Health Insurance, Inc., of New York City, and demonstrated that short-termed psychiatric treatment was both successful and insurable under voluntary health plans. The Federal Employees Health Benefits Program was expanded to include mental health provisions in 1967–1968, and it is now one of the nation's most advanced examples of psychiatric outpatient coverage. Labor unions have begun to negotiate health plans which include psychiatric benefits: the United Auto Workers undertook the pioneering work, followed a few years later by the United Steel Workers. Several large industrial employers have taken the initiative in providing psychiatric coverage in the health care plans they provide for their employees.

It has been estimated that as many as 15 million persons have been covered by new or expanded psychiatric benefits in the past decade[16] and that these are mainly people who earn too much for publicly supported psychiatric services but who cannot afford the out-of-pocket expense of psychiatric care. Psychiatric benefits will no doubt expand in the future, and the goal will be extension to more segments of the population and broadened provisions in the insurance plans. The present ferment regarding financing and delivery of health services generally will inevitably influence resolution of the same issues concerning mental health services specifically.

The Provision of Mental Health Services

Over a long period of history, attitudes toward the mentally ill and provisions for their care passed through several stages. The attitudes toward such persons changed from viewing them as criminals to regarding them as objects of curiosity and finally to recognizing them as being ill and subject to the same humanitarian treatment as that accorded to individuals suffering from physical illness.

The evolution of provisions for the care of the mentally ill has reflected not only the attitudes toward mental disorders that prevailed at a given time, but also society's general sense of responsibility for those afflicted. Thus, at one time it was considered essential to confine the mentally ill and to segregate them from the rest of society; today the goal is to maintain as many of the mentally ill in their own communities as possible. Similarly, in earlier periods of history, no treatment was afforded to any sufferer from mental illness; now the goals of mental health programs include not only the provision of appropriate treatment for all who need it, but also the provision of preventive and rehabilitative measures in order to forestall the onset of illness and to ensure as complete restoration of functioning as possible. Finally, at one time only the mentally ill who were destitute were considered to be public responsibilities; today public responsibility is defined much more broadly and is expressed through the agency of government at local, state, and national levels.

HISTORICAL DEVELOPMENTS IN THE CARE OF MENTAL ILLNESS

In early periods of history, the well-to-do kept mentally ill family members at home or, if they were troublesome, chained or locked them in attics or cellars. They were of legal concern only insofar as their property was affected. The poor and homeless "insane" were public responsibilities and were incarcerated as felons or paupers.

"Madhouses" were established about the thirteenth century. Their purpose was merely to incarcerate the insane, and no treatment was provided. Bethlehem Hospital (Bedlam) in London was one of the earliest of such institutions. Its manacles, chains, locks and keys, and stocks were standard equipment for the inmates. For centuries a visit to Bedlam to watch the antics of the inmates was one of the sights of London.

In 1793, Philippe Pinel was appointed physician to Paris' notorious Bicêtre, where the lunatics were incarcerated. Shocked by what he saw, he freed those in chains, but he was strongly criticized both by the public and by other physicians. In an essay on mania published after the French Revolution, Pinel outlined his theories on the humane treatment of the mentally ill. Subsequent writings laid the foundation for the French School of psychiatry, which was important throughout the nineteenth century.

In the United States in the mid-1800's Dorothea Lynde Dix became interested in various kinds of institutions, made personal investigations of their conditions, and observed the treatment of mentally ill persons. Ultimately, she was responsible for the establishment of 32 new state institutions for the mental patients. As they were built, local authorities very willingly transferred their mentally ill to these institutions because this saved local tax expense. Soon the institutions were overburdened with chronic patients, many of whom were soon forgotten in back wards. The enormous foreign immigration during the latter half of the nineteenth century brought additional persons with physical, emotional, and social problems who further overtaxed various health and welfare institutions. It was not the intent of those who established state mental hospitals to have them become human warehouses, but over the years they did, and overcrowding became a way of life which has persisted to this day.

Early in the twentieth century, the "mental hygiene" movement came into being. This was due in large part to the untiring work of Clifford W. Beers, who had been a patient in private and state mental hospitals between 1900 and 1903. Gathering firsthand evidence of inhumane treatment and lack of therapy, he was later discharged and wrote a book entitled *A Mind That Found Itself*. This led directly to the establishment of the National Committee for Mental Hygiene, a voluntary association that was the forerunner of the National Association for Mental Health. The association established state and local chapters, which pressed for wider public understanding and support of legislation and programs promoting child guidance services and other psychiatrically oriented services. Their efforts were frequently hampered by public apathy and inadequate financial support. Despite this, the association played an important part in obtaining legislative support for necessary programs.

Numerous other developments in the present century have helped to promote understanding and action in the field of mental health. In the 1940's, mass media communications became much more effective in informing the public about the problem of mental illness. Public concern also was aroused by the large number of men (1.75 million) who were rejected for World War II military service because of psychiatric conditions. At the same time, experiences gained during World War II in treatment of psychiatric casualties encouraged radically new treatment methods. Later, the World Health Organization focused world attention on mental health when it included emotional and social well-being of the individual as part of its general definition of health. In the 1950's, newer drugs helped reverse the usual pattern of prolonged institutional treatment. Interest and activity in mental health matters increased among public health, welfare, and education workers, and thus contributed to the general advancement of mental health goals.[17,18]

PREVENTION, TREATMENT, AND
REHABILITATION MODALITIES

Mental health is coming more and more to be viewed as an integral part of public health programs, and basic public health concepts are readily applicable to the mental health field. Thus, in mental health programs treatment is a major concern, but there is a growing focus on early treatment, and in addition, attention is being directed increasingly toward prevention and rehabilitation. Prevention and early treatment of mental and emotional disturbances are the basis for the newly developing subspecialties of community and social psychiatry. New kinds of facilities have also been increasing as part of the effort in prevention, early treatment, and rehabilitation of mental illness, the most significant development in recent years being *comprehensive community mental health centers.*

Traditional Therapeutic Methods. Psychotherapy traditionally has been and continues to be the basic therapeutic method used in psychiatric disorders. It varies from a mild supportive approach to classical psychoanalysis. It includes both individual methods (therapist-patient) and group methods (therapist-patient and family, therapist — several patients simultaneously, etc.). Regardless of the specific technique used, the important therapeutic factor is the therapist-patient relationship and, as an additional dimension in group therapy, the group's interpersonal relationships. Depending on the nature of the mental illness and its degree of tractability, therapy may be of brief duration or may extend over a period of several years.

Somatic therapy for the relief of symptoms has also been used for many years. Certain of the older techniques such as electroshock and especially insulin therapy have given way largely to the use of the psychoactive drugs which, since the mid-1950's, have brought a dramatic improvement in many of the overt manifestations of mental illness. While the tranquilizers and antidepressants do not in themselves cure illness, they often modify a disturbance and help to make additional therapy more effective. A very significant consequence is that considerably more patients can now be maintained in their homes and communities whereas previously they would have had to be institutionalized.

Several kinds of facilities offering therapeutic services have already been mentioned: state and county, private, and Veterans Administration mental hospitals; general hospitals with psychiatric inpatient facilities; and outpatient clinics. Use of the large, long-term mental hospital (principally state and county institutions) has declined and other kinds of facilities have gained prominence. An increasing number of general hospitals have been adding psychiatric screening and acute treatment facilities, and the number of psychiatric outpatient clinics also has been increasing. The growth of these facilities reflect current trends toward detecting mental illness at an early stage and increasing the treatment of patients closer to home.

In an effort to provide immediate psychiatric help to individuals experiencing a sudden emotional crisis, emergency facilities, usually in the form of walk-in clinics, have come into being. The walk-in clinic provides 24-hour, low-cost service with no waiting period. In addition to the initial emergency visit, several subsequent visits are possible, usually up to a total of seven. If the patient needs further treatment, appropriate referrals are made by the clinic staff. In addition to the walk-in clinics which provide general psychiatric service, a similar but more specialized emergency service is also provided by suicide prevention centers.

There are several kinds of modified residential facilities. One consists of day care and night care centers and hospitals. Day care offers a full program of therapy, activity, and rehabilitation for patients who are able to return home at night. Night care is designed for those who are able to work or attend school during daytime hours but need treatment and a place to sleep at night. Halfway houses are a second form of modified residential service. These are institutions in which patients live together after being discharged from a mental hospital and while they are readapting to the community. The patients receive some supervision and gradually resume their life in the community through employment and social activity. Foster homes (sometimes known as board and care homes) constitute a third kind of provision and are available in situations in which the patient is able to return to the community from a mental hospital but has no home to go to.

Community Mental Health Centers. Provisions for the delivery of mental health services underwent dramatic change when, in 1963, community mental health centers were established through federal legislation. The centers have afforded an opportunity to place in action many of the mental health program concepts that have been developing in the past several decades: the importance of prevention, early treatment, and rehabilitation; the avoidance of the harmful effects of isolated institutional residence in long-stay mental hospitals; the provision of mental health services within the community, so that patients could stay at home, be treated at home, and become well at home; the provision of comprehensive services, resulting in a wide range of programs to meet individual needs; and the provision of continuity of care, so that as a patient's needs change he can be shifted easily from one service modality to another without interruption in care.

To be comprehensive, community mental health centers must supply five basic services: (1) inpatient care for limited time periods; (2) outpatient care, including aftercare for ex-mental hospital patients; (3) partial hospitalization such as day, night, or weekend care; (4) emergency care 24 hours a day; and (5) consultation and education service such as counseling schools or police forces, establishing liaison with other community service agencies, and providing mental health education for professional specialists, community service personnel, and the lay public.[19] These are the essential services that are required for federal assistance under community mental health centers legislative provisions. The services may be expanded to include, in addition, diagnostic and rehabilitation services, precare and aftercare services, training of personnel, and research and evaluation.

Services are required to be geographically accessible and available to all persons within a given area and regardless of the individual's ability to pay. The basic units for planning and delivery of services are known as "catchment areas," which consist of geographic divisions containing from 75,000 to 200,000 people.

As of mid-year 1971, about 450 community mental health centers had been funded, with approximately 300 in operating status. Every state has at least one center. Seventeen per cent are in cities of half a million or more; 49 per cent are in cities from 25,000 to 500,000; and 34 per cent serve large rural areas. In calendar year 1969, 205 centers treated an estimated 372,000 persons.[20]

As might be expected of such an ambitious and wide-ranging venture, the community mental health centers program has been experiencing some problems.[21] Inadequate financing mechanisms is one of the most serious problems encountered by some centers which have achieved full programming. Most centers get only a small percentage of their income from patient fees; the bulk comes from federal, local, and private contributions, which, to say the least, are not altogether stable sources.

A second knotty problem has stemmed from trying to apply the sweeping concepts embodied in the program. In effect, those responsible for developing a community mental health center must decide whether to stick to the more traditional, safer, basically clinical kinds of care, or whether also to venture beyond the center's walls and launch bolder, riskier programs outside in the community.

A third difficulty involves geography: in urban regions the catchment areas sometimes arbitrarily cut up neighborhoods and overlap with county services; in rural areas there are problems of vast distances, lack of transportation, and the need for professional personnel to spend much time traveling.

Finally, all centers — urban and rural — have to tackle a basic problem that confronts the health services generally: staffing and manpower shortages. A number of centers are at least partially coping with this difficulty by using paraprofessionals (new health careerists and others) who are drawn from the local communities and given in-service training at the centers.

One promising solution to the financial problems being experienced by some community mental health centers lies in health maintenance organizations (HMO's) described in Chapter 4. For example, it becomes possible for a community mental health center to enter into a contract with an HMO to provide outpatient mental health services. It is also conceivable that a mental health center can be the organizing focus for a health maintenance organization, with other health services built around those of the mental health centers.

For both financial and ideologic reasons some community mental health centers may evolve as the nuclei for future regional, comprehensive systems which include health, mental health, and social services such as welfare, family planning, and legal aid. This trend would be consistent with the current national thrust to plan and provide increasingly comprehensive services to defined populations. A number of community mental health centers even now are exploring and developing linkages with other health and human services programs in their communities.[20]

Community Psychiatry.   Community mental health centers are regarded as the wide-scale application of a particular subspecialty of psychiatric practice, namely, community psychiatry. Community psychiatry includes clinical services of a diagnostic, remedial, and rehabilitative nature, but the services are community oriented, emphasize prevention, and afford a continuum of care.[22] Community psychiatry developed as psychiatrists became less concerned about abnormal behavior and began giving more attention to conditions affecting those who were *not* ill. It attempts to provide for the mentally ill, and for those in danger of becoming so, opportunities for making contact with forces that are favorable to the maintenance or reestablishment of social adequacy.[23]

Emphasis is placed on trying to understand what has reduced a person's effectiveness, and efforts are directed toward early intervention and mitigation of the destructive influences. As part of this process, an attempt is made to establish mechanisms for "crisis intervention." This involves enlisting the understanding and support of those persons in the community who are most likely to have contacts with individuals experiencing an emotional crisis, and who therefore can be providers of aid at the earliest possible stage in mental health problems. Such persons constitute the community's caretaker and caregiver groups and include ministers, counselors, probation and parole officers, public health workers, social agency personnel, teachers, and physicians in fields of medicine other than psychiatry.[18] Community psychiatry focuses on providing consultation to these caregiver and caretaker groups in order to increase their effectiveness in handling persons who come to them with problems of living.

The new concept of treatment may also take the form of environmental change. Thus, a "war on poverty" and a vast array of efforts to alleviate conditions in the ghetto may be attacks on incipient mental illness. Promoting mental health in a community may require the improvement of community schools. Individual therapy may involve altering the patient's personal relationships.

The general shift in treatment philosophy that has given rise to community psychiatry has been stimulated by several factors, including studies by social scientists pointing up the poor therapeutic value inherent in mammoth institutional settings; the gradual acceptance of the fact that increasing numbers of the community population are, or may become, mentally ill; research indicating that brief therapy may be as effective as other methods; the gradual acceptance of appropriately trained personnel—other than psychiatrists—as therapists, including clinical psychologists, social workers, nurses, and rehabilitation specialists.

Community psychiatry has been gaining worldwide acceptance. Many pioneering developments have taken place in other countries. The first international congress concerned with community psychiatric problems met in London in 1964 and attracted psychiatrists, behavioral scientists, and other specialists from 40 countries. The Fourth International Congress of Social Psychiatry, meeting in Jerusalem in May 1972, held symposia on such topics as suicide, drug abuse, alcohol abuse, aging, family planning, student unrest, child rearing, and violence.

THE FEDERAL GOVERNMENT IN MENTAL HEALTH

Traditionally, the United States government has provided extensive, direct mental health services for veterans of the Armed Forces through a system of clinics and hospitals. In addition, in 1855 it established the Government Hospital for the Insane in Washington, D.C., which became Saint Elizabeths Hospital in 1916. The federal government maintains hospitals for narcotics addicts, which are primarily for federal prisoners, but which also have provisions for a limited number of persons from the general population who enter on a voluntary basis. In recent decades, three significant federal governmental actions have given strong impetus to mental health programs and services in the United States: one was passage of the National Mental Health Act of 1946; another was the establishment of the National Institute of Mental Health in 1949; and third was the passage of the Community Mental Health Centers Act of 1963.

The National Mental Health Act of 1946. Congress passed landmark legislation in 1946 in the form of the National Mental Health

Act. One of its significant provisions was the establishment of the National Institute of Mental Health. The act also made assistance available to state and private nonprofit institutions for mental health services, research, and training. Under these provisions emphasis has been on the development of community mental health programs, particularly for the prevention and early treatment of mental disorders. Financing is in the form of grants-in-aid, in which, for example, a state provides two dollars from state and local sources for each dollar of federal funds it receives.

The National Institute of Mental Health.   The principal federal agency responsible for progress in mental health is the National Institute of Mental Health. The institute, it will be recalled from Chapter 2, is now part of the Health Services and Mental Health Administration of the Public Health Service, U.S. Department of Health, Education, and Welfare. From its establishment in 1949 as a fairly modest effort and with a budget of $3 million, the institute has grown to a $640 million program covering a wide range of problems related to the nation's mental health.

The institute conducts and supports interdisciplinary basic, clinical, and developmental research in the causes, prevention, and treatment of mental illness and the improvement of mental health. It supports a variety of training programs—for mental health specialists and auxiliary personnel, for in-service training, and for personnel of other professions. Under the Community Mental Health Centers Act of 1963, the institute is responsible for the administration of grants for the construction and staffing of community mental health centers. The institute assumed responsibility for Saint Elizabeths Hospital in 1967, and is developing it as a national model for the conversion of a large, old-style mental institution into a modern facility, with a community-based mental health center. The institute operates the National Clearinghouse for Mental Health Information, a computerized repository of scientific information related to mental health.

Attention to special mental health problem areas is the responsibility of a series of institute centers which plan and direct research, training, consultation, and service projects. Included are the Center for Studies of Metropolitan Problems (concerned with the quality of urban life and its impact on mental health); the Center for Minority Group Mental Health Problems; the Center for Studies of Child and Family Mental Health; the Center for Epidemiologic Studies (examines the source and spread of mental illnesses); and the Center for Studies of Schizophrenia. Additional centers each deal with a specific type of social pathology: crime and delinquency, narcotic and drug abuse, and suicide. Increased concern about alcoholism led in 1971 to the conversion of another center into the National Institute on Alcohol Abuse and Alcoholism (the new institute remains within the National Institute of Mental Health).

The Community Mental Health Centers Act of 1963. The federal legislation that established a nationwide program of community mental health centers was preceded by almost a decade of study and deliberation. In 1955, Congress created a Joint Commission on Mental Illness and Health, which was charged with studying and making recommendations for combating the increasing mental health problems in this country. In a final, ten-volume report published in 1961, the Commission recommended a broad, comprehensive attack on mental illness.[24] Early in 1963, the President of the United States delivered to Congress a Special Message on Mental Illness and Mental Retardation, proposing "a bold new approach . . . designed . . . to use Federal resources to stimulate state, local and private action." He urged the search for, and eradication of, the causes of mental illness and mental retardation; the strengthening of knowledge and skilled manpower; and the improvement of programs and facilities. He stated that "when this approach is carried out, reliance on the cold mercy of custodial isolation will be supplanted by the open warmth of community concern and capability."

In response to the President's request, Congress enacted the Community Mental Health Centers Act, which authorized the appropriation of $150 million to finance up to two thirds of the cost of construction of community mental health centers. In 1964, Congress amended the act, authorizing support for staffing by professional and technical personnel during the first 51 months of a center's operation. In 1968, the act was further amended to support specialized services to alcoholics and narcotic addicts. The act was again amended in 1970, with special attention to poverty areas and to children. By the close of 1971, the federal government, through the National Institute of Mental Health, had committed about $700 million to the community mental health centers program, matched by an equivalent amount from state and local governments.[21]

STATE AND LOCAL ROLES IN MENTAL HEALTH

Organization and Kinds of State and Local Mental Health Services. All states in the union now provide some kind of mental health service, although the responsible public agency designated for this function varies among the states. For example, Illinois, Massachusetts, and Michigan are among the states that have a separate Department of Mental Health. California has a Department of Mental

Hygiene located within a Health and Welfare Agency (alongside elements of Public Health, Welfare, etc.); Florida has a Division of Mental Health within a Department of Health and Rehabilitation Services; and Georgia has a Division of Mental Health within a Department of Public Health. Placement of the agency in the state governmental hierarchy has various administrative consequences, of course, such as whether or not the agency reports directly to the governor and whether it receives state funds directly or through a superagency.

Over the past years, many states, in exercising their prerogatives with respect to delegating authority to local governments, have adopted legislation which permitted the establishment of a local mental health authority or board with the power to develop mental health programs. Considerable organizational variation is also found on this level. For example, in California, Los Angeles has a countywide Mental Health Services unit (as part of a Health Services superagency), whereas San Francisco has a Community Mental Health Services agency which is part of the City and County Department of Public Health.

The official mental health agency on the state level optimally has responsibility for general planning and coordination and for the provision of several kinds of services and programs. These include hospital services, psychiatric outpatient services, consultation, personnel training programs, public education programs, assembly of operational statistics, and research. The local agency traditionally has carried on activities such as case-finding, diagnosis, treatment, education, consultation, and rehabilitation.

With the passage of the Community Mental Health Centers Act, the states acquired new responsibilities, and local mental health agencies have also been affected, since they are at the site of the action. As a prerequisite for participating in the program, a state was required to develop a comprehensive, long-range, interagency, mental health plan. All 50 states have developed such plans. In implementing the provisions of the Community Mental Health Centers Act, a state designated a single state agency to administer the plan for centers or to supervise administration of the plan. The designated agency must review and approve all proposals for centers that are advanced by any community within the state. The state has an advisory council, composed of representatives of nongovernmental groups, other state agencies concerned with any facet of mental health center operation or administration, and citizens' groups representing consumers of the services to be provided by the centers.

Although the trend is away from the large state mental hospitals as a method of treatment for mental illness and the number of such hospitals has declined, this category of institution undoubtedly will need to remain in existence for some time to come. The state mental health agency responsible for the administration of these hospitals is in a key position to improve the quality of care provided, and considerable effort has been made in this direction in recent years. Thus, the organization of hospital treatment in some states includes placing all patients from one area in the same unit so they can maintain community identity. Other hospitals have been established as "therapeutic communities" with open wards and free movement of patients and staff.[25] Rehabilitation of elderly patients has resulted in the discharge of some who had been forgotten in back wards. Further advances along these lines are being stimulated by provisions of the Community Mental Health Centers Act, whereby funds are made available to state mental hospitals for the improvement of their treatment programs. Anticipated beneficial results include the earlier discharge of many more patients and new solutions to the treatment of patients who in the past have been considered chronically and hopelessly ill.

State Laws Governing Commitments to Mental Hospitals.   A traditional function of the states has been the provision of laws regarding commitments of patients to mental hospitals. The laws of the different states vary as to commitment procedures, but in general the admission of a mentally ill person to a hospital is on one of four bases.

The first is *involuntary commitment,* a long-standing and formal practice which involves petition to the courts (by relatives or others), medical certification, a court hearing, and final disposition. In some states, formal notice must be served on the mentally ill person, and sometimes arrest on a warrant is the required procedure. Practically all states provide that there may be a jury trial if requested by the person concerned or by someone else.

The second method is *emergency commitment,* which is provided if an individual becomes suddenly and seriously disturbed. In these cases the judicial process is waived temporarily, and patients may be admitted to hospitals on the formal certification of the health officer. Such patients can be held only for a few days, pending action for more formal court commitment procedures, if needed.

The third method is *observational commitment,* which is for a period of from one to three months and is for the purpose of diagnosis and planning future care and treatment.

The fourth method is *voluntary admission,* which may also have the concomitant of voluntary release: when such a patient requests release, he must be freed within a specified period—not more than two weeks in most states. In order to detain him longer, formal involuntary commitment procedures must be initiated. Since voluntary admission does not involve court action, the stigma of a legal record of the patient's mental illness is avoided.

In general, there is a growing public and professional concern regarding state laws and procedures involving commitments to mental hospitals. Some view the processes as too legalistic. On the other hand, since the individual is deprived of liberty perhaps for an indefinite period and since he is usually unable to handle his own affairs, definite legal issues are involved, and some means of providing protection through due process of law seems indicated. In an effort to assist the states in revising their laws, the National Institute of Mental Health has provided guidelines that embody the more modern concepts of commitment laws and procedures.

Some states have already proceeded to up-date commitment procedures. In California, the Lanterman-Petris-Short Act (1969) was passed with the avowed intention ". . . to end the inappropriate, indefinite and involuntary commitment of mentally disordered persons and persons impaired by chronic alcoholism, and to eliminate legal disabilities." Thus, the law provides that for both voluntary or involuntary cases *screening and referral* in a local mental health program are necessary preconditions for admission to a state mental hospital. A further condition is *early evaluation* in the screening process, with persons to be released before the elapse of 72 hours if professionally judged to be no longer in need of evaluation or treatment.

Mental Health Manpower

Mental health services have grown at a remarkable rate, and one of the pressing needs—as in the health field generally—is for more manpower to keep pace with expanding programs, to maintain standards of service, and to meet the complex mental health requirements of the population.[26] There has been marked expansion in the total number of trained personnel in the mental health field, but demand still far outstrips supply.

Categories of personnel that are most central to the provision of mental health services are psychiatrists, clinical psychologists, psychiatric social workers, and psychiatric nurses. *Psychiatrists* make diagnoses, supervise the overall treatment plan, treat patients, supervise the treatment carried on by other personnel, and provide consultation. *Clinical psychologists* administer a variety of psychologic tests and assist in diagnosis, evaluation, and therapy. *Psychiatric social workers* are especially trained to deal with relationships—between patient and family, patient and employer, and so forth. They have important responsibilities in rehabilitation and aftercare services such as supervision of foster home placements.

Psychiatric nurses are an essential part of the staff of an inpatient facility, and they are also needed in day and night hospitals and in outpatient facilities. They may serve as consultants for foster homes and nursing homes and have extremely valuable roles in aftercare programs. In some day hospitals, psychiatric nurses on duty wear ordinary street clothes, rather than the traditional nurse's white, and mingle with patients in the kind of interaction that characterizes a therapeutic community.

While each of the mental health professional categories has a traditional focus, the lines separating the different specialties are beginning to be blurred. Thus, all senior staff—in community mental health centers, hospitals, and other settings—are increasingly involved, often as a team, in diagnosis, in treatment, and in consultation.

The National Center for Health Statistics reported that, in 1969, there were 25,076 physicians whose primary specialty was psychiatry or neurology. This was an increase of only 5,000 over the number of such specialists in 1965. There were approximately 6,400 clinical psychologists practicing in 1968, as well as almost 15,000 social workers employed in various kinds of psychiatric facilities. About 27,000 psychiatric nurses were enumerated in a survey conducted by the American Nurses' Association in 1966. Altogether, the numbers appear substantial, but mental health professionals are seriously concerned that the rate of growth is far from rapid enough.

Aside from the four key professional groups, several other cattegories of personnel contribute significantly to mental health programs. *Occupational therapists, physical therapists, recreational therapists,* and *vocational counselors* are important to rehabilitation programs involving patients in all stages of care. *Psychiatric aides* and *psychiatric technicians* perform valuable services, particularly in day/night treatment programs as well as in inpatient facilities. In a number of mental health programs special provisions have been made to recruit and train *volunteers* from the community, and such efforts have been highly successful.

The search for solutions to manpower shortages continues unabated in the mental health field. One promising resource lies in efforts presently being made to define new types of jobs and to recruit and train workers to fill them. Another possible solution is further development of an aspect of community psychiatry in which mental health professionals, who are scarce in number, teach principles of handling mental health problems to the caretakers of society, who are greater in number. A third solution consists of the more extensive participation in mental health activities by private physicians. As in any kind of community health program, the private physician, who is in the front line of service to persons who are ill, can make an invaluable contribution to the prevention, diagnosis, treatment, and rehabilitation effort. This requires, however, a change in emphasis from the more apparent and clear-cut problems of physical illness to the more subtle problems of mental and emotional illness, as well as an orientation not only to the individual but to society as a whole. A fourth solution is inherent in the various mental health training programs being financed by the federal government. These programs include in-service training and also the support of academic work leading to advanced degrees.

Research in Mental Health and Illness

Several broad areas may be singled out as basic concerns in research in mental health and illness. Although the specific subject matter may differ, the areas themselves are essentially the same as those involved in research in the health field generally.[27] One area of research has to do with the amount, distribution, and causes of mental illness, and descriptions of populations at special risk of developing mental and emotional problems. A second area concerns the "pathways" to treatment and involves such diverse matters as availability and visibility of therapeutic services, intake and diagnostic procedures, and manpower. Third, there is the vast area of research concerning different treatment modalities—that is, the actual treatment regimens afforded patients. A fourth area is research to evaluate the effectiveness of the specific treatment employed.

Through many and varied avenues of research, efforts are being made to understand the nature of mental health and illness, to determine the factors associated with a wide range of mental and emotional states from "general adjustment" to severe pathologies, and ultimately to shed light on the causes of mental disorders. The subject of a particular research investigation may be any one or several of the psychologic or mental states along the broad mental health–mental illness continuum; its approach may be biologic, environmental, or social; and it may include the general population or some special segment of the population.

Efforts continue to try to improve estimates of psychiatric illness, which, as suggested earlier, are beset with particularly thorny problems. Research on this subject involves measurement of the number of cases of mental illness present in the population at a given time (prevalence) and measurement of the number of new cases occurring within a specified period (incidence).

Investigations have been made—and still continue—of the relationship between social class and mental illness. Other demographic and epidemiologic studies are assembling information on the so-cioeconomic and cultural characteristics of communities; the extent to which mental disorders occur in the population, and the conditions that bring about their development; the factors that lead persons with specific mental disorders to seek psychiatric care; and the characteristics that distinguish those who seek psychiatric care from those who do not. Additional research on the relationship between mental health and social and cultural factors, including child-rearing patterns, is under way in other countries.

Investigations of abnormalities of the biologic system which may play a role in mental illness are designed to lead to a better understanding of the chemical substances affecting the central nervous system and of the structure, function, and mode of operation of the brain and its relationship to the body as expressed in psychosomatic illness. Also under study are the effects of stress on glandular systems: how they react to messages from the brain, and the part played by hormones known as the corticosteroids, which help mobilize the body's resources. Studies under way in genetics may answer some of the puzzling and conflicting findings on heredity and mental disease.

Great strides have been made in improving the treatment of the mentally ill, but research must still fill many significant gaps in knowledge. A critical need is sound knowledge on which to base the development of programs related to preventive measures or treatment methods that are faster and better adapted to mass application.

References

1. American Public Health Association. *Mental Disorders: A Guide to Control Methods.* The Association, New York, 1962.
2. Opler, Marvin K. *Culture and Mental Health: Cross Cultural Studies.* The Macmillan Company, New York, 1959.
3. Benedict, Ruth F. *Patterns of Culture.* Houghton Mifflin Company, Boston, 1934.
4. Murphy, Jane M., and Leighton, Alexander H. (eds.). *Approaches to Cross-Cultural Psychiatry.* Cornell University Press, Ithaca, 1965.
5. Mechanic, David. *Mental Health and Social Policy.* Prentice-Hall, Inc., Englewood Cliffs, New Jersey, 1969.
6. American Psychiatric Association. *Diagnostic and Statistical Manual of Mental Disorders.* 2nd ed. The Association, Washington, D.C., 1968.
7. Jackson, Don D. (ed.). *The Etiology of Schizophrenia.* Basic Books, New York, 1960.
8. Zax, Melvin, and Stricker, George. *The Study of Abnormal Behavior, Selected Readings.* The Macmillan Company, New York, 1964.

9. Hollingshead, A. B., and Redlich, Frederick C. *Social Class and Mental Illness.* John Wiley & Sons, New York, 1958.

10. Group for the Advancement of Psychiatry. *Urban America and the Planning of Mental Health Services,* Symposium No. 10. The Group, New York, 1964.

11. Plunkett, Richard J., and Gordon, John E. *Epidemiology and Mental Illness.* Basic Books, New York, 1960.

12. Leighton, Dorothea C., Harding, John S., Macklin, David B., Macmillan, Allister M., and Leighton, Alexander H. *The Character of Danger.* Basic Books, New York, 1963.

13. Srole, Leo, Langner, Thomas S., Michael, Stanley T., Opler, Marvin K., and Rennie, Thomas A. *Mental Health in the Metropolis: The Midtown Manhattan Study.* McGraw-Hill Book Company, New York, 1962.

14. U.S. Department of Health, Education, and Welfare, Public Health Service. *Reference Tables on Patients in Mental Health Facilities: Age, Sex, and Diagnosis; United States, 1968.* U.S. Government Printing Office, Washington, D.C., 1968.

15. Conley, Ronald W., Conwell, Margaret, and Willner, Shirley G. *The Cost of Mental Illness, 1968.* Statistical Note 30. National Institute of Mental Health, National Clearinghouse for Mental Health Information, Washington, D.C., October 1970.

16. Myers, Evelyn S. Insurance coverage for mental illness: present status and future prospects. *Am J Public Health,* **60:**1921–30, October 1970.

17. Berlin, I. Learning mental health consultation: history and problems. *Ment Hyg,* **48:**257–66, April 1964.

18. Caplan, Gerald. *Principles of Preventive Psychiatry.* Basic Books, New York, 1964.

19. U.S. Department of Health, Education, and Welfare, Public Health Service. *Inpatient Services* (PHS Publication No. 1624, 1967); *Outpatient Services* (PHS Publication No. 1578, 1968); *Partial Hospitalization* (PHS Publication No. 1449, 1968); *Emergency Services* (PHS Publication No. 1477, 1969); *Consultation and Education* (PHS Publication No. 1478, 1968); *The Scope of Community Mental Health Consultation and Education* (PHS Publication No. 2169, 1971). U.S. Government Printing Office, Washington, D.C.

20. Ozarin, Lucy D., and Feldman, Saul. Implications for health service delivery: the community mental health centers amendments of 1970. *Am J Public Health,* **61:**1780–84, September 1971.

21. Holden, Constance. Community mental health centers. *Science,* **174:**1110–13 and 1219–21, December 10 and 17, 1971.

22. Hume, Portia B. General principles of community psychiatry. In: Arieti, S. (ed). *American Handbook of Psychiatry,* Vol.III. Basic Books, New York, 1966.

23. World Health Organization. *Social Psychiatry and Community Attitudes:* 7th Report of the Expert Committee on Mental Health. World Health Organization Technical Report Series No. 177, Geneva, 1959.

24. Joint Commission on Mental Illness and Health. *Action for Mental Health.* Basic Books, New York, 1961.

25. Denber, Herman C. B. (ed.). *Research Conference on Therapeutic Community.* Charles C Thomas, Springfield, Ill., 1960.

26. Arnhoff, Franklyn N., Rubinstein, Eli A., and Speisman, Joseph C. *Manpower for Mental Health.* Aldine Publishing Company, Chicago, 1969.
27. Wilner, Daniel M. Research and evaluation in social psychiatry. In: Zubin, J., and Freyhan, F. (eds.). *Social Psychiatry.* Grune & Stratton, Inc., New York, 1968.

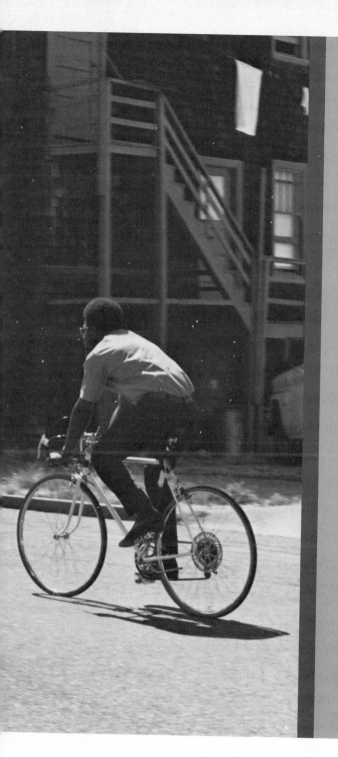

6

SELECTED COMMUNITY MENTAL HEALTH PROBLEMS

CHAPTER OUTLINE

Mental Retardation

Nature and Extent of Mental Retardation
Causes and Prevention of Mental Retardation
Provision of Services for the Mentally Retarded

Drug Abuse

Principal Substances Involved in Drug Abuse
Extent of Drug Addiction
Prevention and Control of Drug Abuse

Alcoholism

Suicide

Courtesy of California's Health, *California Department of Public Health.*
Staff photo.

Mental Retardation

Mental retardation is one of the most handicapping of all childhood and adult disorders. Until the 1940's the problems of the mentally retarded received very little public attention. With the exception of the provision of large, overcrowded residential institutions and special classes for the more educable, little else was done for many years. In the late 1940's and early 1950's, interest in the handicapped increased greatly, and parents of mentally retarded children began to demand that attention be given to their problems. Increasing research, programs, and facilities gradually appeared, and in 1962, the attack on all phases of the problem of mental retardation accelerated markedly.

NATURE AND EXTENT OF MENTAL RETARDATION

The mentally retarded person has, from childhood, unusual difficulty in learning and is hampered from applying whatever has been learned to the problems of ordinary living. Intelligence is sometimes so limited that it interferes seriously with functioning independence in society, either because the person cannot become economically independent or because behavior is not socially acceptable. There is need, therefore, for special training and guidance to make the most of existing capacities, whatever they may be. There is need also for warmth and affection—or at least humane consideration—equal to or even exceeding that preferred persons with other disabilities.

For descriptive purposes the range of mental retardation has been divided into four levels: mild, moderate, severe, and profound. Children who are classified as *mildly retarded,* although limited in scholastic potential, can usually be brought by special educational techniques to a state of self-sufficiency as adults. *Moderately retarded* children have a rate of mental development that is less than half that normally expected, but

TABLE 6-1. Estimates of Mental Retardation by Age and Level of Impairment, 1967

	IQ Range	All Ages	Under 21 Years	21 Years and Older
General population	—	198,100,000	82,000,000	116,100,000
Retardation levels:				
Mild (about 89%)	53–69	5,000,000+	2,000,000+	3,000,000+
Moderate (about 6%)	36–52	354,000	150,000	210,000
Severe (about 3.5%)	20–35	207,000	88,000	123,000
Profound (about 1.5%)	Less than 20	89,000	38,000	53,000

SOURCE: Adapted from National Association for Retarded Children. *Facts on Mental Retardation*, January 1969, p. 15.

nevertheless can learn to care for themselves and to perform tasks in the home or in a sheltered working situation. The *severely retarded* can learn self-care, but their potential economic usefulness is extremely limited, although many are classified as "trainable" for educational purposes. The *profoundly retarded* also respond to training in habit formation, but usually cannot become independent even in eating and dressing, have trouble speaking, and have little sense of personal safety.

It is estimated that there are approximately 6 million mentally retarded persons in the United States (about 3 per cent of the population) and that between 100,000 and 200,000 of the infants born each year are likely to be added to this group. Table 6-1 shows the estimated distribution (1967) of children and adults among the various levels of retardation. About 2.5 million of the retarded were under 21 years of age, according to 1967 estimates. Once a retarded child has lived to the age of five or six he has a good chance of growing up. In fact, the life expectancy at birth of the mildly retarded is probably about the same as that of other people; for the profound and severe levels of retardation life expectancy at birth is considerably less.

CAUSES AND PREVENTION OF MENTAL RETARDATION

Mental retardation can be caused by any condition that interferes with development before birth, during birth, or in early childhood. More than 100 causes have been identified, but these account for only about one fourth of all recognized cases of mental retardation. In the majority of cases, no clear diagnosis of cause can be made, and in most of these there is no evidence of nervous system pathology.

Among the specific identified causes of mental retardation are German measles (rubella) in the mother during the first three months of pregnancy; Rh-factor incompatibility between mother and child; abnormal genes and chromosomal defects, including mongolism; and various childhood diseases, accidents, and other conditions such as meningitis, encephalitis, measles, lead poisoning, glandular imbalance, and metabolism disorders. A broad array of unfavorable environmental and psychologic influences also undoubtedly play a role in causation of this touching syndrome; these include economic, social, and emotional deprivation and physical neglect.

The school setting is sometimes a significant factor in labeling retardation. One example occurs in children with language handicaps who are sometimes judged mildly retarded.[1] The label "retarded" follows the child subsequently in school career and into later life. The tragedy is that the original judgment frequently had nothing to do with intellectual capacity of the child, but resided rather in expectations of teachers and others who applied the label to begin with. This state of affairs has recently been documented in research in which the focus was on the "social system" aspects of mental retardation. The situation arises when judgments are made by teachers and counselors unfamiliar with the language and social behavior of the children, and occurs more often than it should in the case of minority group children.

Some advances have been made in the prevention of mental retardation, but so far only a small fraction of the total problem has been eliminated. Vaccination now protects children against German measles. Rh-factor incompatibility can be detected during pregnancy and corrected by a desensitizing serum for the mother or by a complete blood transfusion in the infant at birth. Corrective surgery can be applied to malformations of the skull or to remove excess fluid from the brain. Phenylketonuria, a metabolic disorder that causes mental retardation, can be detected and can be corrected through dietary restriction.

With the discovery of specific preventive measures, however limited, public health programs to prevent mental retardation have been expanded. These have included the development of diagnostic and case-finding methods for application on a broad scale, as in prenatal programs and programs for the detection of infant disorders such as phenylketonuria. Other mass-attack methods have been used in vaccination programs against measles and campaigns against lead poisoning.

PROVISION OF SERVICES FOR
THE MENTALLY RETARDED

The principal alternative to home care traditionally has been institutionalization of the mentally retarded.[2] In 1969 there were 180 public institutions for the retarded, compared with 96 in 1950. There were 207,716 patients under treatment in these institutions during 1969 at a cost of $765 million in maintenance expenditures. This figure, however, by no means reflects total costs to the nation (for services for care of the retarded, and productivity now lost through handicap), which are estimated at nearly $6 billion a year.

A trend toward new and diversified approaches to the provision of services for the mentally retarded began in 1962 when the President's Panel on Mental Retardation completed a one-year study and reported its assessment of the mental retardation problem, along with a proposal for a comprehensive program.[3]

Federal legislation in 1963 (amended in later years) provided grants to the states for planning coordinated action to combat mental retardation and for the construction of various kinds of facilities. Services offered under these financial provisions include diagnosis and evaluation; treatment; training; clinical nursery school programs; long- and short-term, day- and night-care residential programs; and consultation and education for community groups and professionals. One of the major objectives of the multiple-service approach is to help keep as many retarded children as possible out of the large residential institutions, and to expose them, where appropriate, to socially varied, nonmonotonous environments. In doing so, a child may be expected to reach a much higher level of development as a consequence of the more humane personal attention provided.

Drug Abuse

Drugs that affect the mind and produce changes in mood and behavior have become of considerable concern to mental health professionals as well as to medical and public health practitioners, educators, and government officials. Such drugs have great potential for excessive use, which can lead to both physical and psychologic dependence on them. The fact that the United States is a drug-oriented culture—with a staggering array of drugs and remedies readily available for the purported instant relief of almost anything bothering the individual—provides fertile ground for the development of drug abuse and dependence or addiction.

Numerous substances are involved in the drug problem, and drug abuse involves a wide variety of persons who represent almost every segment of society and adhere to various patterns of drug usage.[4] By and large, however, the drug abuse and dependence problem in the United States has become youth-centered. A large proportion of illegal users of drugs are young, while illegal drug use by older age groups is far less prevalent and thus has less salience as a social problem.

PRINCIPAL SUBSTANCES INVOLVED IN DRUG ABUSE

The drugs that can affect mental processes and behavior are classifiable into three general groups: depressants, stimulants, and hallucinogens. Distinction among the groups is not always sharp; for example, under certain circumstances stimulants and depressants can cause hallucinations; and depressants sometimes may appear to stimulate.

Depressants that are often misused include tranquilizers (e.g., Miltown, Equanil, and Librium), barbiturates ("sleeping pills"), and narcotics, among which heroin is the drug most used by narcotic addicts. Of all the depressants, however, alcohol is the most commonly used and abused. Volatile chemical inhalants (e.g., vapors from glue, solvents, gasoline) also are classified as depressants and show effects similar to alcoholic intoxication: an initial "high" occurs, but with further inhalation may come disorientation, bizarre behavior, and coma. With all depressants, the effects on the central nervous system depend on the concentration of the drug in the blood. Tolerance develops with repeated use, so that larger doses are required to achieve the characteristic effect.

Stimulant drugs misused include the amphetamines ("pep pills"), which in high dosage can cause aggressiveness and hallucinations and can lead to tolerance and psychologic dependence. Nicotine is another strong stimulant to the central nervous system and is the most significant component of tobacco. The dependence of many millions of people on tobacco is a form of drug abuse, and some investigators believe that genuine physical dependence on nicotine develops with prolonged use in large quantities. Unquestionably, the relationship of smoking to lung cancer and heart disease makes tobacco a dangerous substance.

Hallucinogens have been used for centuries to induce visions, but they gained new prominence recently with the development of interest in substances that produce altered states of consciousness. The two principal drugs in use in this category are marijuana and LSD. Marijuana is usually smoked in cigarettes ("joints"), and although there is tremendous variability of response, it may produce a state of consciousness in which ideas flow freely, and time and space perceptions are altered. The long-range effects of marijuana and whether or not its use leads to dependence are subjects of considerable controversy at present. LSD (lysergic acid diethyla-mide) alters sensory perceptions, and its effects are often unpredic-table and uncontrollable, with severe adverse reactions. It can induce mood changes that may be transient, last for long periods, or recur over several months.

Several of the drugs in the various categories have clearly beneficial effects when used under medical supervision to alleviate physical and psychologic problems. For example, amphetamines are used to treat hay fever, certain types of mental depression, and obesity. LSD has been used experimentally in the treatment of psychotic disorders and for the control of severe pain in terminal cancer patients. Morphine and codeine, both narcotics, have long been used for the relief of pain. Recent reports to an international pharmacology conference describe experimental success in the use of marijuana to relieve eyeball pressure in the treatment of glaucoma.

EXTENT OF DRUG ADDICTION

The number of drug addicts of all kinds in the United States is not known. The users of hallucinogens, stimulants, and depressants (except narcotics) are seldom identified unless they are involved in a criminal action and are arrested. Aside from arrest records, only rough estimates of users can be obtained through sample surveys (polls) of particular segments of the population. On this basis there are indications, for example, that in 1972 there were 15 to 20 million adult *marijuana users* (18 years and older) in the United States. This figure is up almost threefold from surveys taken three years earlier. The key word in these statistics is the term *user*, which generally means anyone who has ever "tried" marijuana. In this sense, approximately half the college population have also recently been reported "trying" marijuana. Surveys also reveal that perhaps 5 per cent of marijuana smokers are heavy users, that is, report using marijuana almost every day in a recent period.

Narcotic addicts are reported to the Bureau of Narcotics and Dangerous Drugs (U.S. Department of Justice) by law enforcement authorities and private agencies such as hospitals. In 1962, there were reported 47,000 narcotics users.[5] At the close of 1969 there were about 68,000 persons reported as being physically addicted to narcotics use. Almost half of these addicts were between 21 and 30 years of age, and most were from four states: New York, California, Illinois, and New Jersey. Figures on use of hard narcotics are par-ticularly hard to come by and the preceding figures are almost cer-tainly an underestimation. For example, estimates of true heroin use in the New York metropolitan area range from 150,000 to 250,000; and well over 1,000 opiate-related deaths were recorded recently in a single year. Furthermore, the New York City Narcotics Register shows a sharp rise (in the period 1964–1969) in the proportion of narcotics deaths among young people under 25 years of age. There are particularly tragic cases of heroin deaths among children under 14 years.

Why drug use has spread differentially to younger rather than to older people is not fully understood. One psychiatrist has suggested that the reasons young people give for using drugs seem like attempts to deal with the entire range of adolescent problems—self-discovery, separation from parents, economic stability, sex-role identity, and so on.

Although today's drug problems no doubt have roots in the past, they are also clearly manifestations of social forces unique to the present epoch. To a greater extent than ever before, youth has developed its own, separate segment of society, with peer group influence an extraordinarily important factor. Youth's new values and cultural forms that challenge tradition are to some extent compatible with drug-taking. The new values include concepts such as individualism, self-understanding, immediate pleasure, and sexual freedom. Many of the newer values are found in the counterculture population, and drug use is a significant aspect of that life-style. Indications are that marijuana use among college students is related to many of the new value orientations, and that drug users on college campuses are more likely than other students to be counterculture sympathizers. Among high school students, on the other hand, marijuana appears to be used more for recreational or social purposes than as a symbol of new values.

The culture of the youthful narcotic (heroin) addict is of considerably older origin (starting about the turn of the century) than that of the contemporary counterculture and student drug user, and there are other differences as well. Most young heroin users do not espouse an ideology; the majority are without steady employment or stable family life; and a sizable number are in trouble with the law before they become addicted, while the rest become violators (theft, burglary, prostitution) in order to support their habit. Young heroin addicts are likely to begin drug use as members of juvenile groups or gangs, with language, customs, and codes of their own.

PREVENTION AND CONTROL OF DRUG ABUSE

About 100 years ago, addiction became recognized as a health problem. Since then, federal, state, and local governments have imposed a variety of laws intended to prevent abuse of drugs. The laws include provisions for labeling patent remedies as to alcoholic and other habit-forming content; for establishing the basic distinction between prescription and over-the-counter drugs; for controlling the import and export of narcotic drugs; for regulating the production and distribution of drugs within the United States; and for establishing penalties for illegal possession or sale of dangerous drugs.

Problems of controlling the use of dangerous drugs and preventing addiction are medically and socially complex, and have become highly charged emotional issues. Satisfactory solutions are still being sought. At least some of the difficulty in arriving at enlightened public policy on which to base realistic prevention and control measures arises from a deficit in knowledge concerning the long-range physical and psychic effects of varying dosages of dangerous drugs. Extensive research is required to answer questions such as whether or not—and how much of—a specific drug causes brain damage, birth defects, a particular disease, a change in behavior or personality. In the case of marijuana, which has been the center of particularly heated debate because of its widespread use, research so far has not found—unambiguously—either deleterious physical effects or physical or psychologic dependence resulting from moderate usage of the drug. This does not, of course, rule out the possibility that further research may uncover some seriously harmful physical effects. As to psychologic consequences of marijuana use, answers are presently being sought to complex questions such as whether or not it causes long-lasting changes in personality, behavior, or attitude.

There is growing recognition that legal constraints alone will not prevent drug abuse. Some health professionals feel that wiping out social injustice in addition to understanding and alleviating the frustrations of youth is the only sure method of prevention. Others advocate less sweeping measures such as deglamorizing drugs and attempting to provide meaningful alternative activities to drug use.

At present, educational and informational programs are the principal drug-abuse *preventive* measures that are in wide-scale use, and these occur under both public and private sponsorship at a variety of geopolitical levels. The National Institute of Mental Health is the major source of such programs at the federal level. It has launched a broad public service information campaign aimed at the potential drug user in all segments of society. The institute also maintains the National Clearinghouse for Drug Abuse Information, which collects and disseminates materials and data from federal, state, and local public and private programs and projects.

The most significant growth in drug-related programs so far has occurred in connection with the *treatment* of the drug addict. Most of the efforts fall into four general categories. First, there are community and state hospitals, where inpatient facilities are available to help an addict withdraw. The second category consists of "therapeutic communities," where an addict voluntarily lives with others like himself in an attempt to stay off drugs and eventually return to society.[6] Talk or "rap" centers are a third category, where counseling and referral services are provided for young people with drug problems. Finally, there are methadone programs specifically for heroin users, in which the methadone, although itself addictive, does not produce the "high" of heroin and thus permits the individual to carry on a more normal life while attempting to break the habit. Opinions vary as to whether or not these programs are succeeding, and evaluation of their effectiveness is of major concern.

The crisis nature of the drug abuse problem has led to developments in the narcotics field sometimes outside usual professional channels. One action was the passage of the Narcotic Addiction Rehabilitation Act in 1966. This act, involving the Department of Justice as well as other governmental agencies, sought among several objectives to provide aftercare opportunities in local communities for narcotics users under conditions of civil commitment. Another important action was the establishment in 1971 of a Special Action Office on Drug Abuse—in the White House—for high-level programming in the drug abuse field. One of the first issues attended to by this office was the menacing problem of drug addiction, mainly heroin, among American servicemen in Vietnam and returning veterans. One outcome of these recent events is intensification of efforts to seek cures for addiction to hard drugs, with continued search for both social-psychologic and pharmacologic (e.g., methadone) treatment modes.

One important unresolved issue has to do with the criminal aspects of drug abuse. Is a user of illicit drugs a criminal? Public morals confirm the proposition that drug sellers (pushers) are criminals and should be so treated by police and legal authority. Public outlook regarding users may be undergoing alteration. The first change may well come regarding marijuana. In this connection there is now pressure in several quarters—a President's Commission, some state legislatures, many health authorities—for the decriminalization of marijuana use.

Alcoholism

In the United States, ethyl alcohol is the most commonly abused depressant and the social drug that is in widest use. If consumed in large quantities, alcohol can result in acute intoxication, in which the depression of various elements of the central nervous system seriously interferes with the individual's motor and mental functioning.

For the average, healthy individual, a moderate amount of alcohol can be used without lasting effects on the body, but continuous drinking of large quantities can cause structural damage. Cirrhosis of the liver, ulcers, heart disease, and diabetes are correlated with heavy, continuous consumption of alcohol. Serious nervous or mental disorders or permanent brain damage may also occur with excessive use. Alcohol, like many other drugs that affect the central nervous system, can be addictive, producing withdrawal symptoms (delirium tremens is an extreme manifestation) when alcohol intake ceases.

It is estimated that about two thirds of American adults drink, and of these, 9 million are problem drinkers. Fully half of the alcoholic individuals in the nation are employed; contrary to popular belief, skid-row derelicts comprise only about 5 per cent of the total number. There is some evidence that between the mid-1940's and the mid-1960's the percentage of increase of drinkers among females was greater than among males, that there was an increase in the percentage of drinkers in all age groups, and that the percentage declined with increasing age. A study conducted in 1971 among junior high and high school students in a county in California showed that the students were drinking alcohol even more than they were using marijuana and other drugs.

It has been estimated that alcoholism drains the economy of $15 billion annually—$10 billion in time lost from work; $2 billion for health and welfare services; and $3 billion in property damage, medical expenses, and other costs. Public intoxication alone accounts for one third of all arrests, and alcohol plays a major role in half the highway fatalities, costing 28,000 lives in a recent year. Among young people, 6 of 10 highway deaths involve alcohol.

People drink for a variety of social, cultural, and religious reasons. Although the immediate physiologic and psychologic effects of alcohol are experienced by the person drinking, the pressures to drink have group origins.[7,8] For most people, the use of alcohol is an adjunct to other activities such as visiting, partying, or celebrating with friends; family and religious festivities; or meals. Some individuals, however, use alcohol for its own sake, for the anesthetizing effect it has on mind and body. This characterizes the use of alcohol as a drug and often leads to drinking problems.

There is no exact dividing line between the alcoholic and the nonalcoholic person, but when an individual loses control over his drinking, he is considered to have a drinking problem. The diagnosis of alcoholism remains particularly complex because of the mixed physical and behavioral nature of the symptoms. In 1972, the National Council on Alcoholism drew up a set of guidelines for the purpose of standardizing diagnoses and also to prevent overdiagnosis. The guidelines contained both major and minor criteria for diagnosing alcoholism. The major criteria included presence of withdrawal symptoms; level of tolerance (e.g., high blood levels of alcohol without gross evidence of intoxication); continued drinking in the face of strong penalties (e.g., medical warnings, loss of job, arrest for drunkenness); and major illness usually associated with alcohol. The minor criteria included physical disorders such as irregular heartbeat and behavior patterns such as gulping drinks, drinking on the sly, and drinking to relieve anger, insomnia, or depression. The presence of one or more major criteria would warrant a diagnosis of alcoholism, as would significant combinations of the minor criteria.

Many different factors have been suggested as the cause of alcoholism, but none has as yet been accepted as the single causative agent. Rather, it is generally agreed that alcoholism is likely to arise from a complex interaction of biologic, psychologic, and sociologic factors. Investigations, therefore, are under way to try to determine the role, if any, of a wide range of possible causes, including genetic and chemical abnormalities in the body, poor nutrition, emotional problems, childhood deprivations, and environmental conditions. Professionals who work with alcoholic individuals have reported finding an unusual amount of stress and much deprivation in the lives of these persons.

In spite of mounting evidence as to the seriousness of alcoholism, public attitudes toward the person with an alcohol problem are often indifferent and ambivalent. Jokes about drunkenness and the intoxicated person are commonplace, suggesting denial of a problem or lack of concern for it. The drunken skid-row derelict, on the other hand, is rejected and blamed for his own deplorable state. The image of the "sophisticate" is one who can "hold his liquor," and failure to do so is likely to be viewed with disdain or ridicule. These and other attitudes rooted in culture and tradition hamper efforts to educate the general public about problem drinking and alcoholism.

Services for alcoholics can be found in nearly every community,[9] and include those supplied by physicians for the treatment of acute alcoholics; clergymen who provide counseling; lawyers, courts, and jails that handle alcoholic offenders; Alcoholics Anonymous groups; health and welfare agencies; and private business and industries that provide aid for alcoholic employees.

State and local governmental agencies tend to support treatment services, especially the establishment of clinic facilities. The clinics may provide inpatient care, outpatient treatment, or both, and may be located in general hospitals, in state psychiatric institutions, and sometimes in health departments. Community mental health centers, in particular, provide the structure and resources needed for treatment and prevention services for problem drinkers.

The federal government, late in 1970, established the National Institute on Alcohol Abuse and Alcoholism within the National Institute of Mental Health. The new institute is concerned with research in the biologic, behavioral, and sociocultural aspects of alcoholism; with demonstration projects in prevention, treatment, and rehabilitation; and with training professionals and nonprofessionals to become specialists in the field of alcoholism.

Suicide

Suicide has been among the 12 leading causes of death for at least the past decade. In 1968 there were 21,372 reported deaths from suicide, and in 1969 the number was estimated to be 22,060. Suicide data are based on cause-of-death certification and are suspected of grossly understating the magnitude of the problem. Underreporting undoubtedly results from a general reluctance to admit suicidal intent of relatives and friends and from difficulties in recognizing suicide under certain circumstances. Some estimates place the number of actual suicides at twice the reported figure. Furthermore, there are many attempted or unsuccessful suicides. At least one study has estimated the ratio of unsuccessful suicide attempts to committed suicides at about 8 to 1.[10]

Firearms are used for committing suicide more frequently than any other means, particularly among males, as shown in Table 6-2. The table also indicates the far larger number of males than females who commit suicide—almost 3 to 1. In a detailed study of reported suicides, the National Center for Health Statistics found that suicides

TABLE 6-2. Means of Suicide, 1968, by Sex

	Total		Male		Female	
	Number	Per Cent	Number	Per Cent	Number	Per Cent
Firearms and explosives	10,911	51	9,078	60	1,833	30
Poisoning	5,684	27	2,960	19	2,724	46
Hanging and strangulation	3,099	14	2,265	14	834	14
Other	1,678	8	1,076	7	602	10
TOTAL	21,372	100	15,379	100	5,993	100

SOURCE: Adapted from U.S. Bureau of the Census. *Statistical Abstract of the United States, 1971*, p. 142.

also are more frequent in the white population than in the nonwhite. Suicide rates for white males tend to increase with successive age groups through 85 years and over; for white females they reach a peak in the 45–54 or 55–64 age group.[11] Population subgroups that are considered at particularly high risk of suicide include teen-agers, college students, the aged, American Indians, alcoholics, and the mentally ill.

In recent years the prevention of suicide has become an important concern of health and mental health professionals. Early in the twentieth century in the United States there was very little interest in this area partly because the subject was taboo and partly because suicide was not considered preventable. Gradually, however, it became recognized that a suicidal act frequently is more in the nature of a "cry for help" than a clear desire to die. Furthermore, it became apparent that most individuals experience acute suicidal impulses for only a relatively short period. They also usually communicate their potentially suicidal tendencies in some way. These insights into the nature of suicide gave new hope for prevention and led to programs emphasizing early identification and provision of immediate treatment of the suicidal. Although suicide is still considered taboo in the Western world, education and mental health advances continue to encourage its study. Recognizing that punitive measures are not the solution, state laws outlawing suicide and punishing attempts have largely been revoked, and the remainder are rarely enforced.

Nationwide, more than 150 suicide prevention programs have been started, most of them in the decade of the 1960's. The aims of current programs are to prevent the desire to attempt suicide, to prevent the first suicide attempt, to prevent the repetition of suicidal acts, and to prevent fatal outcome of suicidal acts. Most often, suicide prevention services have been established as separate autonomous units or as crisis clinics which include suicide emergencies. A sizable number of services also are located in hospitals or in some type of community agency.

The Los Angeles Suicide Prevention Center, established in 1958, is a notable example of a full-scale specialized service program. It has a staff of psychiatrists, psychologists, and social workers, plus a number of carefully selected and trained lay volunteers. The center serves primarily as a resource where immediate attention for the emergency crisis period is provided by means of diagnostic and referral services. It maintains close liaison with other resources within the community to whom patients can be sent for appropriate long-term therapeutic, rehabilitative, or environmental care. The center also emphasizes training and educational activities, directed toward various levels of professionals and toward the general community.

The establishment of suicide prevention programs across the country has been aided in recent years by the Center for Studies of Suicide Prevention of the National Institute of Mental Health. This center provides consultation to states and local communities for the development of suicide prevention services. Other aspects of the center's program include improvement of concepts and statistics on suicide; support of training and educational programs for professionals, volunteers, and the public; and support of research on suicidal behavior and means of prevention, intervention, and follow-up.

References

1. Mercer, Jane R. Sociological perspectives on mild mental retardation. In: Hayward, Carl H. (ed.). *Social-Cultural Aspects of Mental Retardation*. Appleton-Century-Crofts, New York, 1970.
2. Poser, Charles. *Mental Retardation: Diagnosis and Treatment*. Harper & Row, New York, 1969.
3. U.S. Department of Health, Education, and Welfare. *The President's Panel on Mental Retardation: A Proposed Program for National Action to Combat Mental Retardation; A Report to the President*. U.S. Government Printing Office, Washington, D.C., 1962.
4. Charalampous, K. D. Drug culture in the seventies. *Am J Public Health*, **61:**1225–28, June 1971.
5. Winick, Charles. The epidemiology of narcotics use. In: Wilner, D. M., and Kassebaum, G. G. (eds.). *Narcotics*. The Blakiston Division, McGraw-Hill Book Company, New York, 1965.
6. Yablonsky, Lewis, and Dederich, Charles E. Synanon: an analysis of some dimensions of the social structure of an anti-addiction society. In: Wilner, D. M., and Kassebaum, G. G. (eds.). *Narcotics*. The Blakiston Division, McGraw-Hill Book Company, New York, 1965.
7. Cross, Jay N. *Guide to the Community Control of Alcoholism*. The American Public Health Association, New York, 1968.
8. Wilkinson, Rupert. *The Prevention of Drinking Problems, Alcohol Control and Cultural Influences*. Oxford University Press, New York, 1970.
9. Cahn, Sidney. *The Treatment of Alcoholics, An Evaluative Study*. Oxford University Press, New York, 1970.
10. Farberow, Norman L., and Shneidman, Edwin S. (eds.). *The Cry for Help*. McGraw-Hill Book Company, New York, 1961.
11. U.S. Department of Health, Education, and Welfare, Public Health Service. *Suicide in the United States, 1950–1964*. Public Health Service Publication No. 1000, Series 20, No. 5. U.S. Government Printing Office, Washington, D.C., 1967.

Additional Reading

Beck, Helen Louise. *Social Services to the Mentally Retarded.* Charles C Thomas, Springfield, Ill., 1969.

Blum, Eva Maria, and Blum, Richard H. *Alcoholism, Modern Psychological Approaches to Treatment.* Jossey-Bass, Inc., San Francisco, Calif., 1967.

Blum, Richard H., and associates. *Society and Drugs,* Vol. I. *Students and Drugs,* Vol. II. Jossey-Bass, San Francisco, Calif., 1969.

Cohen, Sidney. *The Drug Dilemma.* McGraw-Hill Book Company, New York, 1969.

Cooperative Commission on the Study of Alcoholism. *Alcohol Problems.* A Report to the Nation, prepared by Thomas F. A. Plaut. Oxford University Press, New York, 1967.

Durkheim, Emile. *Suicide, A Study in Sociology.* Translated by George Simpson and John A. Spaulding. Free Press, New York, 1951.

Resnick, H.L.P. (ed.). *Suicidal Behaviors; Diagnosis and Management.* Little, Brown & Company, Boston, 1968.

Rothstein, Jerome H. *Mental Retardation: Readings and Resources,* 2nd ed. Holt, Rinehart, & Winston, New York, 1971.

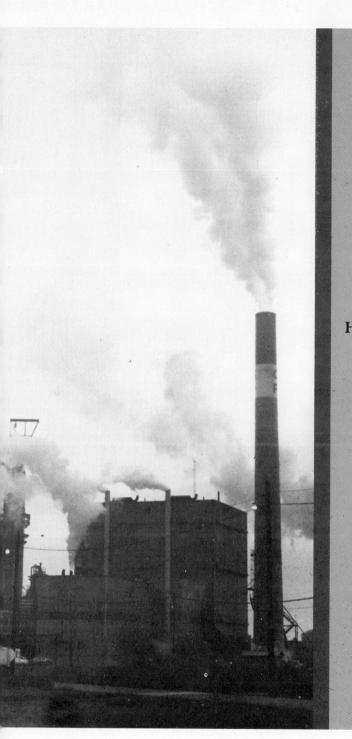

7

HEALTH ASPECTS
OF THE
ENVIRONMENT

CHAPTER OUTLINE

Ecology and the Environmental Crisis

The Science of Ecology
Man's Assault on the Environment
Urbanization and the Environment
The Environment and Health

Air Quality

Water Quality

Sources and Consequences of Water Pollution
Treatment of Public Water Supplies
Water Protection in the Treatment of Sewage

Solid Waste Disposal

Pesticides

Noise

Radiation

Food Sanitation

Rodent and Insect Control

Rodent Control
Mosquito Control
Fly Control

Accidents

Housing and the Residential Environment

Occupational Health and Safety

Categories of Health Hazards
Control of the Working Environment
Control of Hazards to the Worker
Prevention of Occupational Diseases
*The Role of Official Health Agencies in Occupational
Health*

Ecology and the Environmental Crisis

In recent years, the quality of the environment has become an intense and widespread concern among the general public, scientists, and health professionals. Pollution of the environment has become so extensive as to constitute an environmental crisis, and has led to the inception—however haltingly—of an environmental movement to attempt to block the spreading deterioration. Environmental pollution must be considered a real and serious threat not only to health but also to the general quality and fabric of life on this planet.

Environmental problems are as old as history itself, which offers many instances of famines, mass poisonings, and varieties of pollution generated by early industrialization. What particularly sets the present environmental crisis apart is its broad scale, affecting practically all forms of life over a major portion of the earth. Although environmentalists have for years been concerned about the degradation of the environment, it has only been within the past decade that the problem has gained salient public attention. Rachel Carson's *Silent Spring*[1] published in 1962 was a landmark effort to jolt the prevailing apathy with a detailed account of hazards that were developing from the accumulation of pesticides in the food chain. Numerous other insightful and revealing analyses have followed.[2-4]

THE SCIENCE OF ECOLOGY

In an effort to understand environmental pollution and what the environmental crisis really means, attention must be turned to *ecology*, the area of biologic science that is devoted to the study of living organisms in relation to their environment. Ecology is a very old subject, but it did not become a full-fledged science until the end of the nineteenth century. The latter half of the twentieth century has seen a marked upsurge of interest in its concepts and principles.[4-7]

The science of ecology is concerned with

the entire complex of interrelationships between the living and non-living domains. The term *biosphere* refers to the world of living things. It is made up of many *ecosystems*, each of which is the sum total of all the living and nonliving parts that support a chain of life within a selected area.

In an ecosystem, nature provides very specific conditions that are needed to support a variety of plant and animal life, and nature's processes renew these elements so that each form of life is sustained in a healthy state. Thus, a "circle of life" is created which has four principal components. First, there are sunlight, water, oxygen, carbon dioxide, organic compounds, and other nutrients which plants use for their growth. Second, there are plants — on land and in water — which through photosynthesis convert carbon dioxide and water into carbohydrates that are needed both by the plants themselves and by other organisms in the ecosystem. Plants, therefore, are the "producers." Third, there are the "consumers" that feed on the "producers." Herbivores (e.g., cows and sheep) are primary consumers because they feed directly on the plants. Carnivores (e.g., man and other meat-eating animals) are secondary consumers because they feed on the herbivores. Fourth, there are decomposer organisms — bacteria, fungi, and insects — which break down the dead producers and consumers (or their waste material) and return their chemical compounds to the ecosystem for reuse by the plants.

An ecosystem, therefore, constitutes a circle of life in which an animal's waste becomes food for soil bacteria, the bacteria excrete substances that nourish plants, and the animal consumes the plants. Most ecosystems, however, do not consist merely of circular paths. Rather, the circles are crisscrossed with branches to form a complex network or fabric of interconnections. This complexity helps to protect an ecosystem so that in case of abrupt changes alternative relationships can develop in the system. Simplification of an ecosystem — i.e., removal of some of its constituents — seriously weakens it.

As a science, ecology has not yet formulated a complete set of cohesive generalizations. Nevertheless, Commoner[4] has organized an informal series of "laws of ecology" based on the generalizations that are evident at present. The first law ("everything is connected to everything else") states that in the real world all things in the environment are interconnected with all other things. The second law ("everything must go somewhere") holds that there is no such thing as "waste"; what is excreted by one organism as waste is taken up by another as food. The third law ("nature knows best") stipulates that any man-made change in a natural system is likely to be detrimental to that system. The fourth law ("there is no such thing as a free lunch") recognizes that anything extracted from the global ecosystem by human effort must be replaced if the integrity of the system is to be preserved.

Much of what is now known about ecology has been learned from small segments of the complex network of life on earth. In order to learn more about the functioning of entire ecosystems and how they react to man-made stress, the United States is participating in an International Biological Program, a broad multidisciplinary research effort involving over 600 scientists in many countries.[8] In several major habitat types (biomes)—grasslands, forests, deserts, and arctic tundra—the total life web of each environment is being studied closely and the intricate processes are being measured quantitatively.

MAN'S ASSAULT ON THE ENVIRONMENT

The present environmental crisis has arisen because man has in various ways disrupted the circle of life which characterizes ecosystems. In the process, natural endless cycles have been converted into man-made *linear* events.[4] For example, oil is taken from the ground and is converted into fuel, the fuel is burned in an engine in a process that creates noxious chemicals, and the chemicals are released into the air. The end product—given sufficient quantity of emissions and certain atmospheric conditions—is a serious *air pollutant: smog.*

An illustration of the disruptive effect of man-made *waste-disposal* methods on natural processes in surface water is found in the shallows off the coast of southern California. There, sea urchins (small aquatic animals) normally consume kelp (seaweed) as food. Kelp is also the source of man-made products such as iodine. In the past, when the sea urchins overconsumed the kelp, the animals' population declined, thus permitting the kelp beds to replenish. Now, however, the sea urchins are nourished by organic material that is contained in *sewage* being washed out to sea, and they continue also to consume the kelp. The sea urchin population is growing at an unprecedented rate and the kelp beds are fast becoming depleted. In some areas the kelp has disappeared completely.

There are increasing instances in which man-made *toxic agents* are introduced into the environment, make their way into other elements of the life cycle, and eventually return to poison man, himself. Mercury contamination is a case in point. Mercury is used in many ways, including the manufacture of products ranging from paint to pharmaceuticals. In the process, mercury is discharged into the environment where it can be introduced and readily transported in many forms through the air, water, and soil. The human body can absorb the mercury—with deleterious effects—from the air, drinking water, food, and skin contact. Even if all mercury discharges into the environment were stopped immediately, the residual already present from past activities would pose a problem for years to come.

The question of how the present environmental crisis has come about has been the subject of considerable debate, and numerous explanations have been offered of a social, economic, and political nature. There is growing agreement that, of all factors possibly accounting for the increasing array of environmental problems, the most important are *technologic* developments, particularly those occurring since World War II. This view holds that advanced industrial and agricultural technologies, aided by contemporary science, have produced substances that cannot be handled by the cycles of nature because they are alien to ecosystems. Environmental pollution and contamination are the results of these breakdowns in natural systems.

There is hope that technologic and scientific innovation can be applied to helping restore the vital balance of environmental forces and processes. But this can be accomplished only if there is reorientation of national goals regarding technologic development and economic growth. Reform in the production of goods is needed so that useful items can be produced without polluting the environment. This requires a reordering of priorities and a restructuring of industrial growth, a process that will inevitably generate complex social and political problems.

URBANIZATION AND THE ENVIRONMENT

Rural areas are the site of serious environmental problems resulting from agricultural, mining, lumbering, and other exploitative practices. But the epitome of the environmental crisis in concentrated form is found in contemporary large urban areas. Here, pollution and population density interact to create conditions that range from unesthetic to hazardous.

The *inner city* is a product of urbanization that deserves particular attention because severe environmental problems interact with social and economic conditions. The inner city generally includes the decaying, older sections which encircle or are part of the central core of an urban area. Air pollution is likely to be heaviest over the inner city, and problems of noise, sanitation, and congestion are usually worse than in other sections. On the other hand, open space and parks are lacking to a greater degree than elsewhere in the urban complex. Intertwined to form an environmental-social-economic complex of problems are poverty, racial discrimination, inadequate housing, inferior education, lack of recreation, poor health, and other factors.

While the central core of the city suffers from environmental stagnation, the fringe areas suffer from "suburban sprawl." Here, environmental problems are of a different sort, including continuous threats to open space, already in short supply; improper or insufficient sanitation measures; and housing that often appears to be at the one extreme planless, or at the other regimented.

THE ENVIRONMENT AND HEALTH

Long before the emergence of the kinds of environmental pollution and contamination problems that presently cause concern, man recognized certain relationships between his environment and outbreaks of disease. Discoveries in the seventeenth century that microorganisms could cause contagious disease led to the development of environmental activities to curb cholera, typhoid, malaria, typhus, and other epidemic diseases. Such activities became the sanitation aspects of environmental control and are reflected today in programs to ensure, for example, that drinking water is safe, milk is pasteurized, food is hygienically prepared and handled, and waste is disposed of in ways to prevent breeding of insects and rodents.

These environmental sanitation activities are now traditional, but nevertheless require constant vigilance because disease outbreaks occur from time to time even though the sources are presumably well under control. For example, the public water supplies in Riverside, California (1965) and in Delhi, India (1955–1956) were responsible for large-scale outbreaks of salmonellosis (usually a foodborne disease) and of infectious hepatitis, respectively. Both water supplies apparently met acceptable biologic standards at the time, but the water treatment systems did not provide for removal of the harmful microorganisms responsible for the disease outbreak.

Of the pollutants and contaminants that are most salient in today's environmental crisis, some are already known to be health hazards and many others are highly suspect. Most disquieting of all is the suspicion that environmental pollution may harbor an unknown number of hazards to health, of which man is not even aware at this time.

In the category of definitely known environmental health hazards there is lead-based interior house paint, which was used in houses and apartments before World War II. In older structures that are in dilapidated condition, the lead paint peels and chips from wood and plaster surfaces. Small children chew on or eat the paint flakes, ingest the lead, and become high risks for lead poisoning. Although most of the lead ingested is eliminated by the body, ingestion of a few small flakes per week over a period of several months can make a child seriously ill.

Numerous chemicals and commercial products that are commonly used today are now coming under close scrutiny as possible hazards to health. Mercury has already been mentioned as causing alarm because of its accumulation in air and water. It is a health threat because in the human body it tends to concentrate in the brain or other nervous tissue and can cause blindness, retardation, and ultimately death. Another suspect substance is polyvinyl plastic, with numerous uses including automobile upholstery, packaged food wrapping, and containers for storage of blood and other medicinal fluids. Plasticizers used in the manufacturing process to make the plastic flexible have been found to enter the stored blood and subsequently to appear in the blood, urine, and tissues of patients receiving transfusions. Plasticizer contamination of food (from wrappings) and of air in automobiles (from upholstery) is also suspected.

In addition to being responsible for various acute episodes of illness, environmental pollution increasingly is thought to be at the root of certain chronic conditions, either causing them directly or precipitating flare-ups. Regarded as among the most important of these conditions are certain forms of cancer, several lung diseases, arthritis, and "early aging." Chronic and degenerative diseases such as these have, in fact, become known as the "diseases of civilization," and they appear to occur most frequently where industrial technology is advanced and environmental contamination is severe.

In the past, man's adaptive mechanisms have enabled him to survive countless threats to his existence, including the dangers of disease. Thus, it might be hoped that, by adapting further, mankind will ultimately survive modern environmental stresses and the diseases they generate. However, industrial technology has introduced a range of substances and situations that have no precedent in the biologic past of human beings. Furthermore, the evolution of adaptive mechanisms is too slow to keep pace with the rapid technologic and social change in the modern world. Thus, it does not seem probable that man will *ever* be able to adapt to the toxic effects of chemical and other pollutants,[9] and hope for survival rests on efforts to control environmental pollution and contamination.

Air Quality

. . . December 1930, Meuse River Valley, Belgium. This heavily industrialized area covering about 15 miles was blanketed by thick, cold fog. Air pollutants gathered day after day and stagnated. About 6,000 people became ill; 60 died, mostly the elderly and those already ill from heart and lung diseases.

. . . October 1948, Donora, Pennsylvania. In this industrial town of 14,000 population, the pollutant-filled air caused 20 deaths (instead of two that were normal for the period), and almost 6,000 people became ill.

. . . December 1952, London, England. During a five-day period about 4,000 people died in the world's worst air pollution disaster. The lethal component of the smog was sulfur dioxide, which is produced by burning sulfur-containing coal and fuel oil.

The air that envelops the earth is the life-supporting medium in which man lives, just as water is the medium supporting fish. Air is also required in the combustion of fuel to generate heat and power, and is used in manufacturing processes and service activities such as oxidation processes, air cooling, and spray painting. The air supply is always "polluted" to some extent, because used air is constantly generated in the course of natural and artificial ventilation. The *natural* cleansing and rejuvenating process to which used air is subjected is normally sufficient unless the system becomes overloaded. Then, pollution as it is known today results.

There are five main classes of primary pollutants: (1) sulfur oxides, produced mostly by the combustion of coal, fuel oil, and natural gas; (2) particulate matter, such as dust, ash, and soot; (3) carbon monoxide, which can make up as much as 11 per cent of motor vehicle exhaust; (4) hydrocarbons, which are a vast family of compounds containing carbon and hydrogen in various combinations; and (5) nitrogen oxides, which are emitted in motor vehicle exhaust and by power plants. Numerous other noxious gases and harmful particulates also are introduced into the atmosphere from a variety of sources.

The greatest public interest and concern are expressed about concentrations of atmospheric pollutants which have caused deaths and have produced the well-known Los Angeles "smog" and somewhat comparable air pollution situations in various parts of the world. Heavy, widespread concentrations of air pollution are usually associated with meteorologic conditions that do not permit normal dispersion and dissipation of pollutants from an area. The most common condition is known as *temperature inversion*. This refers to the fact that the air temperature normally decreases about 5°F for each 1,000-foot rise in elevation. On some days, for various reasons, a cooler layer of air remains near the earth's surface while the sun warms the air at higher levels. Thus, an inversion occurs when a layer of cool surface air is trapped by a layer of warmer air above it so that the bottom layer cannot rise. Pollutants accumulate in the surface air and cannot escape until the sun warms the lower air mass and breaks the inversion condition. The inversion is accompanied by calm air with very little horizontal or vertical motion. When up-and-down mixing of air currents occurs, it helps to dilute pollutants.

The other factor in some smog formations is a *photochemical process* which promotes chemical reactions that transform nonirritating substances to irritating or tear-producing chemicals and change transparent gases to cloudy materials. In Los Angeles studies, it has been shown that unsaturated hydrocarbons from unburned gasoline or automotive exhaust combine with nitrogen dioxide, ozone, or other oxidants to produce complex chemicals which induce irritation. Control involves attempts to eliminate discharge of unsaturated hydrocarbons by blocking their escape from the engine's crankcase and by developing devices or methods to more completely oxidize or burn the fuel.

In the United States, over 200 million tons of man-made waste products are released into the air each year. Estimates made in 1969 attributed 51 per cent of these pollutants to transportation sources, 16 per cent to fuel combustion in stationary sources, 15 per cent to industrial processes, 4 per cent to solid waste disposal practices, and 14 per cent to forest fires and other miscellaneous sources.

Of the transportation sources, the automobile is the greatest single contributor to air pollution, when measured by pollutant weight. Cars are the biggest producers of carbon monoxide, which outweighs the other four major pollutants combined. There are indications that the level of pollution from automobiles has peaked and may be expected to decline as older cars are replaced by newer ones with pollution-control devices. But in the long run even the effect of these controls could be negated if the number of cars on the road continues to increase at the present rate.

At levels commonly found in urban areas, air pollution contributes to the incidence of chronic ailments such as emphysema, bronchitis, and asthma. Concern is also growing about possible effects that are even more long-range, and studies are being undertaken on such matters as the capacity of chemical agents in the atmosphere to produce mutagenic effects in biologic systems. The adverse economic effects of air pollution range from the waste of fuel and other valuable resources, through the soiling and corrosion of physical structures of all kinds, to damage to agriculture and forests; and by reducing visibility, air pollution no doubt contributes to accidents in the air and on the ground.

Water Quality

. . . 1963, Meramec River, Missouri. Chlorine dumped into the river by well drillers killed approximately 100,000 fish in 18 miles of stream.

. . . 1969, Cuyahoga River, Ohio. The river became so laden with volatile industrial discharges that it caught fire and burned two railroad trestles.

. . . 1971, Lake Erie, United States. This huge inland "sea" has become critically polluted. The natural biologic systems which maintain its economic and social value have largely been killed off. Nearly all beaches are closed by pollution, huge mounds of decaying fish and algae pile up on shore in the summer, the water is thick and discolored, and the lake bottom has a vast accumulation of waste materials that have been dumped into it over the years.

Part of the significance of water in everyday life is suggested by figures on the extent of its use. Each year about 25 trillion gallons of water are consumed in the United States. About 13.1 trillion gallons are used by industry for various manufacturing processes and for cooling; agriculture consumes 6 to 7 trillion gallons for irrigation; and about 5 trillion gallons are used for drinking, bathing, and waste disposal.

SOURCES AND CONSEQUENCES OF WATER POLLUTION

The purification of drinking water has long been a part of environmental control programs and is considered a traditional "environmental sanitation" activity. Yet over 6,000 of the nation's public water supplies, serving 58 million people, do not meet the water quality standards recommended by the federal government, resulting in water-connected disease outbreaks.

Additional and more recent cause for concern comes from the volume and complexity of chemical wastes entering rivers, lakes, oceans, and underground water resources. Increased use of water

TABLE 7-1. Estimated Prevalence of Water Pollution, by Region, 1970

Region	Per Cent of Stream-Miles Polluted	Per Cent of Watersheds Polluted			
		Predominantly Polluted*	Extensively Polluted†	Locally Polluted‡	Slightly Polluted§
Pacific Coast	33.9	14.8	59.3	22.2	3.7
Northern Plains	40.0	37.5	33.3	25.0	4.2
Southern Plains	38.8	27.3	51.5	18.2	6.1
Southeast	23.3	14.3	41.1	16.1	28.6
Central	36.6	23.2	51.8	21.4	3.6
Northeast	43.9	36.1	55.6	5.6	2.8
East of Mississippi River	31.6	23.0	48.7	15.5	12.8
West of Mississippi River	35.5	24.1	47.1	20.7	4.6
United States	32.6	23.7	48.5	17.7	9.9

* Predominantly polluted: ≥ 50% of stream-miles polluted.
† Extensively polluted: 20–49.9% of stream-miles polluted.
‡ Locally polluted: 10–19.9% of stream-miles polluted.
§ Slightly polluted: ≤10% of stream-miles polluted.
SOURCE: Environmental Protection Agency, Water Quality Office. In: The Council on Environmental Quality, *Environmental Quality—the Second Annual Report,* August 1971, p. 220.

for recreation and food production has resulted in greater exposure of man to health hazards because of the unsafe quality of many of these waters.

Today, the nation's surface and underground waters are grossly polluted by a staggering load of waste materials from factory, home, and farm. Estimates for 1970, shown in Table 7-1, classify almost one third of the stream-miles in the United States as characteristically polluted, in the sense that they violated federal water quality criteria, while almost three fourths of the watersheds (the land area from which water drains toward a common watercourse) were classified as "predominantly" or "extensively" polluted.

The pollutants that clog America's waters come from countless sources: (1) some 240,000 water-using industrial plants generate the largest amount and the most toxic of pollutants, and the volume is growing; (2) more than 1,300 communities still discharge their sewage into the waterways without any treatment whatever, and an equal number employ only primary treatment which removes 30 to 40 per cent of some pollutants; (3) oil from vessels and offshore drilling has produced several spectacular spills, and additional thousands of barrels are spilled almost daily in waters across the nation. Still other sources of water pollution or contamination come from the electric power industry, which discharges heated water that threatens aquatic life, and from mining operations, which entail acid and sediment drainage. Agriculture is another source of water pollution, with fertilizer and pesticide runoff from fields; irrigation return-flows containing fertilizer, pesticides, and salts leached from the soil; and animal wastes from feedlots.

All of these activities have a variety of harmful effects on sur- ✎ face waters. Industrial wastes discharged to streams and lakes may deplete the dissolved oxygen, causing fish to die and odors to develop. Some contaminants, which do not kill fish and shellfish outright, render them unfit for human consumption. Oil spills kill fish and water birds, and make beaches unusable for recreation. Certain pollutants, such as phosphates, provide an excess of nutrients in lakes. The nutrients — in a process called eutrophication or overfertilization — promote the growth of algae, which cause cloudy and sometimes odorous water and produce undesirable bottom deposits, as has happened in Lake Erie. In 1969, household detergents became implicated in the phosphate pollution problem because most of them consisted of a substantial proportion of phosphates and were in widespread use. In order to combat this source of water pollution, health officials urged that substitutes replace the phosphates in detergents. Unfortunately, the substitutes turned out to be highly caustic, so that resumption of the use of phosphate detergents was recommended, while the search for a better solution to the problem continued.

TREATMENT OF PUBLIC WATER SUPPLIES

As with all effective control programs, community water supply surveillance involves planning, review, and approval of the various components of the system — sources, treatment, storage, and distribution; periodic inspections; and routine laboratory examination. Water supply sanitation supervision procedures are outlined in the Public Health Service Drinking Water Standards.[10] The standards suggest the number of samples per month to be collected from various points within the distribution system in order to conduct tests for microorganisms of the coliform group.[11] Standards also are given for color, turbidity, odor and taste, total solids, chlorides, and various chemicals and materials that may be toxic or objectionable.

Community water supplies taken from rivers and lakes are normally filtered. The most common method is by the rapid sand filtration process. A coagulant, usually alum of ferric chloride, is mixed with the water, and slow agitation causes a precipitate to develop, most of which settles out in a few hours and takes with it much of the suspended materials. The water then flows through a layer of sand a few feet thick, at a rate of 2 or 3 gallons per minute for each square foot of surface area. Next, the water is chlorinated and flows to a final tank where it remains for about 30 minutes, during which time the chlorine acts on remaining microorganisms. Special treatment is sometimes applied for taste and odor control, usually by use of activated carbon. Some water requires softening or removal of objectionable minerals.

Some water supplies, such as the main supply to Los Angeles, may come from mountain streams and reservoirs which are protected from sewage or industrial wastes. Such supplies are not filtered, but they are chlorinated. Community wells are sometimes used without any treatment if they are built to exclude surface drainage, are located remote from subsurface sewage disposal systems, are over 50 feet from any sewer line, and derive water from sand, sandstone, or a good filtration medium. However, if the water is derived from cavernous or open-jointed limestone, there is hazard of contamination traveling from quite distant sources, and therefore such supplies are usually chlorinated.

Water supply reservoirs are normally designed to exclude all surface drainage and are screened to exclude birds and animals. When a water supply is stored in an open reservoir which may be contaminated by surface drainage, birds, and other sources, the water flowing out should normally be chlorinated before entering the distribution system.

The distribution system must be periodically surveyed to eliminate the hazard of contamination by cross-connections. For example, there may be a direct connection between the public distribution system and an industrial water supply piping system delivering untreated water from a river, canal, or an otherwise unapproved source to be used for processing, cooling, or fire fighting. When the pressure in the unapproved supply exceeds that of the public supply and the interconnecting valve leaks or is opened, serious contamination results. This type of condition has caused several serious outbreaks of waterborne illness. Control is accomplished by prohibiting such direct connections or by special check-valve arrangements which permit the potable water to enter the unapproved water system but prevent flow in the other direction.

One of the most common water treatment processes is softening by zeolite. This is sometimes done for an entire public supply such as in the treatment plant of the Metropolitan Water District of Southern California. It is also the method used in most household and commercial softeners. Hardness is caused by the presence of bicarbonates and sulfates of calcium and magnesium in the water. When these chemicals pass through a mass of zeolite crystals, they exchange their calcium or magnesium for sodium from the zeolites, thus producing sodium bicarbonate and sulfate, which do not cause hardness effects. The increase in sodium is not a health factor except for a person with a strict limitation on sodium intake.

An optimal amount of fluoride ion in the water supply has been shown to reduce dental caries by over 60 per cent in persons consuming such water since childhood. While the fluoridation of water is a subject of public controversy in some communities, optimum amounts of fluoride ion produce no ill effects and there is no technical difficulty in adding the appropriate amount to a public water supply. In the Public Health Service Drinking Water Standards, the optimum amount is given according to the mean annual daily maximum temperature and ranges from slightly under to slightly over 1 mg per liter or part per million (ppm).

WATER PROTECTION IN THE TREATMENT OF SEWAGE

The degree of treatment provided for community sewage and liquid industrial waste depends on the use of the receiving water and the quantity of waste in relation to the quantity of water available for dilution. For example, the degree of removal of potentially pathogenic microorganisms should be much higher when the effluent is discharged into a stream or lake used as a source of a public water supply than when it is discharged into the ocean at a point remote from recreational areas or shellfish beds.

In Los Angeles, sewage is discharged into the ocean through multiple outlets a few hundred feet deep and miles from shore. This procedure meets requirements after only "primary" treatment to remove suspended and floating solids. The removed material (sludge) is digested in a closed, heated tank to break down grease and organic solids, producing a large quantity of gas used for power generation. The digested sludge is then discharged to the ocean from the treatment plants.

For more complete treatment to discharge into fresh water or ocean water near beaches or shellfish beds, large cities and many towns use the activated sludge process to produce a much more highly purified effluent. This process includes introducing air bubbles into sewage held in tanks for 6 to 12 hours or longer, thereby promoting the growth and multiplication of aerobic organisms which feed upon sewage constituents and convert nitrogenous material into stable nitrites and nitrates. These organisms then clump together, or flocculate, to produce a brownish "activated sludge," which settles out in a final settling tank. Part of this sludge is returned to the aeration tank to maintain that desired concentration of microorganisms needed to accomplish good treatment, the balance disposed of, usually by drying after digestion. The effluent may be further "purified' by chlorination or chlorination plus filtration and may be used for irrigation, recreational lakes, recharge of underground water supply "basins," industrial processing, and other purposes.

Simple and efficient sewage treatment also is accomplished by a process applicable to small communities and some industrial wastes. The sewage is simply discharged into one or a series of "stabilization ponds" about 3 feet deep in algae, which in the presence of sunlight liberates oxygen that, in turn, is used by microorganisms to stabilize and purify the waste. About an acre of water surface is required for each 200 to 1,000 population. While originally used only in warmer climates such as California and Texas, the process now operates even in cold northern states. It is especially suitable for developing countries.

Solid Waste Disposal

. . . 4.3 billion tons of solid wastes a year are produced in the United States.

. . . Of this annual total, 190 million tons are picked up and hauled away for disposal. By 1980 the quantity is expected to reach 340 million tons per year.

. . . Throwaways, annually, include 48 billion cans, 26 billion bottles and jars, 4 million tons of plastic, 7.6 million television sets, 7 million cars and trucks, and 30 million tons of paper.

The traditional way of considering the solid waste problem has been to concentrate on the collection and disposal of wastes from households, principally as food wastes. However, in present-day circumstances solid wastes come from a variety of sources and are of numerous kinds. Of the 4.3 billion tons of solid wastes produced annually, an estimated 360 million tons come from household, municipal, and industrial sources; 2.3 billion tons are agricultural wastes; and 1.7 billion tons are mineral wastes.

The most commonly used solid waste disposal methods are sanitary landfills and incineration. In *sanitary landfills,* the waste is deposited in marshes, canyons, abandoned gravel pits, etc.; compacted by bulldozers; and covered with earth before fly breeding or rat feeding can occur. The land reclaimed by the filling operations may provide much-needed parks and "open space." Care must be taken to locate sites where they will not pollute underground water supplies, and to locate and operate them to minimize neighborhood nuisances from blowing papers, dust, and odors. *Incineration* of refuse and garbage in well-designed and properly operated community units costs about five times as much as disposal by sanitary landfills. The incinerator must be designed to predry very moist material, to introduce a controlled amount of air to support combustion, and to provide a combustion chamber of such size and design that it will allow enough time and air mixing (turbulence) to promote complete combustion at a temperature above 1,200°F. Devices to collect "fly ash" from the stack gases prevent neighborhood nuisances from dust and charred paper.

In spite of efforts to control the problem, most present solid waste *disposal* methods pollute either the land, air, or water. A national survey has revealed that less than 6 per cent of 12,000 landfill sites meet minimum federal sanitary standards. Almost all municipal incinerators are obsolescent in terms of today's needs. The problems of disposal are aggravated by widespread and increasing use of elaborate packaging, disposable containers, and materials that do not burn or decay. Municipal waste *collection*, which costs $4.5 billion per year, all too frequently is inadequate and results in waste accumulations that breed disease, rats, and accidents.

Aside from offending the eye and assaulting the nostrils, studies indicate that there is an association between poor solid-waste practices and more than 20 human diseases. Although these health hazards rarely cause mass, acute illness, they do represent slow, cumulative impairment to health and life, involving traces of chemicals, air pollution, drug residues, and other detrimental elements.

Another growing concern has to do with the recovery and reuse of valuable and often irreplaceable resources that form part of solid wastes. Vast quantities of nonrenewable resources, such as ferrous metals, are lost in the waste-generating process and represent an unnecessary economic drain and loss of natural resources.

In order to cope with these problems, new concepts of solid waste management are emerging. They envision a social-technologic system that will control the quantity and characteristics of wastes, adequate collection of wastes that must be removed, recycling of those that can be reused, and proper disposal of those that must be discarded.

Pesticides

. . . In Iraq (1972), an estimated 1,000 persons died from an outbreak of mercury poisoning used as a pesticide on grain imported from the United States or Canada. The grain was intended for planting only. But some of it was made into flour

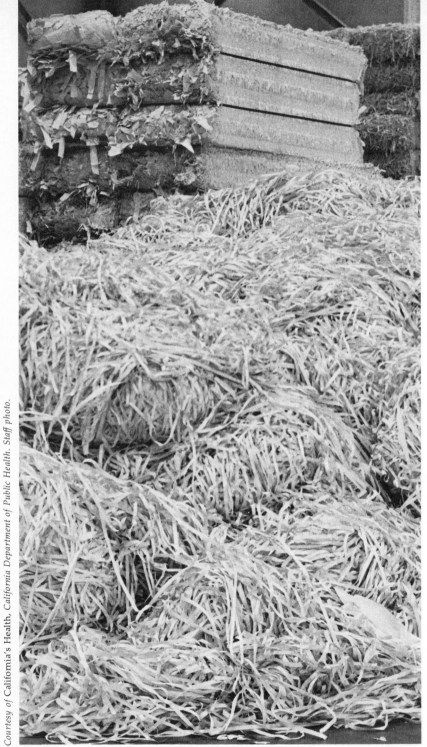

Courtesy of California's Health, California Department of Public Health. Staff photo.

210

and some was fed to cattle which were subsequently used as meat. After the poisonous nature of the grain was discovered, some of it was dumped into rivers, contaminating the fish.

. . . In New York City (1969) the Food and Drug Administration seized nearly 2 million pounds of imported cheese which was either returned to the originating country or destroyed because of excessive pesticide content.

. . . In a California-Nevada wooded area, a scale insect became extremely abundant on the pine trees. It was discovered that a pesticide used to control mosquitos had also killed tiny wasps that were the natural predators of the scale insects. Excessive deaths of the wasps allowed the scale to reproduce uncontrollably.

Pesticides constitute one group of the ever-increasing number and variety of chemicals to which man is exposed today. The term *pesticides* means such substances as insecticides, fungicides, rodenticides, herbicides, worm killers, and plant regulators. Although pesticide chemicals were known and used before World War II, their use has increased significantly. In 1969, production of pesticides in the United States totaled 1.13 billion pounds. Of this amount, 409 million pounds were exported, making a net usage, domestically, of about 730 million pounds. About half the pesticide production in the United States was insecticides, among them chlorinated hydrocarbons, of which DDT is no doubt the best-known example.

Worldwide there have been tremendous benefits from the use of pesticides. Increased food production through the control of insect pests and prevention of vectorborne diseases such as malaria and encephalitis are undeniable gains resulting from the use of pesticides. However, side-effects have emerged which are reaching critical proportions as such chemicals continue to enter the environment.

The principal concerns regarding the effects of pesticides have to do with actual or possible acute, chronic, or delayed toxicity to humans, and with adverse effects on the natural environment. It is now known that some pesticide compounds are present in the tissues of humans, birds, fish, and other wildlife. A concentrating effect takes place as one species feeds on another and passes the pesticide from one link to another in the food chain. The average American now carries about 12 ppm (parts per million) of DDT in his fatty tissues, but there is as yet no direct evidence that this concentration has a harmful effect. However, there is evidence that concentrated pesticide residues have adverse effects on some birds—their reproduction, physiology, and perhaps their very survival. Marine fish are almost universally contaminated with pesticide residues, and declining production of shellfish in certain areas is believed to be directly traceable to pesticide contamination.

Ironically, in spite of man's heavy reliance on insecticides, more and more insect species have developed immunity to the pesticides that had kept them under control. Showing tremendous capacity for adaptation and survival, they are thriving again, including some that carry human disease.

The furor that has developed in the past decade over pesticides, particularly DDT, has led to a search for solutions to alleviate the problem. Banning certain pesticides is one means of reducing the immediate dangers from the most harmful chemicals, but the problem does not end there. Some method of pest control to prevent vectorborne diseases and to provide an adequate food supply for the world's population will probably always be needed. The question of alternative methods is a pressing one.

One solution being attempted is the development of pesticides with new chemical bases. Among the newer types of chemical families are the organophosphates and carbamates, which are less persistent (i.e., remain in the environment for a shorter time) than the chlorinated hydrocarbons. However, they are much more toxic and have been responsible for the accidental killing of both wildlife and human beings.

Another solution resides in the development of methods of more selective application of pesticides. This would overcome present deficits where—in agriculture, for example—spraying by aircraft or ground rigs results in less than 10 per cent of the material being applied to the target. The remainder is released into the air to drift and deposit in the area. The home use of pesticide aerosol sprays is similar in pattern, although much smaller in scale, of course.

A third promising solution is biologic control. This consists of the use of natural enemies (such as predators and parasites) to keep pest populations within bounds. Such a practice would, of course, reduce reliance on chemical control of the environment. However, much research is still needed before this technique achieves widespread application.

Noise

. . . Noise has a measurable degree of impact on about 80 million people in the United States, or about 40 per cent of the population.

> . . . At an international meeting of scientists in Geneva (1971), it was predicted that if urban noise continues to increase at its current rate, every city dweller would be stone deaf by the year 2000.

As an environmental contaminant, noise is as unwanted and unnecessary as smog, polluted water, and littered landscapes. Noise, which is sound that is physically hurtful or psychologically disturbing to man, has increased dramatically in volume in the past 30 years. The overall loudness of environmental noise seems to be doubling every decade.

Noise pollution is, of course, concentrated in the big cities, not only in the United States but also in cities in many other parts of the world. Throughout the United States, an estimated 130 million people are living in urban areas which are becoming steadily noisier. Suburban areas have become involved, also. A survey of suburban residential sites in 1967 revealed noise levels that were considerably higher than those noted 13 years earlier.

Basically, sound is a form of energy. The decibel (dB) is the unit used to describe the intensity of sound, 1 dB being the weakest sound level detectable by the healthy human ear under very quiet conditions. When sound reaches a level of 165 decibels, it can kill small animals: the energy of the sound waves is converted to heat in the animals' bodies. The decibel scale is logarithmic (rather than linear), so that for every increase of 10 decibels, loudness is increased by two times. For example, 110 decibels is two times louder than 100 decibels. Sounds of 120 decibels reach the level where they become uncomfortable to the ear and include noise generated by heavy earth-moving equipment.

Noise pollution comes from such urban phenomena as increased crowding and traffic congestion, construction activity, and large-scale manufacturing. Specifically, the sources of noise are many and wide-ranging, including jet planes, jackhammers, diesel trucks, motorcycles, powermowers, radio and television sets, and household electrical appliances.

Table 7-2 shows sound levels for various sources of noise encountered in three different environmental situations: industrial, community or outdoor, and home or indoor. It is evident that noises in *mechanized industries,* as a group, have higher levels than those in the other two environmental settings. Furthermore, it is likely that in industrial operations there is more sustained exposure to various types of high noise levels during the typical 8-hour workday. It has been estimated that 7 million industrial workers in the United States are exposed to occupational noise levels that could damage their hearing. Absenteeism and lowered working efficiency

TABLE 7-2. Sound Levels of Some Noises Found in Different Environments

Overall Level dBA*	Industrial	dB	Community or Outdoor	dB	Home or Indoor	dB
130						
Uncomfortably loud 120	Oxygen torch	121				
	Scraper-loader	117				
	Compactor	116				
110	Riveting machine	110			Rock-n-roll band	114–108
	Textile loom	106	Jet flyover @ 1000 ft	103		
Very loud 100	Electric furnace area	100				
	Newspaper press	97	Power mower	96	Inside subway car, 35 mph	95
			Compressor @ 20 ft	94		
			Rock drill @ 100 ft	92		
90			Motorcycle @ 25 ft	90		
	Cockpit, prop aircraft	88	Prop aircraft flyover @ 1,000 ft	88	Food blender	88
	Milling machine	85	Diesel truck, 40 mph @ 50 ft	84		
	Cotton spinning	83	Diesel train, 40–50 mph @ 100 ft	83		
	Lathe	81				

Overall Level dBA*	Industrial	dB	Community or Outdoor	dB	Home or Indoor	dB
80	Tabulating	80	Passenger car, 65 mph @ 27 ft	77	Garbage disposal	80
					Clothes washer	78
					Living room music	76
					Dishwasher	75
Moderately loud 70					TV-audio	70
			Near freeway auto traffic	64	Vacuum	70
Quiet 60			Air conditioning unit @ 20 ft	60	Conversation	60
Very quiet 50			Light traffic @ 100 ft	50		
Just audible 30						
Threshold of hearing 0						

* Noise levels are expressed as decibels measured on the A-network of a sound level meter (dBA). Noise readings in dBA are weighted measures approximating the human ear's sensitivity to different sound frequencies when heard at moderate intensities.

SOURCE: Adapted from Bureau of Community Environmental Management. *Environmental Health Planning*, Public Health Service Publication No. 2120, 1971.

resulting from excessive industrial noise are estimated to cost the nation $4 to $5 million a day.

Serious though the problem is in industry, certain noises intruding in *community* (outdoor) or *home* (indoor) environments can reach levels comparable to those noted for noisier workplaces, as illustrated in Table 7-2. For example, residents living under the flight paths of a nearby airport or those who frequent discotheques may experience the same noise levels as produced in riveting operations or around textile looms. A home powermower produces a noise level close to that of a newspaper press. The noise of a home food blender may even exceed that of an industrial milling machine.

Exposure to noise can affect people adversely in a variety of ways. First, there is hearing loss, which is believed to be the most serious physical health hazard posed by excessive noise. Generally, the danger level for hearing loss for most people is above 80 decibels. The magnitude of the problem among industrial workers, which has already been mentioned, has prompted the passage of regulations to curb noise in certain occupational settings. With regard to community noise, the effects on hearing have not been established as yet. However, it has been found that some 20 per cent of the population of the United States (in addition to those exposed to excessive occupational noise) suffer measurable hearing impairment by their fifties, whereas people in nonindustrial societies experience no such loss.

A second category of noise pollution effects consists of physical and mental disturbances. It has been demonstrated that noise can trigger changes in cardiovascular, endocrine, neurologic, and other physiologic functions, with associated feelings of distress. However, it is not yet clear whether repeated noise-induced changes of this nature ultimately result in a disease process, although some physicians believe there is a direct link between noise and heart disease, peptic ulcer, colitis, high blood pressure, and migraine. Long-term experiments with laboratory animals have demonstrated that high noise levels can boost cholesterol levels and increase hardening of the arteries. The association between noise and mental disturbances is also highly speculative at this time, although some residents living in communities subjected to intense aircraft and highway noise have claimed they suffer from nervousness and assorted other mental difficulties.

Other adverse effects of noise (some demonstrated and some suspected) include interference with voice communication, disruption in job performance, and interference with rest, relaxation, and sleep. Thus, noise that reaches a level where it interferes with talking and listening can be annoying and even hazardous—for example, in case of failure to hear a warning shout. Noise effects on job performance are most evident in tasks that require concentration, and work on jobs requiring close attention has shown improvement with the introduction of noise control. Interference with rest and sleep has been cited as one of the major causes of annoyance and complaints in communities exposed to intense aircraft flyover noise. Studies have also shown that greater annoyance results when sleep and rest are disturbed by noise than when other activities (e.g., listening) are similarly interrupted.

In the past there has been a tendency to accept noise as a phenomenon that is essentially beyond control. Present views, however, hold that enhancing the quality of life necessarily includes a consideration of noise and how its deleterious effects on man can be prevented or minimized. Many noise suppression techniques are, in fact, already available, but have not been fully utilized. For example, technology exists today to curb noise from construction equipment, railroad equipment, cars, trucks, and buses. Much can be done to reduce noise from aircraft and from machinery used in factory, office, or home. Buildings can be constructed so there is insulation from noise both outside and inside.

Radiation

. . . Beneficial uses of radiation include the application of x-ray and radioisotopes in clinical diagnosis and therapy; radioisotopes in industry for measuring, testing, and processing; electric power generation; lasers in science, industry, and medicine.

. . . But harmful effects on the body of exposure to relatively large doses of ionizing radiation may include leukemia and other types of cancer, reduction in fertility, cataracts and other eye damage, acceleration of the aging process, and damage to reproductive cells.

There are two basic categories of radiation to which human beings are exposed. One consists of *natural background radiation*, which comes from cosmic rays and radioactive material naturally existing in the soil, water, and air as well as within the human body. This background radiation constitutes about 55 per cent of the total radiation to which the average American is exposed each year. The second category consists of *man-made radiation*, which comes from a variety of sources, including x-rays, the operating of nuclear power plants, and electronic devices in the home and workplace.

Public interest and concern over radioactive contamination

reached a peak during the period when nuclear bomb test explosions were releasing huge quantities of man-made radioactive pollution. Radioactivity was easily detected by simple geiger counters in the visible dust accumulations that occurred. Much of the concern had to do with the possibility that genetic damage might affect millions of people in posterity. Another concern was for strontium-90, which accumulates in the bones, including the backbone, and emits ionizing radiation to bombard blood-forming body substances. A further concern was for iodine-131, which was found in milk, water, and food shortly after nuclear blasts. It may accumulate in the thyroid and thereby increase the risk of cancer of the thyroid or other conditions. These problems were alleviated in the early 1960's by the moratorium on nuclear weapons tests in the atmosphere, which reduced radiation levels markedly. At present, fallout from weapons-testing prior to the atmospheric nuclear test ban treaty contributes about 3 per cent of the man-made radiation to which Americans are exposed.

The average level of natural background radiation is between 100 and 125 millirems per year. One millirem is one one-thousandth of a rem; rem stands for "roentgen equivalent man" and reflects the amount of radiation absorbed in human tissues. Current radiation protection guides provided by the federal government call for maximum limits of exposure from all man-made sources for individual members of the general public as well as for special population groups.

Unlike other environmental pollutants, the hazards associated with radiation were apparent long before there was widespread commercial application of radiation-producing technology. As a result, governmental controls were imposed early, and the establishment and enforcement of standards for protection against ionizing radiation have been the most comprehensive of any applied to environmental hazards. Nevertheless, keeping exposure levels as far below accepted standards as possible remains a constant problem.

There are two sources of man-made radiation exposure that currently cause the most concern in the United States. One comes from medical uses of radiation, and the other from nuclear power plants.

At present, *medical uses of radiation,* particularly x-rays, constitute the largest source of man-made radiation. Such uses represent about 94 per cent of all exposure to man-made radiation, or about 40 per cent of all radiation sources to which the average person is exposed. A variety of measures have been developed to control or minimize this type of radiation hazard. Thus, there are devices to limit the size of the x-ray beam so it exposes only the area required for the desired film or treatment. Lead-containing aprons can be worn in order to shield the gonadal region. "Filtration" of the beam through aluminum removes soft, useless, but somewhat undesirable rays. Fast film, more sensitive fluoroscope screens, better fluoroscopic techniques, and more efficient units all aid in that objective. Shoe-fitting fluoroscopes and similar appliances which produce long exposure for relatively useless purposes are outlawed in most places.

Nuclear power plants, which use nuclear energy to generate electric power, increasingly have become the focus of concern as a source of environmental radiation. Radiation emissions released into the environment from reactors and from fuel reprocessing plants constitute only about 0.003 per cent of all man-made radiation to which even those persons living near the plants are exposed. Thus, the contribution of nuclear power plants to environmental radiation is relatively small at present. However, there are now only some 20 of these plants in operation in the United States. By 1990, in order to keep pace with increasing demands for electricity, it is anticipated that about 450 nuclear power plants will be in operation. Furthermore, the disposal of radioactive wastes from nuclear power generation, which is already a problem, may be expected to increase with the growth of the nuclear industry.

Besides the hazards that may come from specific radiation sources, there is also concern regarding the long-term effects of repeated low-level exposure to all forms of radiation. The effects on human health of protracted release of even very low levels of long-lasting radioactivity from an increasing number of man-made sources are little understood as yet and will continue to be the subject of intensive study.

Food Sanitation

. . . Inspectors estimated (1971) that serious potential or actual food adulteration existed in 1,000 out of 4,550 food manufacturing plants in 21 states, with less serious insanitary conditions existing in 800 additional plants.

. . . An estimated two to ten million people in the United States contract some form of foodborne disease annually; food poisoning ranks second only to the common cold as the most frequent cause of illness.

The protection of food and milk from contamination has, traditionally, been an important environmental health concern. There are a staggering number of sites in the United States to be monitored for possible food and milk sanitation problems, including 45,000 food processing establishments; 25,000 manufacturers, warehouses, and similar firms; about 500,000 food service establishments; and approximately 350,000 dairy farms.

Food sanitation and other food-related problems are of three prinicipal kinds. The first consists of microbiologic contamination. Salmonellosis; shigellosis; illness due to *Clostridium perfringens, Vibrio* and viruses; and food poisonings caused by *Staphylococcus* and *Clostridium botulinus* toxins are transmitted through contaminated foods. The development of new foods, changing distribution and delivery systems, centralization of food processing, and widespread use of new technologies and procedures result in increased potential for foodborne illness. Problems of food sanitation are complicated by the use of unclean or decomposed raw materials or by insanitary conditions in food manufacturing, processing, and delivery systems.

A second food-related problem is chemical additives contamination. The average American is said to consume five pounds of chemical additives in his food each year. There are two main classes of food additives, direct and indirect. Direct additives are deliberately used in food processing to enhance or conserve nutritional value or to improve or maintain flavor, color, texture, consistency, and so on. Indirect additives enter and remain in food as a result of their use as pesticides or fertilizers, after addition to animal feed, from synthetic or chemically processed packaging material, or through chemical changes brought about by processing methods. Indirect additives are essentially contaminants and are cause for concern as health hazards, although in recent years the health effects of direct additives also have been coming under close scrutiny.

The third main category of food-related problems has to do with protection of foods from nutritional deterioration and protection of the public from deception and fraud. Food may suffer nutritional loss due to improper storage, excessive shelf life, or poor handling during preparation. Deceptive and misleading claims about the nutritional value of food products is a major concern, costing American consumers as much as $500 million a year. Economic frauds, of which the consumer is also the victim, include slack fill, substitution of cheaper ingredients, or low drained weights.

There are specific kinds of food sanitation activities conducted by official agencies at federal, state, and local levels. The Food and Drug Administration and the U.S. Department of Agriculture largely control interstate, wholesale food processing, packaging, and distribution operations. These programs are primarily concerned with labeling, adulteration, misbranding, control of botulism, regulation of meat and poultry slaughter and wholesale processing, long-range effects of toxic or carcinogenic ingredients, and control of sanitation and insect or rodent contamination of such foods. State and local programs are more directly concerned with administration of laws and ordinances governing food service, preparation, processing, sale, and distribution on a local level. The objectives of the programs are to minimize food poisoning and infection; to provide clean, sanitary, and vermin-free establishments; to provide foods that are sanitary, safe, and wholesome; to provide sanitary utensils; and even to regulate, to a degree, the esthetic conditions of food establishments as they broadly relate to health and sanitation.

Local food sanitation programs cover restaurants, markets, bakeries, bakery distributors, vending machines, caterers, food demonstrators, itinerant restaurants, food service operations at carnivals and festivals, bars, soda fountains, and a wide variety of other types of businesses and establishments.

A food sanitation program for food establishments is most effective if a license or permit, or a grading placard, must be obtained and displayed before operations begin. This is issued only after it is determined that the establishment is designed and equipped to facilitate proper maintenance. A food establishment should have design features to exclude rodents; screens or self-closing doors to exclude flies; lighting to facilitate sanitary operation; surfaces and materials that can readily be kept clean; and equipment to protect foods from contamination by leakage or by customers, including protective devices for unpackaged food displays. Special provision should be made for hand-washing facilities convenient for the employees, preferably in food preparation areas. There should be equipment such as drainboards, garbage disposers, and preflushing devices, and sinks or dish-washing machines for utensil and equipment washing. The provision of facilities to permit orderly storage of foods at safe temperatures is particularly important. Facilities should be provided to prepare foods properly, including washing of fruits and vegetables to be eaten raw; cutting boards and slicing machines capable of being kept clean; and arrangements to keep utensils, containers, and surfaces used for raw foods such as meat, fish, and poultry separate from those used for ready-to-eat products. Instructions and training should be provided to assure capability to operate in compliance with health standards.

The customary measurement of the effectiveness of a sanitizing process is the "rim count" test (standard plate count) indicating a recovery of less than 100 microorganisms from each utensil "swabbed" in a prescribed manner. To meet this requirement it is usually necessary to expose utensils to hot water at about 180°F in a sink or spray-type machine or to immerse them in a 100-ppm chlorine solution or in an equivalent iodine or quaternary ammonium compound solution.

In markets, precautions are necessary to ensure safe preparation of poultry and meats. In such establishments, facilities may be inadequate; raw products may contaminate finished foods; inadequate temperatures may permit salmonella to survive the cooking process; and food "warmers" may be so designed, loaded, or used that foods are held at temperatures that favor multiplication of microorganisms.

Other food service operations that present special problems include central commissaries which distribute food to several establishments or schools. The main concern in such cases is maintaining temperature control during the distribution process. Similarly, catering of foods to special private parties may be hazardous unless properly regulated. Modern lunch trucks which serve industrial plants and carry full meals of both hot and cold foods also have temperature control problems unless proper equipment is provided. A special danger may exist if leftover perishables are kept overnight on a truck that is not equipped with electrically or gas-operated refrigerators and hot-holding units.

"Food poisoning" investigation is an important program of official agencies, especially when results of such studies are used in developing preventive programs through education of the public, agency staffs, and the food industry. One study found that over 80 per cent of foodborne illness from meals in the United States was due to meat or meat products. A second most common cause was found to be custard made of egg and dairy products. Prevention of staphylococcus "food poisoning" is principally accomplished by temperature control, since staphylococcus organisms practically stop multiplying at below 45°F and above 118°F. Codes usually require perishable foods to be kept at below 45°F or above 140°F, except during processing. Salmonella infection is commonly traced to food handlers, unpasteurized egg products, and inadequately cooked poultry. Since symptoms do not occur until 12 to 24 hours after eating, this illness is very inadequately reported, with probably less than 1 per cent of the cases being made a matter of official record.

Milkborne disease is controlled mainly through pasteurization followed by processing and packaging in a manner to prevent recontamination. Pasteurization is heat processing which destroys all organisms that may be pathogenic when ingested. It does not destroy spores or heat-resistant organisms, but these are not pathogenic when ingested. Pasteurization of fluid milk is accomplished under a wide variety of time-temperature conditions. Currently, the most common method is the high-temperature, short-time method , 161°F for 15 seconds, in a unit that employs heat exchange principles to utilize the hot pasteurized milk to warm the cold incoming milk and vice versa. Controls and recorders, checked periodically by the health official, assure conformance with time-temperature requirements. Other temperature-time combinations include 145°F for 30 minutes, and 194°F for 1 second.

Pasteurization is checked by the phosphatase test, which is based on the fact that the enzyme phosphatase, naturally present in raw milk, is inactivated by pasteurization. Standards limit coliform organisms to 10 per milliliter on the presumption that the presence of this organism is evidence of improper pasteurization or of contamination subsequent to pasteurization; the coliform organism is destroyed by pasteurization. The rickettsial organism that causes Q fever is also destroyed by pasteurization; this disease is thought to be transmitted by air as well as by contaminated milk.

The Public Health Service code provides detailed explanations of all important features of dairy farm and milk-processing sanitation. The most common test is the standard plate count, which indicates, principally, improper cleaning of equipment and inadequate refrigeration. Tests that health departments perform on milk samples include the following: tests to discover watering of milk; butterfat tests; nonfat solids tests; bioassay tests for vitamins; tests for radionuclides (most significant when nuclear bombs were being tested); microbiologic growth-inhibiting tests for presence of antibiotics used to treat cows; and insecticide residue tests to determine that milk meets the "zero tolerance" requirement for chlorinated hydrocarbons. Tests of milk-processing procedures include timing tests to be sure milk is held at pasteurization temperature for required time; control-valve tests to see that milk cannot leave the pasteurizer except at required temperature; pressure tests to be sure pasteurized milk in heat exchanger units is always at higher pressure than raw milk, so that the latter cannot leak into pasteurized milk; and total plate counts of milk cartons to check for compliance with microbiologic standards.

Although most municipalities in the United States require milk to be pasteurized, some allow raw milk if it is "certified," which means it is produced under the additional supervision of a Medical Milk Commission and is subject to additional tests. In the production of certified raw milk, cows and milk-handling employees are subject to special health examinations and total plate counts must be low (5,000 to 10,000 per milliliter compared with over 100,000 permitted for raw milk that is to be pasteurized). Most health officials believe modern pasteurization does not destroy or adversely affect any significant component of milk and that pasteurization is the best process to assure milk that is free of pathogens. The Public Health Service code no longer makes provision for raw milk.

Pasteurization of dairy products, other than milk, is also important. This applies to ice cream, butter, cottage cheese, many other cheeses, etc. Dry milk, to meet Public Health Service standards, must be made from "grade A" pasteurized milk. Unfortunately, some dry milk products are made from raw, manufacturing-grade milk and may not be properly pasteurized if dried under a vacuum which permits "boiling" at relatively low temperatures.

Milk plant inspection includes checking recording devices that indicate pasteurization temperatures and setting and sealing pasteurizer pumps to assure that milk is processed slowly enough to provide the required holding time. Proper cleaning and bactericidal rinsing of most pipelines and equipment, both in the modern dairy and at the plant, are by clean-in-place methods which surge rinse water, detergent, and sanitizing solutions through all equipment. This does a satisfactory job, avoids contamination by hands, and saves labor. Much of the milk industry's effort is directed toward quality control. This includes control of off-flavors from the cow's feed, oxidation, overpasteurization, etc., and reduction of psychrophiles (cold-thriving organisms) in order to prolong the "shelf life" of milk.

Rodent and Insect Control

The control of insects and rodents is commonly called vector control because of their disease transmission potential. The rodent is the host for the flea, which is the vector, or carrier, of plague and endemic typhus; anopheles mosquitoes transmit malaria. Vector control is normally most effectively achieved by modifying and regulating the environment to reduce or prevent propagation. This is particularly applicable in cities and developed areas.

RODENT CONTROL

As in nearly all health programs, rodent control involves cooperative work of many groups, organizations, and the public. Buildings should be constructed to prevent rodents from entering and from nesting inside. Food wastes should be stored and disposed of so that they are inaccessible to rats. When necessary, extermination measures through poisons, trapping, and gassing should be undertaken.

Trapping is relatively slow and difficult. Suitable poisons, mixed with the rodent's favorite food or water supply and placed along runways, are most effective. This is done by commercial pest control operators and some public agencies, including health departments. Some poisons are deadly to man, and their placement must be carefully controlled. Some, such as anticoagulants mixed with cereals, are quite effective and, since feedings are required over several days, are less hazardous to children than the faster-acting poisons. A reasonably effective material, when properly used, is red squill, which kills rodents because they cannot regurgitate, but acts as an emetic to human beings, poultry, and animals other than rodents. To be effective, rodent control programs require constant community education and periodic inspection visits and consultations.

An estimated 14,000 cases of rat bite occur annually in the United States, often involving secondary infections. In an effort to combat this problem, a federally financed rat control program was undertaken in 1968, in which 25 cities were participating by mid-1970. Funds were awarded to state, city, and voluntary agencies in these locales for the purpose of reducing the rodent population and the conditions conductive to rodent infestation.

MOSQUITO CONTROL

Since mosquito eggs hatch and the larvae and pupae develop only in quiet water and under certain conditions, mosquito control is most effectively accomplished by eliminating or modifying these waters. Each species has a special preference for the type of water accumulation in which it develops. Anopheles mosquitoes prefer clean, shallow water. *Aedes aegypti,* which transmit yellow fever and dengue, prefer small quantities of water near concentrations of people, including rainwater accumulations in discarded containers. *Culex tarsalis,* the vector of encephalitis, breeds in a variety of non-salty waters including surplus irrigation water. A vicious daytime-biting *Aedes* species lays its eggs on dry salt marsh flats where it remains until submerged in salt water. *Culex fatigans,* which causes urban filariasis, prefers water heavily contaminated with human wastes.

Control programs include draining and filling marshes and low areas; planting a species of fish (*Gambusia affinis*) which eats the larvae; fluctuating water levels to cause larvae and pupae to be exposed to waves and currents; applying larva-killing sprays; improving irrigation practices; designing better gutters and drainage systems for new subdivisions; and conducting public education programs on control procedures.

Some health departments have active mosquito control programs. However, in New Jersey, California, and some other states, mosquito control is the responsibility of well-organized mosquito abatement districts which operate heavy grading and ditching equipment, airplanes for spraying, and special vehicles to spray the water in gutters and catch basins. Ponds are also maintained to stock *Gambusia* fish for planting where needed and for distribution to persons who maintain garden pools in which mosquitoes may breed.

FLY CONTROL

As with mosquito and rodent control, fly control is most effective when the breeding habits are understood and the program is directed toward eliminating conditions favorable to fly development. With but few exceptions, the fly's eggs must be deposited in moist organic material on which the emerging larvae can feed. After about three or more days of feeding, the larvae leave the very moist material, burrow into the ground or reasonably dry material, where they develop shells to become pupae, and then, a few days later, emerge as adults. The housefly, *Musca domestica,* prefers animal manure; the lesser housefly commonly develops in chicken manure; and the shiny "blowflies" prefer garbage and decomposing meat.

Fly control involves keeping flies from their preferred larvae-developing materials; disposing of such materials before the larvae are fully developed; arranging and operating poultry and animal-raising facilities to dry the manure before the larvae are fully developed; and substituting units to dispose of garbage in the sewer instead of in garbage containers. Adult flies are excluded by screens and self-closing doors.

Extermination of adult flies requires continuous attention. As new insecticides are developed, the fly develops resistance, so that new products must constantly be developed. Strict control to prevent contamination of milk and certain foods with DDT-like compounds has reduced the use of these chemicals on dairy farms and in food establishments. Lindane vaporizers are not favored because they may cause contamination of foods and are a suspected cause of a few cases of aplastic anemia. Pyrethrum sprays have been used for many years, are effective if the mist strikes the fly, and are relatively nontoxic.

Accidents

Accidental injuries and deaths are a health and medical problem of major significance. Accidents are the fourth greatest killer in the general population of the United States, but the leading killer of persons 1 to 35 years of age. In 1968, there were almost 115,000 deaths from accidents, as shown in Table 7-3. Almost half these deaths (55,000) resulted from motor vehicle accidents.

About 50 million accidental injuries occur annually in the na-

TABLE 7-3. Deaths and Death Rates from Accidents, United States, Selected Years*

	Number of Deaths	Rate per 100,000 Population
1950	91,249	60.6
1955	93,443	56.9
1960	93,806	52.3
1965	108,004	55.7
1968	114,864	57.5

* Prior to 1960, excludes Alaska and Hawaii.
SOURCE: Adapted from U.S. Bureau of the Census. *Statistical Abstract of the United States, 1971*, p. 57.

tion, with many of the victims permanently disabled. Table 7-4 shows that in 1969 more injuries occurred at home than at places of employment: 10.0 injuries per 100 population were incurred at home and 4.2 while at work. Compared with females, males have an overall higher rate of accidental injuries, the difference being accounted for by a higher injury rate while at work and from other sources, including motor vehicles; the rate of home accidents is similar for both sexes (Table 7-4). Annually, injuries account for 100 million visits to private physicians; 80,000 hospital beds for care and treatment; 200,000 hospital personnel required for care and treatment of victims confined to hospital beds for an estimated 22 million days.

Since motor vehicle accidents account for such a sizable proportion of accidental deaths and injuries, they have been the cause of increasing concern in recent years. Driver-training courses in schools, other kinds of educational programs such as those conducted by the National Safety Council, and the accident prevention programs of official health agencies are all directed toward reducing motor vehicle accidents. There is also a growing national

TABLE 7-4. Rates of Persons Injured, by Class of Accident and Sex, United States, 1969*

	Rate per 100 Population		
	Male	Female	Both Sexes
While at work	7.3	1.2	4.2
Home	11.1	9.0	10.0
Other (incl. motor vehicle)	14.6	8.6	11.5
Total	31.4	18.5	27.4

* Data refer to the civilian noninstitutionalized population.
SOURCE: Adapted from U.S. Bureau of the Census. *Statistical Abstract of the United States, 1971*, p. 76.

participation by health professionals in programs to improve automotive safety. This includes such diverse activities as conducting studies to aid in developing safe traffic arrangements in new residential areas, participating with others in learning the causes of automotive accidents and injuries, and developing corrective measures. Health authorities are conducting research to learn what automobile design factors will minimize injury from collision and what human reactions are related to the causes of accidents.

Accident prevention is an integral part of any industrial-plant or residential-housing program that has inspection, enforcement, and educational provisions. Institutions and housing for aged and handicapped persons are target sites for accident prevention and the development of corrective programs involving construction and maintenance.

Health departments have in some places stimulated development of good accident-reporting and analysis programs in what is known as the epidemiology of accidents. This provides factual data for use in educational and control programs such as the prevention of accidental poisonings of children by various causes, the most common cause being improper storage of drugs and chemicals.

Housing and the Residential Environment

. . . There are 63.4 million occupied dwelling units in the United States (1970).

. . . About 6.7 million occupied dwellings are substandard: of these, 4 million lack one or more essential indoor plumbing facilities, and 2.7 million are in such poor condition that they cannot be rehabilitated without major repair.

. . . About 4 million dwellings of standard quality are overcrowded.

The term *housing*, in the narrow sense, usually refers to physical structures that provide shelter. There are also broader meanings, however, and these are encompassed in the term *residential environment*, which refers to both the dwelling (physical structure) and all aspects of its neighboring environs. The environs and the dwelling are usually functionally interrelated with respect to problems affecting both physical health and mental health. Fifty years ago, principal concerns were for the sanitation aspects of housing as a means of preventing physical illness. Now it is recognized that housing and the residential environment should also promote and contribute to a state of positive physical and mental health and to general social well-being.

Taken as a whole there is substantial evidence of the relationship between health and the quality of the residential environment.[12] It has been found that acute respiratory infections are related to housing deficits such as poor heating or ventilation and inadequate or crowded sleeping arrangements. Digestive tract diseases are associated with crowding, inadequate water supply and sewage, and multiple use of toilet, water, sleeping, and food-handling facilities. Other health hazards associated with poor housing include lead poisoning in children (from ingestion of lead-based paint), carbon monoxide poisoning (from improper heating devices), rodent-transmitted diseases, rat bites, and accidents. Housing also appears to have some influence on family and social relationships. Substandard housing is often part of a complex of problems such as unemployment, school dropout, illegitimacy, alcoholism, drug addiction, crime, and delinquency. This complex is, of course, very likely to be found in inner-city slums. The quality of the residential environment is of great concern in slum areas, therefore, but is not restricted to them. The broad target area actually consists of any place where people live.

Master plans, zoning regulations, and building codes and standards are intended to ensure that new housing is properly located, designed, built, and equipped. Provisions include space for light and ventilation; freedom from avoidable traffic hazards, noise, and air pollution; separation of housing from undesirable industrial and commercial activities; and provision of requisite community services and facilities such as water, sewers, drainage, play and recreational facilities, greenbelts, refuse collection services, and other elements of a good neighborhood. Special consideration also is given to establishing standards for legal conversion of large, old homes to multiple occupancy for apartments, "light-housekeeping" units, rooming houses, or boarding homes; occupancies intended for the aged; mobile home parks; condominiums; and multistoried buildings, especially those intended for large numbers of families with children. The American Public Health Association has long been active in promoting and developing standards for healthful housing by providing goals and guides for designing new housing and by developing codes and evaluation procedures for existing housing.[13]

Housing code administration and enforcement should emphasize the prevention of deterioration in housing and the residential environment, as well as the correction of such conditions. Local official agencies generally are responsible for enforcing state laws regulating sanitation, maintenance, ventilation, and occupancy of all housing. Unfortunately, code enforcement, alone, does not completely correct unsatisfactory housing conditions, and citations and fines are not particularly effective in producing lasting results.

Authority to require vacating of grossly unfit housing is a valuable administrative tool when suitable substitute housing is made available through cooperative programs among health officials, public housing authorities, welfare officials, relocation specialists of community redevelopment agencies, and other agencies or groups with resources for relocating displaced families. In some cases, occupants must be educated and motivated to properly use and maintain housing.

In the past several decades, a number of large-scale programs have come into being to provide new housing and to rehabilitate existing housing and residential environments. Thus, federal financial assistance has helped many communities to provide new *public housing* for low-income families at rents they can afford to pay. Proper utilization of such programs provides acceptable housing for that segment of the population which cannot otherwise afford suitable quarters. In some communities this program is well accepted and supported, while in others groups have objected to such an extent that little or no public housing is being built.

There are a wide variety of federal financial assistance programs available for improving housing and the environs. Some must be administered by a special housing agency authorized by state law and organized by local government. To qualify for such programs, the community must first adopt a "workable program" with several requisite elements, including adequate codes and ordinances; acceptable administrative procedures and financing; assistance for displaced families to find "decent, safe, and sanitary housing at rents they can afford to pay"; citizen participation through communitywide and neighborhood housing committees; a program to evaluate and appraise existing housing; and a master plan to guide future development and redevelopment.

When its program is approved, a community is eligible to receive federal financial aid in various forms. For instance, two federal dollars are available for each local dollar to finance an approved *community renewal project,* which is a comprehensive study of physical, social, and economic factors to plan and program future community improvement programs.

Community redevelopment programs provide federal financial assistance for the acquisition of areas so unfit or poorly planned that they should be cleared, replanned, and rebuilt. The cleared land is sold to private developers who build according to the local agency's plans. *Assisted rehabilitation* is a program in which federal funds are available for a staff to administer and operate area improvement programs and to help property owners plan improvements. Qualifying property owners may obtain government-insured financing to make improvements, and completely unfit units may be purchased and demolished to make room for play areas, parks, or automobile parking. *Code enforcement* assistance is available to pay for extra inspection staff and to finance surface improvements such as paving and street lights.

In the mid-1960's, federal funds became available to qualifying cities to undertake programs to upgrade depressed neighborhoods and improve the lives of the people living in them. Advocating the total attack approach on slum problems, the effort at first was called the Demonstration Cities program, but now is known as the *Model Cities program*. A significant characteristic of the program is that cities are given a free hand—and more responsibility—in deciding how to make the best use of the federal funds they are awarded. There are now 147 Model Cities projects underway across the country. New York has the nation's largest, with a $65 million annual federal grant.

A promising method of influencing the quality of urban growth is the construction of *new towns,* the building of entire communities, including some mainly for older persons.[14] New towns provide a group of goods, services, resources, and facilities needed by the residents, ranging from on-site industry and jobs to complete health care provisions. Between the east and west coasts of the United States, there are about 200 sites, variously called "new towns," "new cities," or "new communities," which are under construction or planned. Each occupies 5,000 or more acres, but only a few so far appear to have serious aspirations of providing jobs and a balanced economy as well as housing. Among the best-known typical new towns at present are Reston, Virginia; Columbia, Maryland; and Irvine, California.

Occupational Health and Safety

. . . More than 14,000 workers in the United States are killed annually in industrial accidents.

. . . Over 2.2 million workers suffer disabling work injuries each year.

. . . Workmen's compensation claims amount to about $3 billion per year.

The target population of occupational health and safety programs is the entire United States work force of over 80 million persons. Some large industries have well-organized, well-staffed, full-time occupational health programs covering medical, nursing,

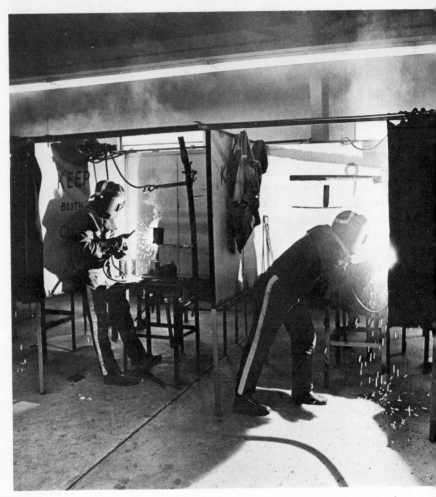

Courtesy of U.S. Department of Labor, Manpower Administration. Robert Moeser, photographer.

engineering, environmental, radiologic, physiologic, and psychologic problems of workers. Industry spends an estimated $320 million annually for these services, but no more than 25 per cent of the total work force is employed in plants where such services are provided. The remainder—75 per cent of those employed—work in approximately 3 million small industries, businesses, and farms, which have fewer than 500 workers each and, with few exceptions, provide little or no health services.

Comprehensive occupational health programs include, first, environmental control of health and safety hazards at the workplace and, second, preventive health maintenance of workers. "Industrial hygiene" is primarily concerned with industrial sanitation and control of those specific materials that are known to produce particular occupational disease.

The earliest industrial hygiene programs resulted from the discovery that workers who were exposed to certain substances, usually over an extended period of time ranging from hours to years, developed specific symptoms which came to be associated with such exposures. Breathing lead fumes or ingesting lead produced peculiar conditions such as the blue line of the gums and wristdrop recognized as symptoms of lead poisoning. Years of exposure to silica dust as in "hard-rock" mining and sandblasting reduced the oxygenation capacity of the lungs and accelerated the ill effects of tuberculosis and other lung diseases. Mercury compounds used in preserving rabbit furs for felt hats produced a nervous irritability which led to the saying "mad as a hatter." Workers not adjusted to exposure to zinc oxide developed a nighttime chill known as brass founder's ague.

In the field of occupational health, the concentration of deleterious material in the worker's environment which produced no demonstrable injury to workers was, for years, called the "maximum allowable concentration." In recent years, the term was redesignated "threshold limit value"[15] to avoid the assumption that an exposure to such material is acceptable if its harmful effects are not now demonstrable. Periodically, new information is developed to show harmful effects from concentrations that had been considered safe. In addition, attention is being directed toward reducing concentrations of pollution in the occupational environment which are irritating or seriously unpleasant, even though the physiologic effects are not yet measurable.

CATEGORIES OF HEALTH HAZARDS

Occupational health hazards to which workers may be exposed are usually classified into four categories. First, are *toxic chemical agents* such as solvents, dusts, gases, metallic compounds, plastics and synthetic resins, and pesticides. Second, there are *physical agents or energy stresses* such as excessive noise, temperature extremes, vibrations, pressures, and laser, ultraviolet, and ionizing radiations. The third category consists of *biologic hazards* such as infectious agents and enzymes. Fourth, are *other work-related stresses* such as rigors of the work process, equipment design, and workplace layout, as well as the relationship between the capabilities and tolerances of the individual worker and the demands and stresses of the job.

As a rule, skin conditions are the most prevalent occupational diseases. Pneumoconioses are the most costly diseases from the standpoint of workmen's compensation, and occupational poisonings persist despite the availability of knowledge for controlling them.

CONTROL OF THE WORKING ENVIRONMENT

A good occupational health program includes checking plans for new plants and new proposed processing operations in order to identify potential hazards and to "build in" appropriate controls. New chemicals are checked and tested for deleterious effects before workers are exposed to them. This kind of industrial hygiene should be carried out in conjunction with all other interested environmental control program administrators. For instance, processes are checked to assure that discharges from workroom ventilation systems meet air pollution control requirements. The source of water supply is checked to be sure that it is safe, and water-piping plans are checked to assure no cross-connections will contaminate the supply. Industrial liquid and solid waste-handling proposals are reviewed. Proposed installations of x-ray units or facilities for use of radionuclides are reviewed. Plans for lighting, ventilation, air conditioning, noise control, first aid, drinking fountains, toilet rooms, dressing rooms, special safety eye showers, and all other items related to health are checked.

A well-rounded program establishes a planned, periodic inspection program for most places of employment. This should cover the entire working environment, including water supplies and cross-connections, stream and air pollution potentials, sanitation, and housekeeping as it relates to safety.

CONTROL OF HAZARDS TO THE WORKER

Control to limit worker exposures to injurious materials is effected by a combination of procedures. Thus, harmless substances are substituted for those that have a deleterious effect, as in the case of the substitution of a nontoxic glue for liver-damaging benzol as a rubber adhesive. Particular kinds of processes are isolated, such as the handling of all lead oxide for batteries in a closed, vacant, glass-sided room until mixed and made into the dust-free battery plate. Local exhaust ventilation is provided in order to draw contaminants away from workers, such as in paint spray booths. Various personal protection devices are used such as aprons and gloves to protect against acids and air-line respirators for sandblasters who cannot be otherwise protected.

In the decade from 1953 to 1963, the number of hearing-loss claims filed by workers against their employers rose dramatically. This started with a New York court case in which, for the first time, substantial compensation was awarded for partial hearing loss, a condition for which such awards previously had been limited to medical costs and lost wages. Awards of over $20,000 have since been made in certain cases. Control of industrial noise exposure includes reduction of noise at its source, isolation of noise-producing operations in sound-proofed areas or rooms, and use of suitable noise-reducing earplugs or muffs. Regular hearing tests are advocated for all employees subject to sound levels that approach 85 decibels for a considerable part of the working day.

Since workmen's compensation laws make occupational diseases compensable (as explained in Chapter 4), physicians report suspected cases. Investigations and tests are made to determine whether a cause-and-effect relationship is demonstrated, and suit-able corrective measures are recommended as required.

PREVENTION OF OCCUPATIONAL DISEASES

Preemployment and periodic examinations are part of a good occupational health program and include special tests to enable measurement of incipient, adverse health effects from the working environment. Such examinations include special blood and urine tests, x-rays, hearing tests, and whatever else may be necessary to learn whether exposure to dusts, fumes, chemicals, noise, and special stresses are producing measurable deleterious effects. Beyond this, the program may tie in with a total preventive and case-finding health program for the worker and his family. Some exemplary programs bring together the entire applicable resources of the employer, the unions, and the official health agency.

Occupational health physicians and nurses observe workers for symptoms of specific diseases. Special effort is made to reduce exposure to excessive temperatures or repeated motion which causes strain. Facilities are provided to make the employees' environment as healthful and pleasant as practical. For outdoor workmen such as telephone linemen, advice is offered on controlling exposure to, and effects of contact with, poison ivy or poison oak. Agricultural workers are given information on methods of protection from toxic sprays—not always effective—and mechanics are advised on skin-damaging effects of various solvents, cutting oils, and chemicals.

Industrial medical, nursing, and consultation services may be operated in conjunction with other official health agency, private agency, or labor organization programs. Programs of this kind may include case-finding for tuberculosis or more broad medical provisions similar to those now existing under certain private and government sponsorship. There must be close collaboration with the workmen's compensation and safety officials of labor departments and with industrial safety experts so that all understand and agree on systems of referrals and avoid conflict and overlapping. While officials of public health agencies are interested in accident prevention, that program is largely the responsibility of labor or industrial welfare agencies, with whom health officials collaborate.

Mental health services are considered to be an important part of comprehensive occupational health programs. Such services cannot, of course, be developed by every company independently, particularly the smaller ones. But large companies or small, the mental health needs of employees are equally important. One solution that is gaining prominence is the utilization of community-based mental health programs, particularly those found in comprehensive community mental health centers (as described in Chapter 5). A center can, in effect, be the mental health service for occupational health programs in a variety of work settings regardless of size. Among the advantages of such arrangements are the quality of mental health care that can be provided and the fact that both the employee and his family can be served.

THE ROLE OF OFFICIAL HEALTH AGENCIES IN OCCUPATIONAL HEALTH

Occupational health units are maintained in 42 states, the District of Columbia, and Puerto Rico as well as in 32 local jurisdictions. Staffing and activities of these programs vary widely, and resources have never been commensurate with size and needs of the work force. Personnel assigned to occupational health duties, either full or part time, in state and local governments numbered 702 in 1969. All state and local expenditures for worker health protection total about 5 cents a year for each member of the nation's work force.

The staff of the occupational health units of those state and local health agencies that have a formal program usually includes one or more physicians, engineers, nurses, chemists, industrial nurse consultants, and a number of industrial hygienists and field inspection personnel. Some occupational health inspection and survey programs are operated only on a consultant basis, responding to requests of other governmental agencies, industry, and labor. Good support has been given, however, to those agencies that make routine visits to all places of employment, comprehensively survey the total working environment, and require necessary corrections. Local health departments sometimes combine this type of program with sanitation inspections of food service, general sanitation, and cross-connection control in places of employment. They then refer observed suspected occupational hazards to industrial hygienists, engineers, nurses, or physician for follow-up or consultation.

State programs vary according to what department is assigned primary responsibility for occupational health. In some states, rather full legal authority is assigned to health departments. In most, the primary legal authority is assigned to another agency, with the health agency serving in a consulting role. However, there is need for an occupational health unit in every state health department in order to provide advice, at least, on health problems of industrial, agricultural, transportation, mining, and construction programs.

The nation's first comprehensive job-safety law became effective early in 1971. Known as the Occupational Safety and Health Act of 1970, it was hailed as the most important legislative item ever for occupational health in the United States. The law is designed to assure safe and healthful working conditions for the nation's work force, and it provides broad authority to the Department of Labor and the Department of Health, Education, and Welfare to accomplish its aims. During the first six months of the act, federal inspectors found violations in four out of every five of the 9,300 workplaces inspected. Three out of every four violations were serious enough to warrant issuing citations against the employers. There were 19,578 alleged violations of safety and health standards involved in the citations.

References

1. Carson, Rachel L. *Silent Spring.* Fawcett Publications, Inc., Greenwich, Connecticut, 1962.
2. Graham, Frank, Jr. *Since Silent Spring.* Houghton Mifflin Company, Boston, 1970.
3. Linton, Ron M. *Terracide.* Paperback Library, New York, 1970.
4. Commoner, Barry. *The Closing Circle: Nature, Man, and Technology.* Alfred A. Knopf, New York, 1971.
5. Odum, Eugene P. *Ecology.* Holt, Rinehart, & Winston, New York, 1966.
6. Sears, Paul B. *Where There Is Life.* Dell Publishing Company, New York, 1962.
7. Storer, John H. *The Web of Life.* Mentor Books, New York, 1961.
8. Hammond, Allen L. Ecosystem analysis: biome approach to environmental research. *Science,* **175:**46–48, January 7, 1972.
9. Dubos, René. Human ecology. *WHO Chron,* **23:**499–504, November 1969.
10. U.S. Department of Health, Education, and Welfare, Public Health Service. *Public Health Service Drinking Water Standards, 1962.* Public Health Service Publication No. 956. U.S. Government Printing Office, Washington, D.C.

11. Senn, C. L., Berger, B. B., Jensen, E. C., Ludwig, H., and Shapiro, M. A. Coliform organisms as an index of water safety. *J Sanit Eng Div Am Soc Civ Eng*, **87**, No. SA6, November 1961.
12. Wilner, Daniel M., Walkley, Rosabelle P., Pinkerton, Thomas C., and Tayback, Matthew. *The Housing Environment and Family Life: A Longitudinal Study of the Effects of Housing on Morbidity and Mental Health.* The Johns Hopkins Press, Baltimore, 1962.
13. American Public Health Association. *Housing: Basic Health Principles and Recommended Ordinances.* The Association, Washington, D.C., 1971.
14. Walkley, Rosabelle P., Mangum, Wiley P., Jr., Sherman, Susan R., Dodds, Suzanne, and Wilner, Daniel M. *Retirement Housing in California.* Diablo Press, Berkeley, California, 1966. Also, Wilner, D. M., Sherman, S. R., Walkley, R. P., Dodds, S., and Mangum, W. P., Jr. Demographic characteristics of residents of planned retirement housing sites. *The Gerontologist*, **8:**164–69, 1968.
15. American Conference of Governmental Industrial Hygienists. *Threshold Limit Values of Industrial Atmospheric Contaminants.* The Conference, published annually.

Additional Reading

American Public Health Association. *Accident Control in Environmental Health Programs — A Guide for Public Health Personnel.* The Association, New York, 1966.
American Public Health Association, Subcommittee on Radiologic Health. *Ionizing Radiation.* The Association, New York, 1966.
Environmental Protection Agency, Water Quality Office. *A Primer on Waste Water Treatment*, revised ed. U.S. Government Printing Office, Washington, D.C., March 1971.

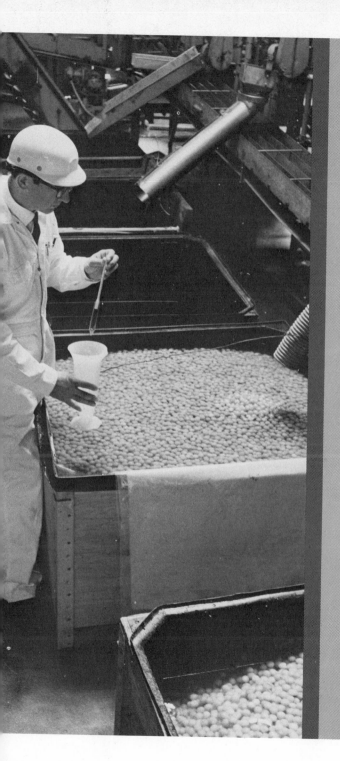

8

ORGANIZATION
OF
ENVIRONMENTAL
PROGRAMS

CHAPTER OUTLINE

The Impetus for Organizing Environmental Programs

The Role of Government
Federal Legislation
Federal Programs
State and Local Activities

The Role of the Private Sector
Action by Industry
Action by Citizens

The Conduct of Environmental Programs
Standard-Setting and Enforcement
Economic Considerations in Pollution Control

The Outlook for Achieving Pollution Control

Manpower for Environmental Programs

The Impetus for Organizing Environmental Programs

In the United States, the year 1970 marked a beginning of unprecedented awareness of and concern with environmental quality in the nation. Federal, state, and local governments, industry, citizens, and international bodies began vigorous activity to restore and protect the environment. There were concerted efforts to organize for such action. Regulatory agencies were strengthened and accelerated the tempo of their programs. Citizens voted for environmental improvements and gave their own time to certain program developments. Industries increasingly made financial commitments to comply with pollution control standards. International institutions entered more forthrightly into the area of environmental action.

Several concepts underlie and provide impetus for the recent organizational and action efforts. First, there is the growing awareness of man's dependence on the intricate web of nature of which he is a part. The realization has grown that man's continued existence depends on the functions of a vast number and variety of other organisms and on the natural cycles that, with great sweep, govern the flow of elements through the earth's environment. Much of the present concern about environmental problems stems from the knowledge that man has disrupted natural cycles and has been responsible for polluting, contaminating, and degrading the environment (see Chapter 7).

Second, as greater concern is being directed toward the quality of the natural environment, there is also an awareness that increased attention must be given to the quality of the *man-made* environment in its totality. If life is to be satisfying, the environment must do more than merely sustain it. The environment must, in addition, provide the esthetic satisfaction and the sense of human dignity that give meaning and purpose to existence.[1] The impact of the total environment on man is suggested in the following statement by René Dubos: "Man is in general more the product of his environment than his genetic endowment. The health of the people is determined not by their race but by the conditions of their life."[2]

Third, there is recognition of the need to develop a broad approach to environmental problems, rather than one limited to the now outmoded concept that an environmental effort must be justified in terms of disease control. Concern is no longer limited to direct and long-range microbiologic, toxic, or carcinogenic effects; now attention is additionally directed toward all other stresses and forces that affect man. Clean water, decent housing, pure air, and pleasant surroundings are objectives and programs that need not be "sold" on the basis of disease control.

The Role of Government

There have been federal and state laws to protect the environment for many years, with new measures to regulate water and air pollution on the books since the end of World War II. Recent years, however, have witnessed a far greater commitment to environmental preservation on the part of governments at all levels. The efforts have taken two forms: first, organization for a comprehensive approach to the total environment; and second, strengthening the control and management of individual segments of the environment. The measures provide for centralization of administrative authority, greater fiscal aid to local projects, and increased regulatory control.

Since 1969 at the federal level, a *national environmental policy* has been established, a comprehensive environmental policy-making agency has been created, and many former operating agencies have been consolidated. There were also gains in setting water quality standards, in air pollution control regulation, and in solid waste management.

Parallel activities took place at the state level, with efforts at reorganization and consolidation as well as new approaches to financing pollution control and strengthening regulation of water quality. In addition, states began to take long-range views of environmental quality, with moves toward land-use planning and efforts at environmental education.

FEDERAL LEGISLATION

National concern about the quality of the environment was reflected in activities of the United States Congress early in the

1970's when environmental bills constituted fully 20 per cent of the congressional workload. The bills ranged from severe restrictions on open burning and ocean dumping to reclamation of strip-mined land and noise controls on jet planes. Significant federal legislative enactments in this period included two measures dealing with broad policy and organizational matters (the National Environmental Policy Act of 1969 and the Environmental Quality Improvement Act of 1970) as well as three major antipollution laws in the areas of air, water, and solid waste (the Clean Air Act Amendments, the Water Quality Improvement Act, and the Resource Recovery Act).

The National Environmental Policy Act of 1969 (signed into law on January 1, 1970) established a national policy to "maintain conditions under which man and nature can exist in productive harmony, and fulfill the social, economic, and other requirements of present and future generations of Americans." The act created a Council on Environmental Quality to coordinate environmental activities at the federal level and to serve as the principal advisory body to the President in such matters.[1] Under another provision of the act, all federal agencies and all state and local governments applying for federal aid are required to file a statement on the impact of proposed projects on the environment.

The Environmental Quality Improvement Act of 1970 strengthened the Council on Environmental Quality by establishing an Office of Environmental Quality to supplement council staff, to assist federal agencies in coordinating environmental programs, and to develop interrelated federal environmental quality criteria.

The Clean Air Act Amendments of 1970 is an omnibus measure amending earlier federal legislation. The first federal program on air pollution was developed in 1955 when the Public Health Service conducted a modest air pollution research program and offered technical assistance to state and local governments. In 1963, Congress passed the Clean Air Act, which constituted landmark legislation and included authorization for financial assistance to state and local governments to initiate and improve control programs as well as provisions for federal-interstate abatement actions. The Air Quality Act of 1967 provided for the designation of a system of nationwide air quality control regions and required states to establish air quality standards and implementation plans for the regions designated.

The 1970 Clean Air Act Amendments authorized establishment of national ambient air quality standards specifying the maximum levels to be permitted in the ambient air of the principal and most widespread classes of air pollutants. States must carry out approved implementation plans for limiting the emission of pollutants, and the federal government is authorized to act if a state fails to do so. The legislation provides for the formulation of motor vehicle emission standards and provides grants to state agencies for developing and maintaining systems for testing motor vehicle emission devices. Provision is made for issuance of aircraft emission standards and for study of possible noise standards. The legislation also permits class action suits against any public or private air pollution offenders.

The Water Quality Improvement Act of 1970 included important new authorizations to fight pollution, thus stepping up federal clean water efforts which had begun formally in 1956 with passage of the first pollution control measures. In 1965, the Water Quality Act provided for establishing water quality standards for all interstate and coastal waters. The standards specify stream-use classification (whether for recreation, fish and wildlife propagation, public water supplies, industrial uses, or agricultural purposes); the quality of water required to support these uses; and plans for achieving and enforcing the desired levels of quality.

A significant mechanism for achieving clean water was provided in 1966 when a federal court decision held that the Refuse Act of 1899 outlaws industrial discharges of pollutants into navigable waters or their tributaries without a permit. In the Water Quality Improvement Act of 1970, Congress clarified liability for oil pollution in coastal areas and set stiff penalties for deliberate or negligent oil pollution. It also directed the President to prepare a National Contingency Plan to enable swift and effective mobilization of federal, state, and local resources in case of major oil spills. Other provisions of the act included formulation of national standards for marine sanitation devices, assessing needs for and training of manpower for waste treatment operations, and demonstration grants for water pollution control projects in mine areas and in the Great Lakes region.

The Resource Recovery Act of 1970 constituted an omnibus amendment to the Solid Waste Disposal Act of 1965, which had marked the first significant interest by the federal government in the problems of solid waste management. The 1965 act offered assistance to state and local governments and others involved in managing solid wastes. It provided financial grants to demonstrate new technology, technical assistance through research and training, and encouragement of proper planning for state and local solid waste management programs. The Resource Recovery Act of 1970 provided a new focus on recycling and recovery of valuable waste materials. It also authorized a study of potential sites for the storage and disposal of hazardous wastes, and it provided for the training of personnel in waste disposal occupations.

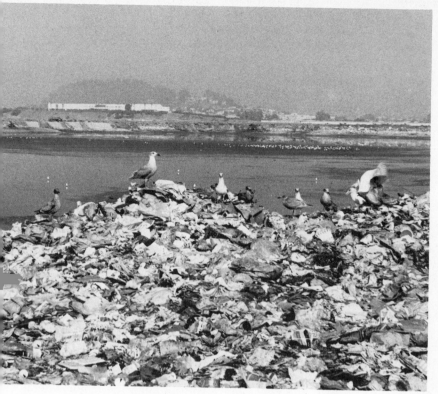

Courtesy of California's Health, *California Department of Public Health. Staff photo.*

FEDERAL PROGRAMS

Prior to 1970, efforts at the federal level to control pollution through environmental programs were hampered by the scattering of responsibilities through numerous federal agencies. The resulting piecemeal approach to environmental problems inhibited progress and sometimes merely substituted one form of pollution for another. In order to launch a more comprehensive attack, federal programs dealing with the environment were reorganized and strengthened in 1970.

Environmental Protection Agency. The United States Environmental Protection Agency was established and designated an independent entity reporting directly to the President, and is responsible for the environmental problems of air pollution, water pollution, solid waste management, pesticides, radiation, and noise. Created to lead a broad, comprehensive attack on pollution, the Environmental Protection Agency brings together for the first time in a single organization the major environmental control programs of the federal government. The agency has regulatory responsibilities, establishing and enforcing environmental standards within the limits of its legal authority. It also conducts research, monitors and analyzes the environment, and undertakes studies of the causes and effects of pollution as well as the techniques of pollution control. In addition to research carried out in its own laboratories located throughout the nation, the agency supports studies in universities and other research institutions through grants and contracts.

The Environmental Protection Agency provides technical and financial assistance to regional, state, and local jurisdictions. It maintains regional offices in ten major cities. These offices are empowered to act for the agency and to give assistance to state and local authorities, industries, and citizens in the solution of technical problems. The agency also provides a training program to help develop the skilled manpower needed to combat environmental problems. It serves as a source of information to the public, disseminating scientific data bearing on environmental problems.

National Oceanic and Atmospheric Administration. The second major organizational innovation in the federal government's stepped-up attack on pollution was the National Oceanic and Atmospheric Administration. Established within the Department of Commerce in 1970, the new agency consolidated the major federal programs of oceanic and atmospheric research and monitoring, including the United States Weather Bureau and the Coast and Geodetic Survey. The administration is responsible for research on long-range effects of pollution on the physical environment. It monitors the impact of pollution on the marine environment; describes changes in the oceans, estuaries, and the atmosphere; and establishes ecologic baseline data and models.

Public Health Service. Several programs related to environmental quality are the responsibility of the Public Health Service within the U.S. Department of Health, Education, and Welfare. The oldest and perhaps the best-known programs are those of the Service's Food and Drug Administration (which began its functions in the 1920's in the U.S. Department of Agriculture). The Food and Drug Administration has regulatory responsibilities for sanitary conditions, raw materials used, and controls exercised in the production, packaging, and labeling of products destined for interstate shipment. The FDA undertakes research in the characteristics, safety, efficacy, and toxicity of a wide variety of consumer products; controls the marketing of new drugs; establishes food standards; monitors the safety and/or efficacy of food additives, antibiotics, coloring agents, and household chemicals; and conducts educational programs to bring about compliance with legal requirements.

The Health Services and Mental Health Administration (in the Department of Health, Education, and Welfare) has two units with responsibilities for environmental programs. One is the Bureau of Community Environmental Management, which is concerned with the man-made or built environment plus the sociocultural aspects of neighborhoods and communities. The bureau's emphasis is on environmental problems of the inner city, but it also has basic concern with broad concepts of human ecosystems. The bureau recommends and promotes a policy of comprehensive long-term planning by local communities to define their problems and needs, set priorities for action, and carry out successive improvement of projects of several years' duration. Specific program responsibilities include urban rat control, lead poisoning eradication, health aspects of housing, control of accidental injuries, and recreational and general sanitation.

The second environmental unit within the Health Services and Mental Health Administration is the National Institute for Occupational Safety and Health. Under the Occupational Safety and Health Act of 1970, the institute is responsible for extensive research and training programs and makes evaluations of the hazards of workplaces on written request from employers and employee groups. The institute also administers the health activities of the Federal Coal Mine Health and Safety Act of 1969, which includes the development of mandatory health standards for coal mines and the provision of a medical examination program for underground coal miners for the detection of pneumoconiosis ("black lung disease").

As one of the National Institutes of Health (in the Department of Health, Education, and Welfare), the National Institute of Environmental Health Sciences conducts a program of long-term scientific inquiry into the mechanisms by which environmental factors produce injurious effects on exposed persons. It investigates the circumstances that make these factors operative, the nature of bodily responses to the factors, and the consequences for health, longevity, and productivity of human beings. The institute conducts its own research studies and supports research and research-training activities in educational institutions and other public and private nonprofit organizations.

STATE AND LOCAL ACTIVITIES

States, like the federal government, began to reorganize and expand their environmental programs in the 1969–1970 period. For many years prior to that time every state conducted at least basic sanitation programs which usually included water, food, milk, and drug purity; waste treatment and sewage disposal; rodent, insect, and other vector control; and housing and institutional standards. States also have generally had provisions for occupational and radiologic health programs and for limited air and water pollution control activities. The local programs associated with these state provisions have usually consisted largely of periodic inspections of a wide variety of businesses and activities, and involved code enforcement as well as issuing of health permits and licenses. At both state and local levels, environmental programs have traditionally been scattered among several agencies, boards, and commissions. Scattering of responsibilities still exists, but the new thrust to preserve and enhance the environment has led to action on state and local levels to overcome the confusion of multiple jurisdictional authorities.

In line with current trends, state and local governments are carrying out organizational reforms, increasing their enforcement activities, augmenting funds and manpower for environmental programs, tightening pollution control standards, and proposing and enacting a wide range of new legislation. Although local governments are vital in pollution control, federal legislation has been placing more and more responsibility on the states. Increased state involvement is thought to be the key to more effective pollution control particularly because it can be a first step in the direction of comprehensive, *regional* efforts.

Recognition at the state level of the need for a broad approach to the environment has coincided with a general trend to modernize state government management and increase executive accountability. The result has been a wide-ranging move to consolidate environmental functions into a single broad-based state agency, frequently a department for the environment in new cabinet-style state executive systems. New York set up one of the most comprehensive programs in 1970. It consolidated all environmental and resource programs into a Department of Environmental Conservation, which has responsibility for developing an overall environmental plan, administering all the programs, assessing new threats to the environment, conducting research, and carrying on public education. Similar reorganization-consolidations have been made in Washington and Illinois, and other major actions have taken place in more than a dozen additional states.

State increases from 1970 to 1971 in funds and manpower for two categories of pollution control—air and water—are shown in Figure 8-1. The amounts reflect spending for standard setting and enforcement, monitoring, planning, and training; they do not in-

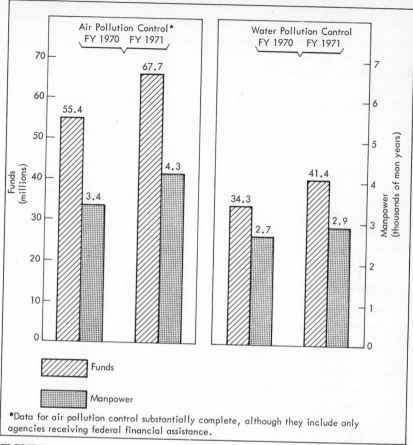

FIGURE 8-1. *Funds and manpower for state and local air and water pollution control agencies (includes federal financial assistance).* [Source: *Environmental Protection Agency. In: The Council on Environmental Quality.* Environmental Quality: The Second Annual Report, *August 1971, p. 40.*]

clude substantial expenditures (primarily at the local level) for pollution control facilities such as waste treatment plants. The states in general have broadened their fiscal support of environmental efforts through a variety of traditional and new monetary devices. A sizable number of states have undertaken bond issues. To encourage industries to control pollution, many states have granted tax exemptions on control equipment. Maryland and New York have created full-scale environmental finance corporations to aid localities with a wide range of projects. In spite of these and other efforts, however, financing of programs and manpower shortages continue to be grave concerns.

Many states have tightened their pollution control standards or have expanded coverage to new pollutants or activities. It has been estimated that states and localities have passed more than 1,000 laws and ordinances aimed at air, water, and solid waste pollution. Many states also have intensified antipollution enforcement activities.

State governments have been taking a closer look at the important area of land use regulation. Under the United States Constitution, states have the authority to regulate land use, but most have delegated the authority to local governments, which in turn generally consider it largely a problem of controlling urban development through zoning systems. However, traditional local zoning systems are not considered adequate to deal with today's environmental problems, and expanding state intervention in land use regulation is aimed at controlling the use of land to meet the needs of preservation as well as development.

The Role of the Private Sector

Accelerated action by government to restore and protect the environment has been accompanied by activity in the private sector, notably on the part of industry and private citizens. Industries, partly on their own initiative and partly from outside pressure, are undertaking the development and application of technology for pollution control, as well as assuming some of the financial burden entailed. Private citizens throughout the nation have shown concern and taken action through a variety of organizations and by political and legal means.

ACTION BY INDUSTRY

Industrial processes have been major contributors to the nation's pollution problems, in both quantity and toxicity. Therefore, large-scale reduction in the levels of the most serious pollutants requires an effective and sustained effort by industry. Such efforts include installing pollution control equipment and other facilities, developing new technology, and making major changes in management policies.

Although industrial spending for pollution control is difficult to assess, it has been estimated that the nation's utilities, oil companies, paper mills, steel plants, nonferrous metal producers, and chemical works invested about $2 billion in equipment alone to meet stricter government standards in 1971. In general, industry's expenditures for pollution control appear to have risen significantly in recent years, but authorities agree that even higher rates of spending will be required by some industries if they are to meet standards established under current laws.

A number of technologic innovations by industry have already helped to solve certain pollution problems. The electrostatic precipi- tator, which was developed years ago, has made possible virtual elimination of all fly ash and dust emissions from fuel-burning facilities. More recently, a process has been developed to remove sulfur oxides from stack gases. The pulp and paper industry is developing a closed system for water recycling in order to avoid waste water discharges which pollute. Many firms have undertaken complex research and development to provide new solid waste recycling technology. Despite progress, however, there still remains a pressing need to develop better technology to control a wide range of toxic substances and other environmental pollutants — without, in the process, introducing new hazards.

Industrial management has a vital role to play in abating pollu- tion and enhancing environmental quality. Management decisions regarding major actions such as location of new plants and pur- chases of heavy equipment have import for pollution control. In- vesting in abatement facilities and participating in community environment programs are other facets of management policy that affect the total effort to improve the environment. Some companies have reorganized to give increased emphasis to pollution control, including the designation of executives charged with environmental responsibilities. In some cases these responsibilities include ad- vance review of the company's designs and plans from the stand- point of their impact on the environment.

ACTION BY CITIZENS

The American public has become involved in environmental issues through several routes, one being participation in local and national environmental organizations. There were an estimated 3,100 of these organizations in the United States in 1971. *Local envi- ronmental organizations* often form to concentrate on a single project such as saving a particular area from degradation by pollution or poorly planned development. Concern for the problems of the urban environment and particularly those of the inner city has been the focus for a growing number of these local citizen groups. *Na- tional environmental organizations* have traditionally promoted con- servationist interests, and they have now expanded their activities to include new areas that had previously received little attention. Chief among them are programs to examine urban and interna- tional environmental issues. *Civic and social groups* have provided another avenue of citizen involvement in activities to control pollution and enhance the environment. Many of these groups have launched cleanup projects and conservation programs, with the effort sometimes national in scope.

Citizen interest in the environment has become evident in *political action* of various kinds. One way has been at the polls, voting for bond issues to finance environmental measures. In 1970, voters in four states alone (California, Illinois, Oregon, and Wisconsin) approved $1.3 billion in state bonds for pollution control facilities. Environmental quality has also become an issue in election campaigns for public office. The records and positions of candidates on environmental matters were of considerable importance in a number of campaigns in 1970. Although it is difficult to attribute specific defeats and victories solely to a candidate's stand on environmental issues, it appears in some cases to have been an important factor.

Citizens and environmental groups have also turned to *legal action* as a remedy for environmental degradation. Citizen-initiated court cases can halt actual or potential instances of pollution and may also lead to more comprehensive and rational planning by focusing public attention on a problem.[3] Known as "public interest" litigations, these court actions have challenged specific government and private activities that were environmentally undesirable. They have speeded up court definition of what is required of federal agencies under environmental protection statutes. The suits have forced both government and industry to be more aware of environmental considerations, and they have educated lawmakers and the public in the need for new environmental legislation. The court cases often have been handled by "public interest lawyers" and supported by biologists, urban planners, and other professionals who donate their time to study the technical aspects of the issue and appear before the court to offer expert testimony.

The Conduct of Environmental Programs

STANDARD-SETTING AND ENFORCEMENT

The most common strategy to deal with environmental problems is to set and enforce environmental quality standards. This applies whether the problem involves a sanitation program (e.g., milk purity) or a pollution control program (e.g., river contamination). Standards are based on available scientific knowledge, and target levels of quality are established according to what is known about the toxicity, persistence, and other effects of contaminants.

Pollution Control. In pollution control, the discharge into the environment of materials that are extremely hazardous to health may need to be entirely forbidden. For other waste discharges not crippling to human health, it is more reasonable to curtail but not outlaw them.

Enforcement, once pollution standards have been established, can be laborious and time-consuming. Public agencies charged with enforcement must locate and prove violations of standards, and some companies and municipalities that have been ordered to undertake specified control action have been able to delay or circumvent compliance. However, the fact that enforcement authority can be used effectively was illustrated by the Environmental Protection Agency within the first year after its establishment. For example, the agency was instrumental in closing 23 large industrial plants for about 24 hours in order to relieve an air pollution crisis in a major southern city. In other action enforcing water quality standards, the agency issued 47 violation notices to municipal or industrial polluters. By mid-1971, more than 50 civil or criminal actions had been brought against industrial polluters of water.

Strategies other than enforcement are possible in achieving environmental goals. One is persuasion—relying on a sense of community pride and responsibility. This technique often works in prodding individual actions, such as antilittering or beautification, but it is less likely to be effective with a manufacturer who is concerned with competition and profits. In the latter cases, economic incentives are considered to be more successful. One promising possibility in this category is the "pollution charge," the levying of financial charges for dumping waste materials into the environment.[4] Under this plan, charge levels can be set to stimulate each discharger to take positive and effective action to curb pollution. Pollution control officials consider that standard-setting and enforcement in combination with economic incentives can provide powerful tools to achieve a high-quality environment.[1]

Sanitation Measures. Several agencies and organizations, notably the Public Health Service and the American Public Health Association, have prepared model codes for use in promulgating standards for milk, drinking water, food service, housing, swimming pools, and other areas where sanitation provisions are a public responsibility. The purpose of the model codes is to enable state and local jurisdiction to achieve a high degree of uniformity of regulations, thereby overcoming the confusion that can arise when communities have widely differing codes and standards.

In most large communities, there are usually several kinds of abatement provisions. These include legally requiring quarantining contaminated foods, providing emergency treatment of water, abating overflowing sewage, and vacating unfit housing. Other provisions may pertain to closing grossly substandard swimming pools and beaches, abating heavy rodent or insect infestations, and correcting serious occupational health hazards.

The first step in enforcement of sanitation codes usually consists of periodic inspections during which defects are noted and instructions or check sheets are issued indicating what improvements are required. This technique used alone, however, is not as effective as might be hoped because, too often, the same or similar unsatisfactory conditions are found repeatedly or are only temporarily corrected.

Various other methods are often used, therefore, to obtain compliance with standards. One of the most important is to make certain that new construction and equipment meets code requirements from the beginning.

Another method is the conduct of organized training programs for persons with operational responsibilities (e.g., food handlers, milk plant operators, water treatment plant operators). The goal is to educate the persons responsible so that they understand what is desired and to stimulate them to want to do what is necessary to meet standards. Sometimes various categories of operating personnel are required to be certified or licensed.

Issuing of health permits or grades is an additional effective regulatory method. The health permit usually is legally established; it is withheld, denied, or revoked until standards are met; and it is subject to suspension for significant violations of requirements. The grading system is sometimes applied to food establishments and milk supplies. The grade—"A," "B," or "C"—once it is assigned as the outcome of inspection, must be prominently posted on the food establishment premises or printed on the milk container.

ECONOMIC CONSIDERATIONS IN POLLUTION CONTROL

Environmental pollution problems to a large extent are rooted in the way the nation's economy operates, as has been suggested earlier. At the same time, efforts to alleviate these problems have almost inescapable impact on the economy. The magnitude of the cost of pollution control is one aspect of this impact. It has been estimated that total spending required for the six-year period of 1970–1975 for the major sources of environmental pollution—air, water, and solid waste—will amount to more than $105 billion. Figure 8-2 shows the relative contribution to this total of the costs of air and water pollution control and solid waste management.

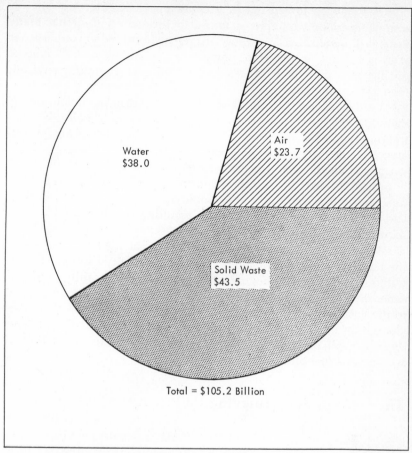

Water
$38.0

Air
$23.7

Solid Waste
$43.5

Total = $105.2 Billion

FIGURE 8-2. *Estimated cumulative expenditures for air, water, and solid waste pollution control, 1970–1975.* [SOURCE: *Environmental Protection Agency. In: The Council on Environmental Quality.* Environmental Quality: The Second Annual Report, *August 1971, p. 113.*]

The largest share, $43.5 billion, will be needed for solid waste abatement, followed by $38.0 billion for water pollution control.

Reducing the harmful effects of pollution will require adjustments in the nation's economy.[1] Some businesses and industries, particularly those that must absorb large costs of pollution control, will be hard hit. Pollution abatement requirements are likely to fall with different impacts on single plants within an industry, even though the same control requirements may apply to all. Some weak or poorly situated plants or companies will unquestionably have difficulty gearing to environmental requirements, and a number may be forced out of business. The brighter side of this somewhat gloomy picture is found in the expectation that many firms will benefit because they will replace outmoded technologies with new ones. In addition, new firms and industries will emerge during the adjustment process in response to changing environmental requirements.

Public agencies and lawmakers are turning attention to methods of dealing with the transitional impacts of pollution control on businesses and industries, and several strategies are considered feasible. These include greater use of tax devices, particularly various kinds of exemptions; direct federal grants to meet all or part of industry's costs for pollution control; loans to businesses and industries; and retraining and reemployment programs for workers laid off because of plant close-down resulting from pollution control requirements.

In general, those concerned with national policy consider that the nation's commitment to environmental quality can be achieved without sacrificing the goal of maintaining a healthy dynamic economy.[1] It is felt that American business and industry will adjust to the costs of pollution control just as they have adjusted to other changes in the costs of doing business. The most difficult problems to solve will obviously be those arising from the dislocation of workers made jobless by plant closings.

The Outlook for Achieving Pollution Control

There are those who hold that efforts to alleviate environmental degradation are too late—that man is helpless to control the technologic forces he has set in motion and life on this planet is already doomed. Others believe that claims about environmental deterioration are considerably exaggerated and that most of the problem consists of the sound and fury created by the alarmists. Even while these debates have been going on, however, it is clear that new understanding, planning, and action have been emerging in both public and private sectors.

The scattered concerns of a few years ago have, more recently, coalesced into a broader understanding of the relationship of the environment to man's total well-being, as well as an appreciation of how complex and multifaceted the problems are. Governmental institutions, the law, and the economy have begun to adjust to a new set of goals which take environmental quality into account. Much of the stimulus for environmental improvement must come from the citizen, who in the long run decides how much he is willing to pay for pollution control. The extent to which pollution control and other environmental enhancement activities become part of the organization, policies, and cost decisions of business and industry also will be significant factors in the nation's ability to achieve environmental goals.

Although important starts have been made, there remain — in both the public and private sectors — many deeply ingrained habits that must be reformed and attitudes that must be reshaped if environmental quality is to be improved. Some very basic and traditional notions of growth, autonomy, and individualism are involved. Long-standing ideas about jurisdictional boundaries will undoubtedly need to give way to regional or other areawide concepts. There is, for example, little to be gained if one city passes laws to stop polluting its river, while another city upstream runs sewers into it.

There seems little doubt that the pursuit of environmental quality has become a firm national commitment. Perhaps the most significant new element in the nation's outlook is the emergence of what has been called the *environmental ethic*. It is a reflection of a change in individual and collective values, and there are signs that it will become a genuine force in guiding environmental action.

Manpower for Environmental Programs

The many different programs in the broad area of environmental enhancement and pollution control require numerous categories of personnel representing a wide variety of professional and technical skills. Three basic and general categories of workers are distinguishable: environmental engineers, categorical program specialists, and sanitarians. Specific types of personnel are far more numerous and complex than this grouping would indicate, however. For example, there are several different kinds of environmental engineers; and each categoric program (e.g., air pollution control) includes a number of different types of occupational specialties. In recent years, the trend has been to utilize technicians and aides for certain routine inspections, sample collection, and monitoring. More highly qualified administrative and technical personnel are thereby freed to organize, plan and manage programs, handle special problems, undertake research, conduct demonstration projects, and perform the more technical inspectional and educational activities.

Environmental engineers apply engineering and scientific principles and practices to the prevention, control, and management of environmental factors that may influence man's physical and mental health and general well-being. Prior to the last decade, engineers in the health field were engaged primarily in environmental sanitation activities, but with the broadening of environmental concerns the diversity of tasks for engineers has also broadened considerably.

Air pollution control personnel are one example of *categoric program specialists* and include engineers, chemists, meteorologists, statisticians, physicists, biologists, sanitarians, technicians, inspectors, and a variety of other occupational designations. Radiation protection personnel, as another example of categoric program specialists, include health physicists, engineers, chemists, biologists, and other scientific and technical occupations with special training in the health aspects of radiation. Their work is conducted mainly in industrial, medical, research, or educational institutions that use radiation sources, and in health agencies that have responsibility for health protection. A third example of categoric program specialists consists of industrial hygiene personnel and includes industrial hygienists, engineers, chemists, toxicologists, physiologists, occupational hygienists, dermatologists, environmental hygienists, technicians, and other related occupational designations. In workplaces that offer a comprehensive preventive health program for their employees, occupational health programs may also be staffed with physicians, nurses, toxicologists, x-ray technicians, and laboratory personnel.

Sanitarians perform a broad range of duties, including the conduct of inspection programs in food manufacturing and processing plants, dairies, water supply systems, and so on. They seek compliance with local regulations and with state and federal laws relating to environmental health. They also plan and conduct sanitation programs, administer environmental health programs, and promote the enactment of health regulations and laws.

As environmental protection programs have increased, there has also been increasing need for trained technicians and aides. Environmental technicians assist professional personnel in the conduct of a variety of environmental control programs. Specific tasks may include inspections, surveys, and evaluations to determine compliance with laws and regulations; collection of samples and performing of tests; and operating environmental sanitation facilities such as water purification systems. Environmental aides assist professional personnel and environmental technicians, performing a variety of routine tasks under supervision.

Although there is great need for personnel to staff environmental *service* programs, there is also pressing demand for professional specialists who have appropriate training and background for the conduct of environmental *research* programs. One of the most urgent research needs is the investigation of deleterious effects resulting from long-term exposure to low levels of chemical, physical, and biologic substances, alone or in combination. Other areas of needed research include environmental monitoring and surveillance, methods of recycling wastes, and the development of nonpolluting industrial processes. Many of the categories of personnel just enumerated participate in these and other research efforts on environmental quality and pollution control. Present trends increasingly are toward a multidisciplinary approach in the conduct of environmental research—several persons from different professions and academic disciplines pooling their knowledge to solve a research problem.

References

1. Council on Environmental Quality. *Environmental Quality: The Second Annual Report.* U.S. Government Printing Office, Washington, D.C., August 1971.
2. Dubos, René. *Man and His Environment.* Pan-American Health Organization Scientific Publication No. 131. Washington, D.C., 1966.
3. Levi, Donald R., and Colyer, Dale. Legal remedies for pollution abatement. *Science,* **175:**1085–87, March 10, 1972.
4. Freeman, A. Myrick, III, and Haveman, Robert H. Residuals charges for pollution control: a policy evaluation. *Science,* **177:**322–29, July 28, 1972.

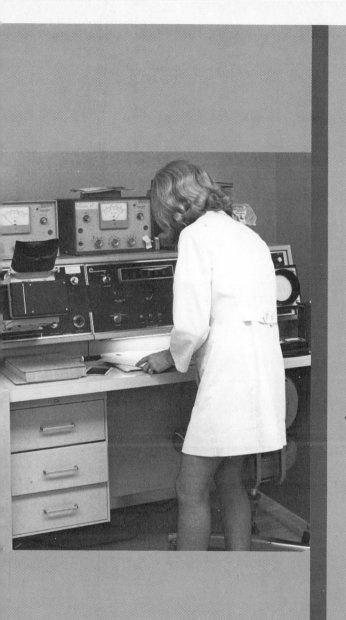

9

MEASUREMENT
OF
HEALTH STATUS
AND
THE SEARCH FOR
DISEASE
CAUSATION

CHAPTER OUTLINE

Courtesy of California's Health, *California Department of Public Health.*
Staff photo.

The commonest measures of the health status of a population are illnesses (how many and what kind) and deaths (how many and from what causes). Other measures that help further to illuminate health status include whether the population, numerically, is growing, declining, or staying about the same; whether it is young or old; how it is distributed geographically; how mobile it is; and the extent of births, marriages, and divorces.

The Components of Demographic Data and Vital Statistics

Demographic data consist of numbers that describe (a) population size and characteristics, and (b) vital events of birth, death, marriage, and divorce. Information on population size is derived from census enumeration of the number and characteristics of persons living in a specified area at a particular time. Information on vital events is obtained from official registration records of births, deaths, marriages, and divorces. *Vital statistics* relate the total numbers of various kinds of vital events that occur over a period of time (usually one calendar year) to the size of the affected population.

The number of occurrences of a vital event has little meaning unless it is related either to the total population within which the event occurs or to that segment of the population which is subject to the risk of the event. For example, only females age 15 to 49 rather than those of all ages are usually considered to be at risk for the occurrence of pregnancy. Because vital events, to be meaningful, must be related to population size, people within the relevant geographic area must be counted, and each individual's age, sex, and other characteristics enumerated. The resulting information describes the composition of the population, and the evaluation of vital statistics must be made in light of this composition; a population's death rates, for example, are influenced by age distribution, sex ratio, racial components, and other factors.

Although the main sources of demographic information are the records of vital registration and enumeration of the census,* many agencies, institutions, and individuals also conduct sample surveys in order to obtain demographic data. In addition, special health surveys of particular diseases such as coronary heart disease are sometimes used to supplement knowledge in specific areas. These surveys are needed when more detailed information is required from individuals and when that information is not collected in the desired detail from large aggregates of individuals. Frequently sampling techniques are used in a study to gain health information which is then used in connection with census and vital registration data.

Census or Enumeration Information

THE DECENNIAL CENSUS

The Constitution of the United States provides that a regular census be taken of the country's inhabitants, and the first such count was made in 1790. Though the U.S. Census is not the oldest, it has the longest continuous record of any census in history. Originally the count was made to determine the number of representatives each state was entitled to send to the House of Representatives. As time went by, the usefulness of census information to government, business, welfare workers, and numerous other individuals, groups, and agencies became obvious. The volume and variety of information collected have grown tremendously, and the requests for additional data remain unabated.

Kinds of Information Obtained and Methods Used. Every ten years the Bureau of the Census (U.S. Department of Commerce) takes on the herculean task of counting every man, woman, and child in the United States. The age, sex, race, and marital status of each individual are recorded, and data are obtained about the number and make-up of households. Additional information, such as condition of housing, income, education, occupation, distance traveled to and from work, and length of stay in present residence, is acquired from representative samples of the population. In the 1970 census, either a 5, 15, or 20 per cent sample of households was asked these additional questions. Data obtained by the sampling procedures employed by the census may be used with confidence.

* There are other sources, which are demographically interesting, but are not directly relevant to health problems — for example, information from the Immigration and Naturalization Service.

Undoubtedly sampling will be used more and more in future census counts. Among other advantages, it enables the bureau to obtain more information per given cost than could be obtained with complete enumeration. To obtain useful information within small geographic areas, however, complete enumeration is necessary. This is one of the reasons for retaining a complete count of some items in the census.

In the past, an enumerator visited every household to ask for information, which he recorded on the standard census schedule (questionnaire form) of population and housing. In 1960, an "Advance Census Report," mailed to all homes, asked for information about the dwelling and the individuals who lived there. This was to be completed and made ready for the enumerator who transferred the information to the census schedule. The 1970 census relied even more on a mailed questionnaire, particularly in the larger metropolitan areas and adjacent counties. Census forms were mailed to each household, filled out by the respondents on census day, and returned by mail to the census office. Enumerators visited only those households that failed to mail back their forms or omitted items of information that the enumerator could not obtain by telephone.

Much preliminary planning is needed in the conduct of the census. This involves choosing the questions to be asked and checking the legal authority for asking them. Needs of government have top priority, but the needs of businessmen, labor leaders, and research workers in all fields using census data are considered. Attention is given to recommendations of the United Nations, which tries to encourage greater comparability among the population statistics of all nations. Furthermore, the questions to be asked must be pretested and geographic areas must be defined; instructions must be prepared for the enumerators, crew leaders, and district supervisors.

Geographic Units for Data Collection. For purposes of collecting information on population and housing, the United States is divided into enumeration districts. These districts are carefully mapped by the Census Bureau, often after consultation with local authorities. Care is taken that these small, well-defined areas are delineated in such a way as to take account of the boundaries of various governmental units. Local governments rely heavily on census information for such needs as planning health, welfare, and education programs; planning construction and development projects (schools and hospitals, for example); and determining legislative representation. Some federal funds are allocated to states on a per-person basis; the estimated number of persons and thus the amount of money are based on census counts. When the information that has been collected by enumeration districts appears in published form, it is summarized in tables for various geographic and governmental units.

Geographic Units for Tabulating and Reporting. For purposes of tabulating and reporting census information, the United States is divided into a series of progressively smaller units. The largest units consist of four *regions* and nine *divisions* within the regions, as follows:

A. Northeast
   1. New England
   2. Middle Atlantic
B. North Central
   3. East North Central
   4. West North Central
C. South
   5. South Atlantic
   6. East South Central
   7. West South Atlantic
D. West
   8. Mountain
   9. Pacific

Each *state* falls within one of the nine divisions. Information is published for regions, for divisions, and for each state. Within states, information is prepared for *counties* when appropriate. For some kinds of information, an *urban-nonurban* classification may be preferable. Information for the urban areas is available by *census tract* for all areas that have been tracted. Census tracts are small geographic units into which metropolitan areas are divided for purposes of reporting population characteristics, and these characteristics tend to be quite homogeneous within tracts. Requests have been made to the Census Bureau that censuses obtain more detailed information for very small areas, but one of the problems in providing such information, e.g., for a city block, is that of protecting individuals' rights to privacy. Areas must be kept large enough so that data can be made available in aggregates that will not betray information about particular individuals or households.

The census must take account of changing patterns of population distribution and growth while preserving as much continuity and comparability as possible with earlier census data. One of the more obvious patterns of population change has been the move-

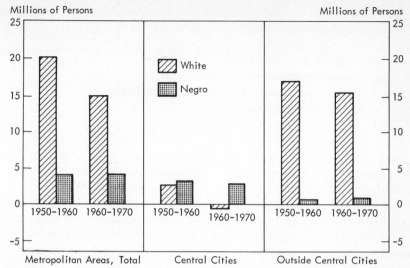

FIGURE 9-1. *Population changes in metropolitan areas by race: 1950–1960 and 1960–1970.* [SOURCE: *U.S. Bureau of the Census.* Statistical Abstract of the United States, 1971, *p. 4.*]

ment of people in large numbers to the densely settled urban centers. An example of a parallel change made by the census is its alteration of the definition of "urban." Before the 1950 census, a number of large and densely settled places were not included in the urban category because they were not incorporated. In 1950, the Census Bureau adopted the concept of the urbanized area and delineated boundaries for unincorporated places. As a result, all the population residing in urban-fringe areas and in unincorporated places of 2,500 or more is now classified as urban.[1]

Shifts of population within urban areas is another type of distribution pattern that the census tracks. Figure 9-1 illustrates changes in racial composition within urban areas for the decades of 1950–1960 and 1960–1970, and shows the shift of the white population out of the central cities. Thus, the white population in central cities *increased* in the decade 1950–1960 by almost 3 million persons; but in the 1960–1970 decade it *decreased* by almost 1 million.

The Nature of Census Data Reporting. Census information is readily available to everyone. Improvements in the speed of processing data have been made so that preliminary information obtained by a census is available within a few months after the enumeration is completed. Data that are compiled for each state are broken down by counties, by urban-rural areas, and by the large metropolitan areas. The census volume published for each state normally includes at least four elements:

1. Number of inhabitants
2. General population characteristics
3. General social and economic characteristics
4. Detailed characteristics

More detailed information, which is not generally demanded by users, is available on computer tapes from the Census Bureau for research or other legitimate needs, with the requirement that information about particular individuals remain confidential.

Census data, like most demographic information, are collected and presented as aggregates of large numbers. To make them comprehensible and useful they must be expressed in statistical terms such as averages, frequency distributions (e.g., age distributions), percentages, or ratios. Some examples of the statistics that can be obtained from census enumeration are given in the remainder of this section. Only those that have some relevance to public health are included in what follows.

AGE DISTRIBUTION

Within a large geographic area, the age distribution of a population will have its impact on almost everything, from television programs to voting patterns. For the United States as a whole, there are two significant aspects of the age distribution. First, the relative number of people in the older age groups has been increasing. This has been accompanied by greater emphasis on old-age social security, including, for example, the provision for medical needs under Medicare. Second, there are also increasingly large numbers of people under 21 years of age (about 80.4 million in 1970).

Table 9-1 provides an example of age distribution derived from census enumeration data; the table shows the relative proportions, or *percentages*, of persons in various age categories in the United States in 1970. Another way to assess age composition is by computing the *median*, which consists of the middle value of the age distribution; exactly half the cases lie on either side of the median. Median age of the total population increased steadily over the years through 1950, but by 1960 a very slight decrease had occurred for the first time since 1820, which is the earliest that appropriate data are available. Thus, for example, median age was 19.4 in 1860, 22.0 in 1890, 25.3 in 1920, and 30.2 in 1950—but 29.5 in 1960 and 28.3 in 1970.[1] Such changes in age composition over periods of time are one of several indicators of changing needs of the population.

TABLE 9-1. Age Distribution of the
Population of the United States, 1970

Age Interval	Percentage Distribution
Under 5 years	8.4%
5–13	18.0
14–17	7.8
18–20	5.3
21–24	6.3
25–34	12.3
35–44	11.4
45–54	11.4
55–64	9.1
65–74	6.1
75 and over	3.8
ALL AGES	100.0%

SOURCE: U.S. Bureau of the Census.
Statistical Abstract of the United States, 1971,
p. 23.

The relative proportions of the young and the old within the population are of interest to public health because they influence the way health and welfare resources are employed and distributed for the country as a whole, for individual states, and for local areas. One would anticipate, for example, rather different public health needs in Alaska as compared with Florida. Similarly, a particular city may have some areas with a preponderance of elderly persons, other areas a large number of housing developments with mostly young married couples and children, and still other areas a preponderance of employed adults with few children. Planning for and meeting the needs of these various areas within the city will be influenced in part by the age distribution of people living there.

The age distribution of a population by sex and race is very useful from a health point of view, particularly when it is related to age distributions of disease incidence and causes of death. For example, the increasing control over causes of maternal death has altered the age distribution of females. Differences between the age distributions of males and females have changed with advances in all fields of medicine, permitting the apparent biologic superiority of the females to assert itself in a longer life expectancy at birth and lower death rates for females in all age groups, both white and nonwhite, in the United States.

SEX RATIO

The sex ratio is the number of males per 100 females. When the ratio is more than 100, there are more males than females; when it is less than 100, the reverse is true. At the time of the 1970 census there were about 98,912,192 males in the United States and 104,299,734 females, giving a total average sex ratio of 94.8, thus:

$$1970 \text{ sex ratio} = \frac{98,912,192}{104,299,734} \times 100 = 94.8 \text{ men per 100 women}$$

The number of males per 100 females has declined steadily over the years. For example, in 1910 the sex ratio was 106.2, in 1930 it was 102.6, in 1950 it was 98.7, and in 1960 it was 97.1.[1] At present, the sex ratio is over 100 in the younger age groups because more male infants are born than female infants, but the ratio declines with age, giving further evidence of the higher death rates of males in all age categories.

DEPENDENCY RATIO

The dependency ratio is related to the age distribution. It indicates, as its name implies, the relative importance of the dependent age segments to the productively active age segments of a population. The dependency ratio takes account of three main age groups: dependent children, the active population, and the dependent aged. The size of the ratio will depend on the numbers in each group and how one chooses to define dependency. In the past, the dependency ratio has usually been defined as the number of persons under age 15, plus the number of persons 65 years and over, divided by the number of persons in the 15-through-64-year age group. The ratio, multiplied by the constant 100, estimates the number of dependent persons for every 100 in the active population, thus:

$$\text{Dep. ratio} = \frac{\text{No. of persons less than 15 years} + \text{no. of persons 65 and over}}{\text{No. of persons 15 through 64 years of age}} \times 100$$

However, when children stay in school longer and many are dependent on parents until the completion of college, the age 15 years may be too low. Some suggest the dependent youth category should include all persons under 20 years. Such an increase in the size of the dependency category in the numerator of the ratio, with an equal decrease in its denominator, would produce an increase in the size of the dependency ratio.

The following example, using 1970 census figures (in thousands), presents information about the size of various age categories and the resulting dependency ratios:

The total number of persons under 15 years of age   57,900
The total number of persons under 20 years of age   76,970
The total number of persons 65 years and over   20,066
The total number of persons 15 through 64 years   125,246
The total number of persons 20 through 64 years   106,176

$$\text{Dependency ratio (when dep. youth is 0--14 yrs.)} = \frac{57,900 + 20,066}{125,246} \times 100 = \text{62 dependent persons per 100 active persons}$$

$$\text{Dependency ratio (when dep. youth is 0--19 yrs.)} = \frac{76,970 + 20,066}{106,176} \times 100 = \text{91 dependent persons per 100 active persons}$$

CHILD-WOMAN RATIO

The child-woman ratio is the ratio of children under 5 years of age to women in the childbearing ages 15 through 44 years (sometimes 15 through 49 years). This ratio gives some indication of the incidence of childbearing. Its greatest advantage is that it depends only on census data. For a country that does take a census but has a poor vital registration system or does not register vital events at all, the child-woman ratio gives a rough estimate of fertility. However, much better measures of childbearing incidence are obtained when the relevant vital registration data on births can be used with census estimates of population in the appropriate age categories.

At the time of the 1970 census, the number of women 15 through 44 years of age was 42,436,894, and the number of children under 5 years of age was about 17,154,337. From these figures, the child-woman ratio is computed as follows:

$$\text{Child-woman ratio (1970)} = \frac{17,154,337}{42,436,894} \times 100 = \text{40 children under 5 years of age per 100 women in the childbearing ages}$$

This reflects a decline in the child-woman ratio from 1960, when there were 56 children under 5 years old per 100 women of childbearing age.

INCOME, EDUCATION, AND EMPLOYMENT

Income, education, and employment are population characteristics often referred to as socioeconomic variables. This information is available from the decennial census. Each variable—for example, income—may be classified by age, sex, race, location, or other characteristics. Such data are frequently considered in connection with indicators of health and well-being, and are useful in planning health and other public programs.

There are relationships between health and socioeconomic status which have been observed for so long that some individuals tend to assign a "causal" relationship, even though the relationship may not persist indefinitely. For example, mortality differences based on income, education, and occupation are much smaller now than they once were and are declining with time.

Vital Registration Data

Historically, there were very early attempts (dating back to the pre-Christian era in Greece, Rome, and Egypt) to count the population, usually for military conscription or for taxing purposes. There are also examples, as far back as the Middle Ages, of records from which crude estimates of vital events can be made. These are the church registers, which recorded, not births, marriages, and deaths, but baptisms, weddings, and funerals and the gratuities that were received for performance of these sacraments. The problem of incompleteness in such records is obvious, as are the other disadvantages of recording ceremonies rather than vital events. The first civil registration in the Christian epoch occurred in the Massachusetts Bay and New Plymouth colonies in the first half of the seventeenth century.[2]

Registration of vital events means legally recording their occurrence in a permanent place. To meet today's requirements, registration of the vital events of birth, death, marriage, and divorce must be compulsory, and the individual responsible for registering each event must be clearly designated. Usually time limits are set within which the individual who is responsible must register the event. Unless these time limits are enforced, events may be forgotten and registration will be incomplete.

Past experience has demonstrated that vital registration is the most effective method of obtaining information about vital events. Attempts to get estimates of births and deaths from early United States censuses were grossly unsuccessful and were abandoned after 1900.

REGISTRATION AREAS OF THE UNITED STATES

Many years ago, the federal government undertook the establishment of a mechanism for collecting data from the states on the occurrence of births and deaths and began to set standards for exactness, completeness, and promptness of reporting by the states. Toward this end, the national government passed model registration laws, and the states were urged to adopt them. Subsequently, as a state developed satisfactory birth and death registration laws and achieved 90 per cent completeness in reporting, it was admitted to membership in the "Registration Area for Births" and the "Registration Area for Deaths."

The death registration area was established in 1880, but the collection of mortality information did not begin until 1900 and then for only ten states, plus the District of Columbia and a number of cities located in nonregistration states. The birth registration area was established in 1915, and also included ten states and the District of Columbia; not all the states were the same as the ten contained in the death registration area. It was not until 1933 that all states in the Union had officially met the minimum requirements for membership in both the birth and the death registration areas.

GOVERNMENTAL REGISTRATION FUNCTIONS

Registration of vital events in the United States has remained a function of the states and of local governmental units. Standard recommended certificates are provided by the National Center for Health Statistics, but the state legislatures must approve them for adoption. States usually modify the proposed standard certificates to conform to state needs and legal requirements.

Certificates of a vital event are filed with a local registrar, whose geographic area may be a city, county, town, or other civil unit. He checks them for completeness and sends them to the state registrar of vital statistics, where they are again checked for completeness. Transcripts or microfilm copies are prepared in the state offices for transmittal to the Division of Vital Statistics of the National Center for Health Statistics (Public Health Service). At the national office the certificates are put on microfilm, and information from them is compiled for publication.

Care is taken in compilation for publication and in making records available to the public that the individual's right to privacy is preserved. There is a confidential section on the certificates of many states where additional medical information is recorded. More detailed information on immediate and underlying causes of death, complications of pregnancy and labor, congenital malformations and anomalies, and illegitimacy, for example, are valuable pieces of information. The great advantages of accurate reporting by physicians and the acceptance by legislatures of a confidential section can be continued only when privacy of the individual is strictly maintained. The confidential sections are among the most useful to the fields of medical research and public health.

BIRTH REGISTRATION

The Certificate of Live Birth.   The physician is responsible for completing and filing the Certificate of Live Birth (see Fig. 9-2). Consulting with the parents, he records demographic and personal information about them; he also records the name and sex of the child, birth order, and place and date of birth. The medical and health sections of the certificate are separate from the rest of the certificate and can be kept confidential. Facts recorded about prematurity, birth injuries, methods of delivery, conditions of pregnancy and labor, legitimacy, etc., provide important information which is used for medical and health purposes.

Definition of Live Birth.   Every infant born alive must be registered as a live birth. If he is born alive, according to official defini-

FIGURE 9-2.

tion, but subsequently dies, the death must also be registered. There is not universal agreement as to how a live birth should be defined, and before taking published birth and infant mortality rates at face value, one should compare the definitions of live birth and fetal death, particularly when comparing rates among different countries.

The following definition of live birth has been adopted by the World Health Assembly and is recommended for use in the United States: "Live birth is the complete expulsion or extraction from its mother of a product of conception, irrespective of the duration of pregnancy, which, after such separation, breathes or shows any other evidence of life, such as beating of the heart, pulsation of the umbilical cord, or definite movement of voluntary muscles, whether or not the umbilical cord has been cut or the placenta is attached; each product of such a birth is considered liveborn."

DEATH REGISTRATION

Death was the first and most adequately registered vital event. In 1953, the United Nations[2] proposed an international statistical definition as follows: "Death is the permanent disappearance of all evidence of life at any time after live birth has taken place. (Post natal cessation of vital functions without capability of resuscitation.) This definition therefore excludes fetal deaths."

The purpose of the definition was not so much to provide criteria of death, per se, but rather to distinguish postnatal deaths — for statistical and registration purposes — from fetal and prenatal deaths, which are separately defined and registered.

The cause of death is also an important element of death registration. In order to standardize the nomenclature as to cause of death, the World Health Organization publishes a manual entitled *International Statistical Classification of Diseases, Injuries, and Causes of Death.* The purpose of the manual is to establish international usage of comparable terms. The manual is revised about every ten years and is used routinely by health departments.

The Death Certificate.   In case of death, the funeral director fills out that part of the certificate (see Fig. 9-3) having to do with demographic facts about the deceased. He takes the certificate to the physician, or other appropriate professional, who completes the medical certification of death and affixes his signature. The funeral director then delivers the completed certificate to the local registrar from whom he obtains a burial permit.

Fetal Death Certification and Definition. In the certification of fetal death, the procedure and roles of funeral director and physician are essentially the same as those in the completion and filing of the death certificate. There are, however, some problems as to what constitutes a fetal death.

In 1950, the Third World Health Assembly approved the following definition of fetal death, which was subsequently adopted by the United Nations Statistical Commission in 1953: "Fetal death is death prior to the complete expulsion from its mother of a product of conception, irrespective of the duration of pregnancy; the death is indicated by the fact that after such separation the fetus does not breathe or show any other evidence of life, such as beating of the heart, pulsation of the umbilical cord, or definite movement of voluntary muscles. . . . If a child breathes or shows any other evidence of life after complete birth, even though it be only momentary, the birth should be registered as a live birth and a death certificate also should be filed."

This definition was recommended for use in the United States,

FIGURE 9-3.

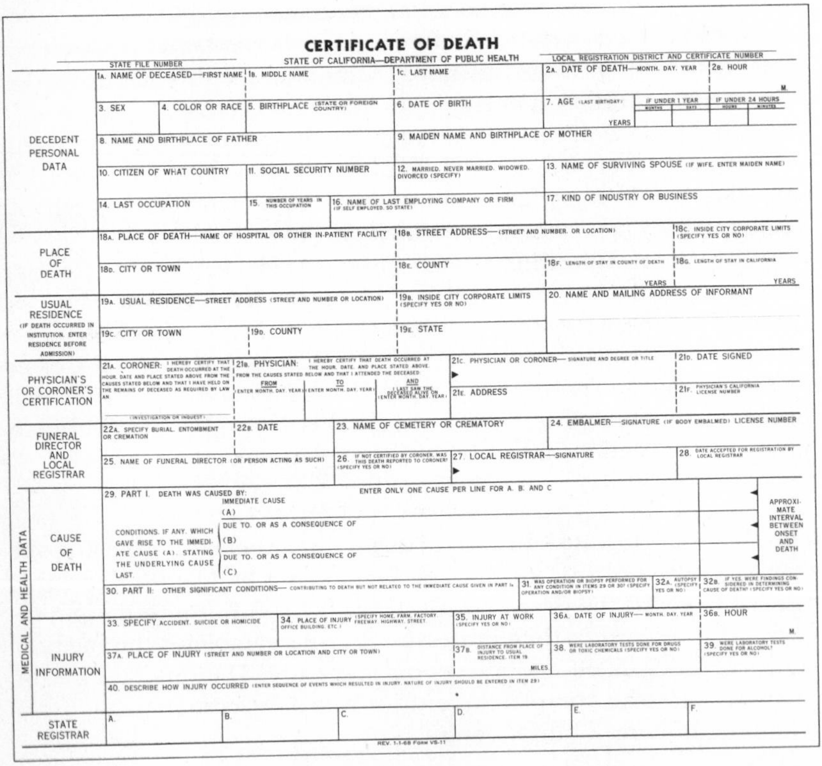

CERTIFICATE OF DEATH
STATE FILE NUMBER
STATE OF CALIFORNIA—DEPARTMENT OF PUBLIC HEALTH
LOCAL REGISTRATION DISTRICT AND CERTIFICATE NUMBER

DECEDENT PERSONAL DATA
1A. NAME OF DECEASED—FIRST NAME | 1B. MIDDLE NAME | 1C. LAST NAME | 2A. DATE OF DEATH—MONTH, DAY, YEAR | 2B. HOUR M.
3. SEX | 4. COLOR OR RACE | 5. BIRTHPLACE (STATE OR FOREIGN COUNTRY) | 6. DATE OF BIRTH | 7. AGE (LAST BIRTHDAY) YEARS | IF UNDER 1 YEAR MONTHS DAYS | IF UNDER 24 HOURS HOURS MINUTES
8. NAME AND BIRTHPLACE OF FATHER | 9. MAIDEN NAME AND BIRTHPLACE OF MOTHER
10. CITIZEN OF WHAT COUNTRY | 11. SOCIAL SECURITY NUMBER | 12. MARRIED, NEVER MARRIED, WIDOWED, DIVORCED (SPECIFY) | 13. NAME OF SURVIVING SPOUSE (IF WIFE, ENTER MAIDEN NAME)
14. LAST OCCUPATION | 15. NUMBER OF YEARS IN THIS OCCUPATION | 16. NAME OF LAST EMPLOYING COMPANY OR FIRM (IF SELF EMPLOYED, SO STATE) | 17. KIND OF INDUSTRY OR BUSINESS

PLACE OF DEATH
18A. PLACE OF DEATH—NAME OF HOSPITAL OR OTHER IN-PATIENT FACILITY | 18B. STREET ADDRESS—(STREET AND NUMBER, OR LOCATION) | 18C. INSIDE CITY CORPORATE LIMITS (SPECIFY YES OR NO)
18D. CITY OR TOWN | 18E. COUNTY | 18F. LENGTH OF STAY IN COUNTY OF DEATH YEARS | 18G. LENGTH OF STAY IN CALIFORNIA YEARS

USUAL RESIDENCE (IF DEATH OCCURRED IN INSTITUTION, ENTER RESIDENCE BEFORE ADMISSION)
19A. USUAL RESIDENCE—STREET ADDRESS (STREET AND NUMBER OR LOCATION) | 19B. INSIDE CITY CORPORATE LIMITS (SPECIFY YES OR NO) | 20. NAME AND MAILING ADDRESS OF INFORMANT
19C. CITY OR TOWN | 19D. COUNTY | 19E. STATE

PHYSICIAN'S OR CORONER'S CERTIFICATION
21A. CORONER: I HEREBY CERTIFY THAT DEATH OCCURRED AT THE HOUR, DATE AND PLACE STATED ABOVE FROM THE CAUSES STATED BELOW AND THAT I HAVE HELD ON THE REMAINS OF DECEASED AS REQUIRED BY LAW AN (INVESTIGATION OR INQUEST)
21B. PHYSICIAN: I HEREBY CERTIFY THAT DEATH OCCURRED AT THE HOUR, DATE, AND PLACE STATED ABOVE FROM THE CAUSES STATED BELOW AND THAT I ATTENDED THE DECEASED FROM (ENTER MONTH, DAY, YEAR) TO (ENTER MONTH, DAY, YEAR) AND I LAST SAW THE DECEASED ALIVE ON (ENTER MONTH, DAY, YEAR)
21C. PHYSICIAN OR CORONER—SIGNATURE AND DEGREE OR TITLE | 21D. DATE SIGNED
21E. ADDRESS | 21F. PHYSICIAN'S CALIFORNIA LICENSE NUMBER

FUNERAL DIRECTOR AND LOCAL REGISTRAR
22A. SPECIFY BURIAL, ENTOMBMENT OR CREMATION | 22B. DATE | 23. NAME OF CEMETERY OR CREMATORY | 24. EMBALMER—SIGNATURE (IF BODY EMBALMED) LICENSE NUMBER
25. NAME OF FUNERAL DIRECTOR (OR PERSON ACTING AS SUCH) | 26. IF NOT CERTIFIED BY CORONER, WAS THIS DEATH REPORTED TO CORONER? (SPECIFY YES OR NO) | 27. LOCAL REGISTRAR—SIGNATURE | 28. DATE ACCEPTED FOR REGISTRATION BY LOCAL REGISTRAR

MEDICAL AND HEALTH DATA

CAUSE OF DEATH
29. PART I. DEATH WAS CAUSED BY: ENTER ONLY ONE CAUSE PER LINE FOR A, B, AND C
IMMEDIATE CAUSE (A)
CONDITIONS, IF ANY, WHICH GAVE RISE TO THE IMMEDIATE CAUSE (A), STATING THE UNDERLYING CAUSE LAST.
DUE TO, OR AS A CONSEQUENCE OF (B)
DUE TO, OR AS A CONSEQUENCE OF (C)
APPROXIMATE INTERVAL BETWEEN ONSET AND DEATH
30. PART II: OTHER SIGNIFICANT CONDITIONS—CONTRIBUTING TO DEATH BUT NOT RELATED TO THE IMMEDIATE CAUSE GIVEN IN PART I. | 31. WAS OPERATION OR BIOPSY PERFORMED FOR ANY CONDITION IN ITEMS 29 OR 30? (SPECIFY OPERATION AND/OR BIOPSY) | 32A. AUTOPSY (SPECIFY YES OR NO) | 32B. IF YES, WERE FINDINGS CONSIDERED IN DETERMINING CAUSE OF DEATH? (SPECIFY YES OR NO)

INJURY INFORMATION
33. SPECIFY ACCIDENT, SUICIDE OR HOMICIDE | 34. PLACE OF INJURY (SPECIFY HOME, FARM, FACTORY, FREEWAY, HIGHWAY, STREET, OFFICE BUILDING, ETC.) | 35. INJURY AT WORK (SPECIFY YES OR NO) | 36A. DATE OF INJURY—MONTH, DAY, YEAR | 36B. HOUR M.
37A. PLACE OF INJURY (STREET AND NUMBER OR LOCATION AND CITY OR TOWN) | 37B. DISTANCE FROM PLACE OF INJURY TO USUAL RESIDENCE, ITEM 19 MILES | 38. WERE LABORATORY TESTS DONE FOR DRUGS OR TOXIC CHEMICALS (SPECIFY YES OR NO) | 39. WERE LABORATORY TESTS DONE FOR ALCOHOL? (SPECIFY YES OR NO)
40. DESCRIBE HOW INJURY OCCURRED (ENTER SEQUENCE OF EVENTS WHICH RESULTED IN INJURY. NATURE OF INJURY SHOULD BE ENTERED IN ITEM 29)

STATE REGISTRAR
A. | B. | C. | D. | E. | F.

REV. 1-1-68 FORM VS-11

and in 1955 the Standard Certificate of Fetal Death was adopted, replacing a certificate which required only the reporting of still-births. However, in spite of the new definition's phrase, "irrespec-tive of the duration of pregnancy," certain states in the United States still retain some minimum gestation period in their specifica-tion of fetal death. For example, fetal death may apply only to prod-ucts of conception having a minimum gestation period of 20 weeks, and no other pregnancy wastage is registered in those states. Es-timates of pregnancy wastage, at best, are very rough. Even states that use the recommended definition of fetal death undoubtedly ob-tain only gross estimates of pregnancy wastage, especially for the early abortions (i.e., prenatal deaths).

VITAL STATISTICS RATES

Most demographic data are collected in the form of actual numerical counts by categories. There are times when it is desirable to know the actual numbers, but sometimes derivative measures are more useful. The earlier section of this chapter which discussed the census used some examples of averages (the median age), distribu-tions (the age distribution of a population), and ratios (the sex ratio, the child-woman ratio, etc.). These illustrated some ways in which enumeration data are systematically compiled and manipulated to make them understandable and useful.

The information about the vital events that occur during a year's time is expressed most meaningfully as vital rates. A vital rate may be defined as the number of occurrences of a vital event that takes place during a year's time divided by the average or mid-year population "at risk" to the event. Vital registration data appear in the numerator; enumeration data are used in the denominator. (There are exceptions to this rule; for example, the infant mortality rate uses vital registration data in both numerator and denomina-tor.) The resulting ratio is multiplied by a constant, usually 100, 1,000, or 100,000. This yields a rate of occurrence per given number of persons per year. The estimated midyear population is used in the denominator of the ratio as the estimated average population for the year.

Death Rates.   There are two basic kinds of death rate, a crude death rate and a rate that is specific for some demographic characteristic. The crude death rate has the advantage of being easy to calculate, and it is understood by most people. It consists of the number of deaths occurring in a given year divided by the estimated popula-tion living on July 1 of that same year, multiplied by 1,000, thus:

$$\text{Crude death rate} = \frac{\text{No. of deaths in one calendar year}}{\text{Midyear population in that year}} \times 1,000$$

In 1968 there were 1,930,082 deaths in the United States, and the estimated population of the country on July 1, 1968, was 199,861,000. Relating deaths to population, the 1968 crude death rate for the United States is calculated as follows:

$$\text{Crude death rate} = \frac{1,930,082}{199,861,000} \times 1,000 = 9.7 \text{ per } 1,000 \text{ population in}$$
the United States in 1968

The crude death rate may give a distorted picture, and so when more refined mortality statistics are desirable, rates may be calculated which are specific for various demographic characteristics. Some examples are death rates specific for different age categories, sex, race, marital status, or any other characteristic for which the appropriate information is available.

The age-specific death rate is frequently of interest, not only at a given time, but for changes that may occur over time. It is also enlightening when comparisons are made among countries having populations with different age structures. It is possible, for example, for country A to have a higher crude death rate than country B, even though country A has lower age-specific death rates at all ages. Differences in age structure could very reasonably account for what at first appears paradoxical. The age-specific death rate is calculated as follows:

$$\frac{\text{Age-specific}}{\text{death rate}} = \frac{\begin{array}{c}\text{No. of deaths in a stated age} \\ \text{group occurring in a calendar year}\end{array}}{\begin{array}{c}\text{Estimated midyear population} \\ \text{of that age group}\end{array}} \times 1,000$$

Thus, for example, in the United States in 1968, there were about 40,796,000 persons of age 45 to 64, and 389,038 deaths occurred among persons in this age group, so that:

$$\frac{\text{Age-specific}}{\text{death rate}} = \frac{389,038}{40,796,000} \times 1,000 = 9.6 \text{ deaths per}$$
1,000 population
age 45–64 years

Death rates may be still further refined by specifying more than one category or characteristic. For example, death rates may be made specific for age, sex, and race simultaneously, as follows (figures for 1967 are approximate):

$$\text{Death rate for white males, age 20–24 years, U.S., 1967} = \frac{\substack{12{,}400 \text{ deaths} \\ \text{in specified} \\ \text{population}}}{\substack{\text{Midyear} \\ \text{population} \\ \text{of } 7{,}389{,}000}} \times 1{,}000 = 1.7 \text{ deaths per } 1{,}000 \text{ white males age 20–24 years}$$

Birth Rates. Data on number of births are used in several vital statistics rates, including the crude birth rate, the general fertility rate, age-specific birth rates, and the infant mortality rate. The best known and most commonly used measure of the incidence of births and fertility is the *crude birth rate.* This consists of the number of registered live births occurring in a specified area during a calendar year, divided by the midyear population, as follows:

$$\text{Crude birth rate} = \frac{\substack{\text{No. of births occurring} \\ \text{during one calendar year}}}{\text{Midyear population}} \times 1{,}000$$

There were 3,501,564 registered live births in the United States in 1968, occurring among an estimated midyear population of 201,152,000, so that:

$$\text{Crude birth rate} = \frac{3{,}501{,}564}{201{,}152{,}000} \times 1{,}000 = 17.4 \text{ live births per } 1{,}000 \text{ population in 1968}$$

Since the crude birth rate relates births to total population, its size will be influenced by such demographic characteristics as age distribution and sex ratio of the relevant population. Crude birth rates tend to be higher among young than among old populations. (An "old" population is one having a relatively large percentage of its population 65 years of age and over.) Relative to total population size, the *total* number of women in the childbearing ages and the number of *married* women in the childbearing ages have an important influence on number of births and thereby on the crude birth rate.

A better measure of the incidence of birth than the crude rate is the *general fertility rate,* which is computed by dividing total live births occurring in one calendar year by the midyear population of women aged 15 to 44 (or 15 to 49) years, thus:

$$\text{General fertility rate} = \frac{\substack{\text{No. of births occurring} \\ \text{during one calendar year}}}{\substack{\text{Midyear population of women} \\ \text{15–44 (or 15–49) years of age}}} \times 1{,}000$$

In 1969 there were an estimated 3,571,000 live births in the United States and an estimated midyear population of 41,612,000 women in the childbearing years 15 to 44, thus:

$$\text{General fertility rate} = \frac{3,571,000}{41,612,000} \times 1,000 = 85.8 \text{ births per } 1,000 \text{ women of childbearing age}$$

If more refined information is required about the fertility of *married* women, the population of women aged 15 to 44 years may be limited to the midyear population of married women in those age groups.

Age-specific birth rates provide information about the distribution of a year's births by age of mother. In computing the rates, mothers are usually classified in five-year age groups. Table 9-2 shows the birth rate in 1968 per age category of mothers; the table also presents birth rates specific for race, i.e., white and nonwhite.

For purposes of comparison among various populations at a given time and for the same population over time, the general fertility rate and the age-specific birth rate are preferable to the crude birth rate. If one assumes there is agreement about the definition of live birth, the specific birth rates are more comparable than crude rates because other influencing demographic characteristics have been eliminated.

Another useful vital rate employing data on number of births is

TABLE 9-2. Live Birth Rate per 1,000 Women in Each Category, by Age and Color of Mother, 1968

	No. of Live Births per 1,000 Women
BY AGE OF MOTHER	
10–14	1.0
15–19	66.1
20–24	167.4
25–29	140.3
30–34	74.9
35–39	35.6
40–44	9.6
45–49	0.6
BY COLOR OF MOTHER, FOR AGES 15–44	
White	81.5
Nonwhite	114.9

SOURCE: Adapted from U.S. Bureau of the Census. *Statistical Abstract of the United States, 1971,* p. 49.

the *infant mortality rate.* It may be defined as the number of deaths occurring among persons less than one year of age, divided by the number of births. Multiplied by 1,000, this ratio gives the rate of infant deaths per 1,000 live births, thus:

$$\text{Infant mortality rate} = \frac{\begin{array}{c}\text{No. of deaths occurring in one}\\ \text{calendar year among persons less}\\ \text{than one year of age}\end{array}}{\begin{array}{c}\text{No. of live births in one}\\ \text{calendar year}\end{array}} \times 1{,}000$$

$$\begin{array}{l}\text{Infant mortality rate} = \dfrac{76{,}263}{3{,}501{,}564} \times 1{,}000 = 21.8 \text{ infant deaths}\\ \text{(U.S., 1968)} \hspace{5.5cm} \text{per 1,000 live births}\\ \hspace{7cm} \text{in the U.S., 1968}\end{array}$$

The infant mortality rate has been relied upon a great deal as an indicator of health and well-being; changes in its size have been used to assess changes in the extent and effectiveness of medical care and public health programs. The relatively high risk of death in the first year of life has made the infant mortality rate sensitive to various circumstances, particularly to conditions of sanitation and other environmental factors, as well as to quality of medical care and to the level of general education and health education.

Morbidity Statistics

Statistical measures of morbidity, or the amount of illness in a population, are useful in public health in assessing the relative importance of a given illness or injury at a particular time or over a stated time period. They also provide measures of change over time in the occurrence of an illness or injury and in its relative importance to all other illnesses or injuries.

Two common measures of the amount of illness are the incidence rate and the prevalence rate. The difference between the two is that the prevalence rate counts all the cases of an illness or injury that exist during a time period, while the incidence rate counts only the new cases that occur. They differ from the rates and ratios described in preceding sections in that they do not use vital registration data in the numerator.

THE INCIDENCE RATE

The incidence rate for an illness is defined as the number of new cases that occur during a given time period, divided by the number of persons exposed to the risk of the illness (the number of persons at risk is often the total population of the relevant geographic area, and thus a "crude" incidence rate is produced). The resulting ratio is multiplied by a constant, 1000 or 100,000, as follows:

$$\text{Incidence rate} = \frac{\begin{array}{c}\text{No. of newly reported cases of a}\\ \text{stated disease or injury during a}\\ \text{given time period}\end{array}}{\begin{array}{c}\text{Population living in stated area during}\\ \text{that time period}\end{array}} \times 1{,}000 \text{ or } 100{,}000$$

Thus, for example, there were 266,222 cases of measles reported in the United States in 1965. These cases occurred among a population of about 194,204,000 persons, so that:

$$\begin{array}{l}\text{Incidence rate}\\ \text{for measles}\end{array} = \frac{266{,}222}{194{,}204{,}000} \times 1{,}000 = 1.371 \begin{array}{l}\text{cases of measles}\\ \text{per 1,000 persons}\end{array}$$

More refined rates of incidence may be computed by age, sex, race, or other demographic characteristics. For some injuries or illnesses it is important to define more specifically the population at risk. An example is the complications of pregnancy, to which only a fairly well-defined segment of the population is at risk.

THE PREVALENCE RATE

The crude prevalence rate may be defined as the number of cases of an illness that exist at a particular time, divided by the number of persons living in the defined geographic area at that time, and multiplied by 1,000 or 100,000. The prevalence rate indicates the relative number of persons who have a stated illness at a given time. For example, an estimated 3,248,000 persons were afflicted with rheumatism or arthritis in the United States for the period July 1965 to June 1967. Using the 1966 population estimate of 196,907,000 persons, the prevalence rate was 16.495. In other words, during the stated time period, an estimated 16.495 persons out of every 1,000 had rheumatism or arthritis. More refined prevalence rates may be computed by age, sex, race, marital status, or some other characteristic that more precisely defines "population at risk" than does the total population estimate.

Uses of Demographic Data and
Vital Statistics in Public Health

UTILIZATION AT THE LOCAL LEVEL

In planning local health programs it is essential to know how many persons need a particular program and, in evaluating the program, how much benefit is being derived from it. In all its activities, the local public health agency must know the size, location, and characteristics of the population. Without this information it would be impossible to estimate personnel needs and to evaluate what proportion of the target population is taking advantage of public health services.

Census data are used to describe the density of various areas of a community, and information on characteristics of the population such as race, age, transiency, and income are used in program planning. Data collected from birth certificates are used to anticipate the need for postnatal care programs for mothers and their children, to plan vaccination and immunization programs, and to develop programs for the congenitally handicapped. Likewise, data derived from death certificates are used by the local public health agencies to plan control programs for specific communicable diseases (especially in countries where epidemics such as smallpox exist); to clear other records such as police, social security, and welfare status of deceased persons; and to plan public health programs for accident or suicide prevention and chronic disease.

Other local groups in schools, hospitals, and businesses use census and birth information in planning facilities and anticipating personnel needs. Voluntary agencies also use the vital statistics records in planning when and where to concentrate their efforts.

UTILIZATION BY THE STATE

On the state level, public health personnel provide a continuing surveillance of reportable diseases in terms of morbidity statistics as an aid to local agencies. If unusually high values occur, action can be taken at the state and local level. These same morbidity and mortality statistics are used to plan campaigns by health educators in deciding when specific diseases peak, so that they can start their campaign at an appropriate time of the year.

Census, morbidity, and mortality information is used by the state for comparison purposes. The incidence rate of a disease such as measles could be plotted year by year to assess trends and compare them with public health program efforts and medical advances in prevention of these diseases. One may think that a disease such as tuberculosis is disappearing, only to find later that there is still considerable incidence among certain population groups. By checking the morbidity and mortality trends over time, the public health programs can be kept up to date.

Census, mortality, and morbidity statistics are also used for in-service training programs, to pinpoint problem areas, and to make administrative decisions as to budgeting and personnel needs. Good planning requires a description of the needs of the various areas and population subgroups of the state. A particular subgroup such as migrant workers might need special health programs at certain times of the year. The need for special efforts in air pollution programs, vector control, inspection of fish or meat, or pesticide control can be evaluated.

UTILIZATION AT THE NATIONAL LEVEL

At the national level, there is a greater emphasis on research, and demographic data and vital statistics are used for this purpose. The data reported by the National Center for Health Statistics are used as basic elements in public health and medical research. The census data are used to estimate the present population and to project the future population. These, combined with the morbidity and mortality statistics, form the guideposts for deciding where research efforts should be encouraged. Besides encouraging research by outside groups, special research teams are formed in the Public Health Service to tackle particular public health problems. As in the states, trends over time in morbidity and mortality statistics are useful in planning future research efforts.

In the future, it is anticipated that with the use of computers, data will be compiled much faster and users will have more current information. Furthermore, it will be possible to match records on the computer from various sources in the government for comparison purposes. If the problems of protection of the rights of the individual can be overcome, then these combined records will be even more useful planning tools for the development of public health programs.

Epidemiology: the Search for Causes of Disease

Epidemiology describes the distribution of human health problems and seeks to establish the causes of these problems. The purpose of investigating and establishing disease causation is to discover and formulate effective control measures.

DEFINITION AND SCOPE OF EPIDEMIOLOGY

Specific definitions of epidemiology vary somewhat, the differences being largely a matter of degree of inclusiveness. In certain definitions, the focus is on the investigation of disease; in others, disease is included as part of a broader spectrum of concern. Thus, epidemiology has been defined as "the study of the distribution and determinants of disease prevalence in man"; [3] or it has been viewed as being "concerned with measurements of the circumstances under which diseases occur, where diseases tend to flourish, and where they do not."[4] The circumstances referred to in the latter definition may be microbiologic or toxicologic, and they may be based on genetic, social, or environmental factors. In the more broadly based definitions, epidemiology is considered to include "the various factors and conditions that determine the occurrence and distribution of health, disease, defect, disability, and death among groups of individuals";[5] or it is "concerned with the study of the processes which determine or influence the physical, mental, and social health of people."[6] In general, these definitions of epidemiology—whether the focus is on disease or on the total health-disease spectrum—share in common an emphasis on *process* and a recognition of the involvement of a *multiplicity of influencing factors.*

The most significant early contributions of epidemiology were in connection with the infectious diseases. These contributions included the discovery of microorganisms as causative agents of disease (thus ushering in the bacteriologic era), the development of immunology, and the acquisition of new knowledge regarding the transmission of disease. Such discoveries did not, of course, occur as an uninterrupted chain of events. For example, in 1854 John Snow proved that cholera was transmitted in water and by personal contact, but the identification of the cholera organism was not made until 27 years later. Similarly, William Budd established the contagious nature of tuberculosis 15 years before the tubercle bacillus was identified.[7] Thus, the contributions of epidemiology have, historically, come about through a series of steps which have sometimes extended over a considerable period of time and in which important epidemiologic facts have sometimes been discovered before specific mechanisms have been identified.

In recent years, the scope of epidemiology has broadened considerably.[8] As a consequence of its early concern with infectious diseases, the principal function of epidemiology for many years was to investigate epidemics of such diseases, including tracing their sources, controlling spread, and initiating measures to prevent recurrences. On the international health scene, there is still great concern with well-known communicable diseases that continue to wrack many regions of the world, including smallpox, typhoid, schistosomiasis, and trachoma. However, in the more developed industrial nations where infectious diseases have largely been brought under control, the concerns of epidemiology have tended to shift to the vast array of *noninfectious* diseases which have gained increasing prominence.

Epidemiologic activity in the noninfectious diseases is by no means new. Even during the eighteenth and early nineteenth centuries, a number of epidemiologic achievements in the noninfectious diseases had occurred, for example, in nutritional disease and occupational disease through investigations of scurvy among merchant seamen and of scrotal cancer in chimney sweeps.[9] Today, the chronic and degenerative diseases such as cardiovascular disorders, cancer, and arthritis, as well as mental illness, nutritional disorders, congenital defects, and accidents, are all considered to be highly appropriate for epidemiologic study and investigation. Conditions in which social pathology is clearly present, such as alcoholism, drug addiction, divorce, delinquency, and suicide, also have aspects to which epidemiology is relevant.

To the present-day public, epidemiology is perhaps best known through reports of investigations of sometimes spectacular disease outbreaks that often have the quality of suspense of an absorbing detective story.[10,11] Usually beginning with a single case of an undiagnosed illness—with a set of puzzling and sometimes bizarre symptoms—the thread of the detection follows a tortuous path to establish the diagnosis and find the source of the disease which, in the process, has been claiming additional victims. Through the course of the investigation, which is often referred to as "shoeleather epidemiology," the epidemiologist struggles with the pieces of the puzzle until they finally fall into place and the problem is solved. Sometimes the illness turns out to have a highly unexpected origin, as illustrated by the following example of an actual occurrence.[11] An 8-year-old boy developed symptoms including pallor, rapid heartbeat, irregular breathing, muscle twitches, diarrhea, nausea, vomiting, abdominal pain, and mental confusion. Before long, several other boys about his age developed similar symptoms. Diabetes was suspected at first and other diagnoses were considered, but the final diagnosis was organic phosphate poisoning due to Phosdrin, a pesticide. Phosdrin concentrate had been stored in a warehouse where one can sprang a leak and contaminated a shipment of boys' blue jeans stored nearby. The blue jeans later were purchased and worn by the boys who became ill, the Phosdrin in the blue jeans having been absorbed into the boys' systems through the skin.

Epidemiology provides both a body of knowledge and a formulation of methods for learning about health and disease status with the goal of ultimately finding solutions to health problems. It constitutes part of the scientific foundation of public health and a basis for public health action.[12] With respect to the distribution of disease, epidemiology provides information on the frequency of occurrence of disease in different populations and in different segments of the same population. This aspect is often referred to as *descriptive epidemiology*. It attempts to answer questions regarding "who," "where," and "when" in terms, for example, of age, sex, race, and various geographic and time dimensions. Such information enables the maintenance of general surveillance of the health status of a population and alerts health workers to outbreaks of infectious diseases and to increases in the occurrence of specific noninfectious diseases. Descriptive epidemiology also provides historical perspective regarding the prevalence of diseases in different epochs of time.

In addition, descriptive information underlies another major concern of epidemiology, namely, the search for causes of disease. Knowledge of the cause of disease, in turn, serves as the basis for preventive measures. In establishing disease causation, epidemiology attempts to answer questions regarding "how" and "why." To do this, two levels of investigative techniques may be employed. On one level, an effort is made to determine the statistical association between a specific factor and a given disease; for example, a great deal of evidence has been assembled that shows a strong statistical association between cigarette smoking and the incidence of lung cancer. This kind of investigation has been called *analytic epidemiology*.[3] On the other investigative level, an attempt is made to determine exact disease causation through controlled experiments using techniques that are also the basis for much clinical research. Such investigations have been referred to as *experimental epidemiology*.[1] The principles and methods of descriptive, analytic, and experimental epidemiology will be discussed in greater detail later in this chapter.

In addition to generating its own knowledge and methods, epidemiology also utilizes those of certain other relevant and important disciplines. *Clinical medicine* and *pathology* contribute to the accurate description and classification of disease, which are important in determining disease frequency. *Biostatistics* provides methods for analyzing epidemiologic data, including the determination of whether variations in disease frequency within or between population groups are chance occurrences or form systematic patterns. Other disciplines such as *microbiology* and *biochemistry* contribute methods of experimental investigation. *Genetics* and the *behavioral sciences* provide information on the characteristics of persons and on the social and cultural characteristics of population groups, respectively, which may influence the occurrence of disease.

BASIC EPIDEMIOLOGIC ELEMENTS

The human population group constitutes a basic element of study in epidemiology. Epidemiologic investigations may involve many different kinds and sizes of groups depending on the nature of particular studies. Once a population group has been defined, however, attention is directed toward the total group, including both its sick and well members. This approach differs from that of clinical medicine and dentistry where the focus is on the individual case and in which the clinician deals with a discrete series of patients and their illnesses.[5]

The concept of the natural history of disease, or the processes through which deviations from health occur and the course and outcome of the deviations, is another basic element in epidemiology. The natural history of a disease describes "its development from the first forces which create the disease stimulus in the environment or elsewhere, through the resulting response of man, to the changes which take place leading to recovery, disability, defect, or death."[13] This process involves the interaction of three different kinds of factors: the causative *agent,* the susceptible *host,* and the *environment.*[5,12] Epidemiologic investigations are concerned with the assembly and analysis of information about these factors for the purpose of describing the occurrence, distribution, and cause of disease.

An agent is usually thought of as a factor whose *presence* causes disease, but it may also be a factor whose *absence* can cause disease. An example of the latter is insufficient intake of vitamin C, which may lead to scurvy. There are several general categories of causative agents. One category consists of *physical agents,* which include various kinds of mechanical forces or frictions that may be the source of injury and several different kinds of atmospheric abnormalities such as extremes of temperature or excessive radiation. A second category consists of *chemical agents,* which can occur in various forms such as dusts, gases, vapors, and fumes; such agents may be acquired by inhalation, ingestion, or contact. A third category consists of *nutrient agents,* which are also chemical in nature, but include the lack or the *over*abundance of one or more of the basic dietary elements. The final and historically most prominent category consists of *biologic agents,* which are living organisms, and include insects (arthropods), worms (helminths), protozoa, fungi, bacteria, rickettsiae, and viruses.

The human host's susceptibility or resistance to a disease agent, and hence the occurrence and distribution of disease in a population, are influenced by many factors. Habits, customs, and characteristic modes of living may serve either to encourage or to inhibit the disease process. Factors in this general category may range from matters of personal cleanliness and food habits to sanitation practices, extent of interpersonal contacts, and degree of crowding. Various population characteristics may also be important factors in determining the onset, type, and course of certain diseases. Such attributes include age, sex, ethnic origin, marital status, and socioeconomic indicators such as occupation and income. The status of various general and specific mechanisms in the host which provide defenses against disease constitute another set of influencing factors in the disease process. These defenses include immunity as well as numerous anatomic structures (e.g., the skin, hair, nails, and secretions) and physiologic processes (e.g., coughing, temperature regulation, and tolerance development) which protect against disease and injury. Other host factors that may contribute to the disease process are heredity and general constitutional make-up.

The environment may, depending on its characteristics, help to suppress disease or assist it to flourish. The total environment consists of several components: physical, biologic, social, and economic. The most prominent aspect of the *physical environment* is geography, to which climate, season, and weather are closely allied. Health status may be directly or indirectly influenced by the topography, the nature of the soil, the availability of water, and the climatic conditions of a particular area. The *biologic environment* includes living animals and plants, some of which, as mentioned earlier, may be agents of disease. They may also harbor disease agents, or they may serve as transmitters of disease. Of the many aspects of the *social and economic environment* which may influence health and disease, economic status is among the most important. The economic status of a population as a whole, as reflected in its general standard of living, may have considerable impact on health level. The range of economic gradation within the population and the extent and severity of economic deprivations in particular population groups may also be of considerable importance. The social environment is characterized by many different kinds of attitudes, beliefs, and behavior, some of which may alleviate the threat of disease while others may foster it, for example, attitudes and beliefs that lead to the use of properly accredited medical practitioners and facilities as opposed to those that lead to the use of untested or quack remedies. In general, as a population develops socially and economically, ideology and practice tend increasingly to support the growth of environmental factors that promote health and minimize disease.

The nature of the interaction between agent, host, and environmental factors determine the relative health or disease status of a population. The process of interaction has been conceptualized as the degree of equilibrium of forces on a scale in which environmental factors are the fulcrum, and agent and host factors are the opposing balances.[5] If the balance is in favor of the host, disease occurrence decreases. However, if the balance shifts because of deleterious changes in environmental factors or the greater "weight" of agent factors, disease occurrence increases until equilibrium is again restored. At any time in a population, groups of individuals are in various phases of this interaction process; the function of some epidemiologic investigations is to identify these groups and analyze the process.

Principal Aspects of Epidemiologic Investigation

As indicated earlier, epidemiology may be viewed as having descriptive, analytic, and experimental aspects which, in effect, represent progressions along a continuum that ranges from an account of disease occurrence and distribution to the establishment of disease causation. At present, the status of knowledge along this continuum varies among diseases. For some diseases such as cancer and heart disease, epidemiologic investigation has provided some knowledge of their distribution in the population, but exact causes are yet to be determined. For others, such as certain kinds of mental illness, neither the exact distribution nor the causes are known. Epidemiologists seek continuously to close these gaps in knowledge in order to further extend the breadth of disease prevention.

DESCRIPTIVE EPIDEMIOLOGY

In investigating and describing the occurrence and distribution of disease in a population, epidemiology customarily deals with three classes of characteristics: those pertaining to the *time* and the *place* in which persons are found affected, and those pertaining to the affected *persons* themselves.[3]

Characteristics Describing Time. Time, as one element in the description of disease distribution, may be defined in many different ways, such as year, season, or day. Disease frequency may be measured over a long period of time and observed for changes in its pattern of occurrence. The change occurring over a period of years is known as *secular change* and is illustrated by Figure 9-4, which shows death rates for tuberculosis and malignant neoplasms over a

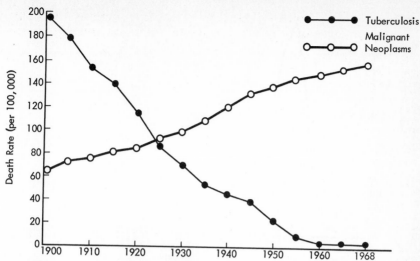

FIGURE 9-4. *Secular change: tuberculosis and malignant neoplasms, 1900–1968. (All forms of tuberculosis. Includes neoplasms of lymphatic and hematopoietic tissues.)* [SOURCE: *Adapted from U.S. Bureau of the Census.* Historical Statistics of the United States, Colonial Times to 1957. *Washington, D.C., 1960, p. 26. Also,* Statistical Abstract of the United States, 1971, p. 58.]

68-year period. Death certificates for cause of death and autopsy reports for incidental pathology have traditionally been the best means of measuring secular change. Data on morbidity that are appropriate for such measurement are at present limited mainly, first, to the infectious diseases that are reportable to health departments and, second, to the cases of mental illness in mental hospitals. In recent years, at least two other sources of epidemiologic information have come into use in the United States and are sometimes found in other parts of the world. These are *registries* (e.g., cancer registries), which attempt to assemble information on incidence and prevalence of a few particular diseases of interest, and *morbidity surveys* (e.g., the U.S. National Health Survey), which systematically screen defined populations for prevalence of illness.

Seasonal fluctuations, cyclic fluctuations, and "point" epidemics are additional ways to describe the time characteristics of disease distribution. In measuring *seasonal fluctuations*, cases are plotted by time of onset using units—hours, days, weeks, or months—that are small enough to show successive variations in the occurrence of the particular disease being investigated. Seasonal fluctuations in acute diseases, especially those of an infectious nature, have received considerable attention in epidemiologic investigations. However, most chronic diseases have not been studied

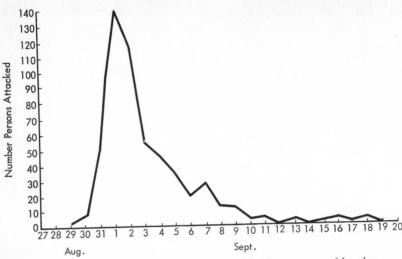

FIGURE 9-5. *"Point" epidemic of cholera, Golden Square area of London, August-September, 1848.* [SOURCE: *Adapted from Snow, John.* On the Mode of Communication of Cholera. *John Churchill, London, 1855.*]

for periodicity of occurrence, partly because of the difficulty in defining the date of onset and partly because the induction period is likely to be prolonged and variable and thus not apt to be related to a periodic factor such as season. Seasonal fluctuation of disease may reflect changes in weather conditions (e.g., cold-induced frost-bite), the presence of plants (e.g., pollen, causing hay fever), the presence of insects (e.g., mosquito-borne encephalitis), or the influence of any one of a number of other kinds of environmental factors. Human host factors may also play a role in seasonal fluctuations, such as increased drownings and exposure to diseases from infected waters as the result of swimming during summer months.

Cyclic fluctuations, or cycles of disease, may be related to the seasons, but they are not limited to annual occurrences. For example, cyclic epidemics of measles every third year are almost predictable in some stable communities. *"Point" epidemics* refer to large but temporary excesses in disease frequency, usually occurring over a period of a few days. Figure 9-5 illustrates a "point" epidemic of cholera in London as identified by John Snow from data he assembled in 1848.

The time relation between exposure and onset of disease provides valuable epidemiologic information in the search for means to prevent disease. A clustering of cases following a medically connectable event often suggests hypotheses of causation, a good case in point being the large number of children born with congenital defects following the use of thalidomide by their mothers during pregnancy. The detection of clustering depends on precise measurement of the time elapsed between the presumed causative event and the onset of disease or other manifestation of pathology. The time relationship is most readily apparent in the infectious diseases (e.g., food poisoning due to salmonella), but it should not be overlooked in those diseases having a long, variable induction period (e.g., myocardial infarction due to arteriosclerosis) or in those diseases occurring only after prolonged exposure (e.g., lung cancer due to smoking).

Characteristics Describing Place. Place, as another element in the description of the distribution of disease, is defined in terms of geographic units, which may vary in size ranging from an entire nation, state, or county to relatively smaller units, including a city or other urban area, a rural area, or a local community. Data on morbidity and mortality are assembled by these geographic units from routinely available sources such as vital records and official records of reportable diseases. Occasionally, information is also obtained through special surveys. There are certain limitations in the use of the routinely available data, one of which stems from the differences that occur from place to place in standards of medical care and in the reporting of diseases. Another difficulty arises from the fact that boundaries of geographic units are, of course, established for administrative or political purposes, and these demarcations may obscure rather than differentiate the geographic factors which could influence the distribution of disease.

In some parts of the world, a good deal is known about the existence of certain infectious diseases from gross epidemiologic observations despite the fact that precise data are often missing. Thus, sometimes not even such basic information as births and deaths is routinely and accurately recorded. For example, the most accurate epidemiologic information in India derives from routine statistics only in "registration" areas surrounding large cities; information elsewhere in India is sometimes reliable only if collected as part of a special "survey."

Geographic units are often compared in order to ascertain variations in disease distribution. The comparisons customarily made are between or among nations, and within countries. It is often desirable to use special techniques in making such comparisons. For example, in state-to-state comparisons, industrial or agricultural areas of one state may be compared with similar areas in the other state. This helps to ensure that the geographic units being compared are generally similar to one another except for the factor being measured, namely, the occurrence of disease. Disease frequency is often compared between urban and rural areas within a state, although variations in standards of medical care between these two kinds of geographic units often make the results difficult to interpret.

In local communities, the distribution of disease is sometimes ascertained by plotting cases on a spot map. This technique is especially likely to be used in the investigation of an outbreak of a disease. In interpreting a spot map, the number of persons in the area must be taken into account since, for example, relatively few cases in a segment of the map may mean only that there are few inhabitants. This problem is overcome by the computation of rates, and such computations are desirable if the population at risk in the area is sufficiently large.

Characteristics Describing Person.   Several attributes of the persons affected are of particular importance in investigating and describing the distribution of disease. Age is perhaps the most important attribute of all. It has been found to be associated with variations in disease frequency more often and more strongly than has any other single factor. As explained earlier, this attribute is used in computing age-specific rates, which measure the association between disease occurrence and age. The association may be measured at one point in time, or it may be measured over a period of time among the members of a specified age group. A special instance of the latter is known as the cohort method, which consists of starting with a group of individuals who were all born in a specified period and subsequently observing the members of the same group at stated time intervals as they grow older.

Sex and race or ethnic group are other important population attributes in describing the distribution of disease. As with age, sex-specific rates or race-specific rates measure the association between disease occurrence and the attribute. Differences between males and females and between white and Negro populations have been demonstrated with respect to the occurrence of certain specific diseases. For example, heart disease and lung cancer are more likely to be found among males than among females. In the United States, mortality rates of arteriosclerotic heart disease and suicide are considerably higher among whites than among Negroes, whereas death rates from hypertensive heart disease, pneumonia, and tuberculosis are higher among Negroes than among whites.

Additional population attributes which are commonly investigated for possible association with disease frequency include occupation, socioeconomic status, and marital status. The first two are to some extent related to one another, but there are problems of definition and measurement in connection with both, and the information is sometimes difficult to obtain or is not available at all. Marital status, on the other hand, has fewer problems of definition and the information is generally more readily available.

ANALYTIC AND EXPERIMENTAL EPIDEMIOLOGY

As indicated in the foregoing discussion, data describing the occurrence and distribution of disease are analyzed for possible relationships between various phenomena in the disease process, such as the association between season and disease, age and disease, or locale and disease. In the analytic and experimental phases of epidemiology, investigation of the disease process is carried forward in greater depth, with the ultimate aim of understanding the determinants and mechanisms of disease. This kind of investigation involves the testing of hypotheses, which are often suggested by descriptive information.

Although information that serves as a basis for the description of disease generally comes from readily available sources, data for more intensive investigations usually must be obtained through special studies. In seeking to ascertain relationships between health-disease states and human and/or environmental factors, two kinds of study designs are commonly used: one design is referred to as a prospective study, the other as a retrospective study.[3,7]

In a *prospective study*, a population group initially free of a disease about which there is concern is generally followed up over a period of time. Particular interest is shown in the disease experience of portions of the population exposed and not exposed to a suspected noxious agent or element in the environment. For example, radiation due to atomic fallout may be suspected of giving rise to leukemia. Communities or other subpopulations initially generally free of the disease are identified as having been exposed to radiation from fallout and are compared with other communities not having been so exposed. If exposure to radiation causes leukemia, the exposed group will contract the disease and the nonexposed group will not. It may turn out that only slightly more of the exposed than of the nonexposed group ultimately contract the disease, which then leads to hypothesizing about possible factors which, along with exposure to radiation, may serve as codeterminants of incidence of the disease (e.g., age or sex). In some investigations, efforts have been made to rule out at least a few possible influencing factors by initially matching the groups on several measurable attributes. However, there still may remain unmatched a multiplicity of factors, both human host and environmental, which may be influential. Moreover, matching of attributes often is not feasible for very large groups.

In a *retrospective study*, a series of cases of a specified disease is compared to a series which is free of the disease for the purpose of ascertaining the factors that are responsible for the two disease statuses. This method generally utilizes what is known as the case-control technique, in which each case is matched to a control on several characteristics such as age, sex, race, and marital status. In order to test hypotheses regarding factors leading to the disease under investigation, information is sought for both groups concerning the frequency of *past* exposure to the suspected cause. Since such information usually must be obtained from the individual members of the two groups, problems of accuracy and completeness of recall become important considerations. The sources of both cases and controls are also of prime importance in a retrospective study. For example, if the cases under study consist of a representative sample of all cases of the disease in the community, the controls should also provide a representative sample of the locale. Similarly, if the cases are drawn from a hospital population, it is usually desirable to draw the controls from the same setting. If two or more hospitals separately provide cases and controls, it must be established in advance that the hospitals are comparable with respect to admission policies or other factors that might serve as a source of bias.

Prospective and retrospective studies utilize what are known as *observational methods*, meaning that a series of measurements are made and conclusions or inferences are derived through a process of reasoning from the evidence. By this means a statistical association may be demonstrated between a specific phenomenon and a specific disease, and it is sometimes possible to infer whether or not the association is causal. However, the most stringent test of an association and sometimes the only way in which it is possible to establish true causality (i.e., the exact determinants and mechanisms of disease) is through an *experiment*.[3,7] Experimental epidemiology was originally developed in the context of colonies of laboratory animals into which disease was introduced and its spread observed in relation to various controlled conditions such as crowding and size of colony.[4,7] In human populations, experiments usually have been undertaken in clinical or institutional settings, but a few experiments have also been conducted on a community basis. The experiments may involve, for example, the testing of the efficacy of a therapeutic drug or of a preventive measure such as a vaccine.

An experiment tests a clearly defined hypothesis stating, for example, that the incidence of a disease will be reduced by the introduction of a specific experimental condition, the latter perhaps consisting of a deliberate alteration of the environment, or the introduction of some preventive measure, or the use of some therapeutic agent. The hypothesis is tested by instituting the experimental condition in one group of individuals (or in a community), but not in a comparable group (or community), and observing the effects over a period of time; an experiment, therefore, is a special kind of prospective study. Those subject to the experimental condition are known as the experimental, or test, group; their counterparts are known as the control group. Such groups may be established by alternate or random assignment of individuals to one group or another or by pairing test subjects to control subjects through strict matching procedures. Ideally, neither those who make the observations nor the subjects themselves know to which group, test or control, any individual belongs. An investigation that adheres to this condition is known as a "double-blind" experiment. The most massive "double-blind" experiment undertaken to date consisted of the field trials conducted in the United States in 1954 to test the effectiveness of the Salk vaccine in preventing paralytic poliomyelitis. More than 400,000 children six to eight years of age received either vaccine or nonvaccine (placebo) inoculations, and neither the observers, the children, nor their parents knew the nature of the inoculation.

There are several instances in which epidemiologic investigations have gone through the entire process of observational and experimental methods.[9] A classic illustration is Joseph Goldberger's studies of pellagra beginning in 1914. Prior to his work, it was generally believed that pellagra was an infectious disease. Goldberger, however, noted that the disease was essentially rural, that it was associated with poverty, and that when it occurred in institutional settings, it was not found among the nurses and attendants. These considerations led him to hypothesize that the disease was caused by a dietary deficiency and that it could be prevented by increasing protein intake. Goldberger first tested the hypothesis *observationally* by demonstrating an association between pellagra and protein-deficient diet in seven cotton mill villages in South Carolina. He next proved the hypothesis *experimentally* by preventing pellagra in institutional patients through an adequate diet and by inducing pellagra in prison volunteers through a protein-deficient diet.

References

1. U.S. Bureau of the Census. *Statistical Abstract of the United States: 1971*, 92nd ed. U.S. Government Printing Office, Washington, D.C.
2. United Nations. *Handbook of Vital Statistics Methods.* The United Nations Statistical Office, New York, 1955.

3. MacMahon, B., Pugh, T. F., and Ipsen, J. *Epidemiologic Methods*. Little, Brown & Company, Boston, 1960.

4. Paul, John R. *Clinical Epidemiology*, revised ed. The University of Chicago Press, Chicago, Illinois, 1966.

5. Clark, E. G. The epidemiologic approach and contributions to preventive medicine. In: Leavell, H. R., and Clark, E. G. (eds.). *Preventive Medicine for the Doctor in His Community*, 3rd ed. McGraw-Hill Book Company, New York, 1965.

6. Cassel, John M. Potentialities and limitations of epidemiology. In: Katz, A. H., and Felton, J. S. (eds.). *Health and the Community*. The Free Press, New York, 1965.

7. Sartwell, Philip E. Epidemiology. In: Sartwell, P. E. (ed.). *Maxcy-Rosenau Preventive Medicine and Public Health*, 9th ed. Appleton-Century-Crofts, New York, 1965.

8. Fox, John P., Hall, Carrie E., and Elveback, Lila R. *Epidemiology — Man and Disease*. The Macmillan Company, New York, 1970.

9. Terris, Milton. The scope and methods of epidemiology. *Am J Public Health*, **52:**1371–76, September 1962.

10. Roueché, Berton. *Annals of Epidemiology*. Little, Brown & Company, Boston, 1967.

11. Roueché, Berton. *The Orange Man and Other Narratives of Medical Detection*. Little, Brown & Company, Boston, 1971.

12. Rogers, Fred B. (ed.). *Studies in Epidemiology: Selected Papers of Morris Greenberg, M.D.* G. P. Putnam's Sons, New York, 1965.

13. Clark, E. G., and Leavell, H. R. Levels of application of preventive medicine. In: Leavell, H. R., and Clark, E. G. (eds.). *Preventive Medicine for the Doctor in His Community*, 3rd ed. McGraw-Hill Book Company, New York, 1965.

Additional Reading

Kessler, Irving I., and Levin, Morton L. (eds.). *The Community as an Epidemiologic Laboratory — A Casebook of Community Studies*. The Johns Hopkins Press, Baltimore, 1970.

Petersen, William. *Population*. The Macmillan Company, New York, 1961.

Roueché, Berton (ed.). *Curiosities of Medicine — An Assembly of Medical Diversions, 1552–1962*. Little, Brown & Company, Boston, 1963.

U.S. Bureau of the Census. *The Methods and Materials of Demography*, Vols. I and II, by Henry S. Shryock, Jacob S. Siegel, and associates. U.S. Government Printing Office, Washington, D.C., 1971.

U.S. Department of Health, Education, and Welfare, Public Health Service, National Center for Health Statistics. *Physicians' Handbook on Medical Certification: Death, Fetal Death, Birth*. Public Health Service Publication No. 593-B. U.S. Government Printing Office, Washington, D.C., 1967.

U.S. Department of Health, Education, and Welfare, Public Health Service, National Center for Health Statistics. *Vital Statistics of the United States*. Four volumes, annual.

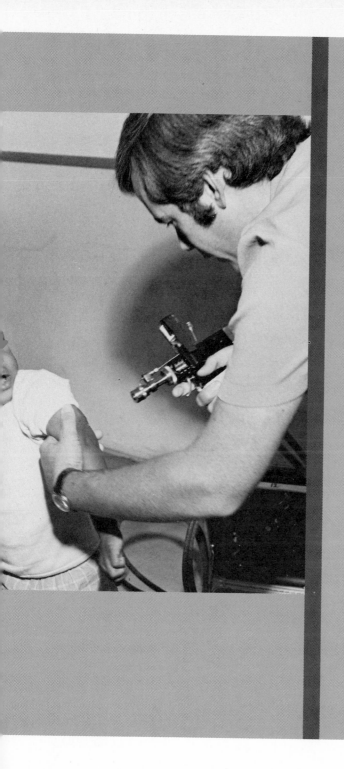

10

CONTROL OF
COMMUNICABLE
DISEASES

CHAPTER OUTLINE

The Significance of Communicable Disease

The Communicable Disease Process

Causative Agents (Pathogens)
Reservoirs of Causative Agents
Means of Escape from Reservoirs
Means of Transmission from Reservoirs
Means of Entry into New, Susceptible Hosts

Principal Prevention and Control Measures

Immunization
Quarantine
Environmental Control Measures
Control of Human Carriers

Public Health Roles in Communicable Disease Control

Objectives of Communicable Disease Control Programs
Responsibilities for Control Programs
The Role of Epidemiology in Control Programs
Nationwide Surveillance
Research
Prevention

Principal Classes of Communicable Diseases

Selected Communicable Diseases

Venereal Diseases
Tuberculosis
Rubella (German Measles)
Infectious Hepatitis (Epidemic or Catarrhal Jaundice)
Serum Hepatitis (Homologous Serum Jaundice)
Staphylococcal Infections
Malaria

Courtesy of Los Angeles County Health Department, Division of Public Health Education.

Communicable diseases have always afflicted mankind and influenced important turns in human history. For example, leprosy resulted in the phenomenon of "social outcast" and the obligation for the diseased person to give verbal warning that he was "unclean." Epidemics over the centuries have killed more soldiers than weapons of war and turned victories into defeat. The Black Death of the Middle Ages carried off intellectual and artistic communities that might have contributed to the earlier enlightenment of the Western world. Pandemics hastened decay of the older civilizations. Tropical fevers such as malaria inhibited development of Asia, and yellow fever had a vivid connotation in "the white man's grave" of West Africa.

The control of these diseases was largely empirical for many centuries. Thousands of years before proof of the germ theory of disease transmission, the enforced requirement for lepers to separate themselves from the rest of the population was an early form of quarantine. The establishment of Adriatic quarantine stations by the Venetian maritime powers in the sixteenth century was the direct forerunner of the present international quarantine covering the pestilential diseases: smallpox, cholera, plague, louseborne typhus, louseborne relapsing fever, and yellow fever.

Jenner's observation of the protective power of cowpox inoculation in 1798 led to the practice of vaccination decades before the basic principles of microbiology and immunology were even contemplated. Louis Pasteur, a century ago, applied the new objective scientific methods of observation and controlled experiment to establish the modern science of microbiology. As a result, he successfully dealt with rabies, a problem that today still challenges the most sophisticated virologic and immunologic techniques and public health practice. Sir Patrick Manson, Sir Ronald Ross, and Walter Reed established the principles of arthropod transmission of filariasis, malaria, and yellow fever.

Provision of pure water supply, sewage disposal, and drainage has been the basis for development of Asia and Africa in the past century. The introduction of these controls for infectious diseases has been responsible for the emergence of many of the newly developing nations of the world today, although the attendant problems of disease control have by no means been completely successful.

Modern means of communicable disease control have contributed so significantly to the current human population explosion that some of the frightened beholders of the results have even suggested withholding means of disease prevention from those most in need. However, history has shown that the intelligence of man has adapted new boons to his own social betterment and that serious trouble results when people selectively judge who will survive.

The Significance of Communicable Disease

Communicable disease saps the well-being and productivity of individuals, communities, nations, and societies of human beings. A primary goal of public health is to prevent occurrence of recognized communicable diseases and to avoid potential diseases that threaten to intrude from elsewhere. Therefore, the priority objective in any acute communicable disease program is prevention. This involves application of the most up-to-date means of sanitation, immunization, and quarantine. Although present-day healthy communities, which are largely free of pestilential diseases of the past exemplify extensive success of such measures, the relentless threat of parasitism requires continued awareness.

In the United States even in relatively recent years, communicable diseases have shown a variety of patterns in frequency of occurrence. Several specific diseases have declined, but others have increased, or remained fairly constant, or fluctuated. Table 10-1 illustrates a few of these patterns, showing the number of cases of several reportable communicable diseases in selected years from 1945 to 1969. Thus, whooping cough, diphtheria, undulant fever, and typhoid fever have declined markedly since 1945. Following upward trends from 1945, poliomyelitis and measles declined after 1950 and 1955, respectively; in fact, poliomyelitis had almost disappeared by 1969 (Table 10-1). Salmonellosis, on the other hand, increased steadily and strikingly from 1945 to 1969. Malaria has had a variable pattern, with peaks in cases coinciding with the return of servicemen from tropical areas overseas. Streptococcal sore throat and scarlet fever began climbing after 1950, and by 1969 had among the highest number of cases of all the reportable diseases (being exceeded only by the venereal diseases, as described in a later section of this chapter).

TABLE 10-1. Selected Reportable Diseases — Cases Reported, United States, Selected Years

	1945	1950	1955	1960	1965	1969
Pertussis (whooping cough)	133,792	120,718	62,786	14,809	6,799	3,285
Diphtheria	18,675	5,796	1,984	918	164	241
Brucellosis (undulant fever)	5,049	3,510	1,444	751	262	235
Typhoid fever	4,211	2,484	1,704	816	454	364
Poliomyelitis, acute	13,624	33,300	28,985	3,190	72	20
Measles	146,013	319,124	555,156	441,703	261,904	25,826
Salmonellosis	649	1,233	5,447	6,929	17,161	18,419
Malaria	62,763	2,184	522	72	147	3,102
Streptococcal sore throat and scarlet fever	185,570	64,494	147,502	315,173	395,168	450,008

Source: Adapted from U.S. Bureau of the Census. *Statistical Abstract of the United States, 1971,* p. 77.

In newly emerging nations throughout the world, one of the greatest problems is the development of a healthy and productive people by conquering the communicable diseases which have vitiated capability to learn and work competitively with those who have largely achieved such control. Communicable diseases are still the number-one health problem of the majority of human residents of the earth. Figure 10-1 shows graphically the far larger contribution of communicable (infectious) diseases to causes of death in a developing country than in a highly developed one. Economic self-sufficiency will not be within reach of emerging nations until communicable disease control and prevention effectively reach all their people.

Since communicable diseases are a worldwide concern — and a critical one in developing countries — they are an important area of activity for international health authorities. Thus, the World Health Organization and the Pan-American Health Organization have attacked certain communicable disease problems such as malaria and smallpox through specific technical assistance programs. However, effective application of knowledge to many problems such as yellow fever and schistosomiasis has not been possible because of limited resources. Localized or epidemic problems are dealt with by provision of expert consultation or participation in investigation and control efforts. Communication of information is through frequent epidemiologic reports of quarantinable and other diseases, general information in periodic chronicles, and outlets for scientific advances and research through technical publications. In addition, comprehensive presentation of specific areas of knowledge is pro-

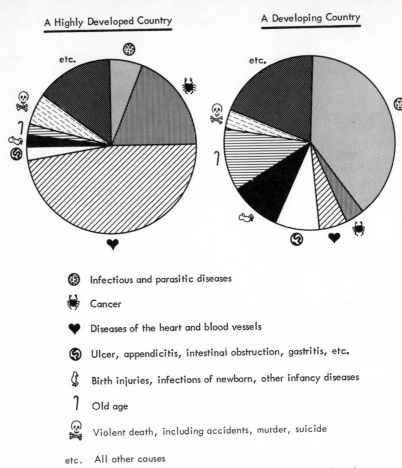

FIGURE 10-1. *Patterns of causes of death: a highly developed country and a developing country.* [SOURCE: World Health Organization, Geneva, 1967.]

vided through special technical reports and monographs. Orientation and general education are provided through widely distributed publication of interesting and readable elementary information in brochures and periodicals.

Possibly the most dramatic reminder of the insidious and potentially global nature of communicable disease is the cholera pandemic of 1961–1971 (a pandemic is an epidemic spread over a vast geographic area). From a remote section of Indonesia where it had been localized for some time, cholera suddenly began spreading in 1961, traveling north to Korea, Taiwan, and the Philippines. After that the disease moved westward, reaching West Pakistan, Afghanistan, Iran, Iraq, and the southern Soviet Union in 1964. In 1970 it invaded Africa, which was particularly hard hit. The World Health

Organization sent special cholera teams to several African states where crash programs were initiated to train health workers to cope with the disease. In 1971, cholera touched Spain and late the same year appeared in Lapland. Not since the great cholera outbreak of 1899 had so much of the world become involved in the disease.

The Communicable Disease Process

A communicable disease is an illness caused by a specific organism that is capable of producing infection or infectious disease. Every case of such disease represents the result of a process—that is, the operation of a series of factors, all of which lead to an outcome manifested in the case. Thus, disease ensues only if a particular chain of events occurs and if the chain is unbroken and completed.

There are five factors that are essential parts of the process that characterizes communicable disease:[1] (1) an etiologic or *causative agent* (pathogen); (2) a *reservoir* or source of the causative agent; (3) a *means of escape* from the reservoir; (4) a *means of transmission* from the reservoir to a new host; (5) a *means of entry* into the new, *susceptible host*.

CAUSATIVE AGENTS (PATHOGENS)

Infection begins with the invasion of the body (human or animal) by a living organism which constitutes the causative or etiologic agent of the disease in question. The agent is usually parasitic since it lives in, upon, and at the expense of the body it has invaded. Sometimes there is a balance between the parasitic agent and the body so that, temporarily at least, no illness appears. For example, the colon bacillus is harmless as long as it is confined to the intestinal tract.

The generally recognized categories of invading parasitic agents or pathogens are viruses, rickettsiae, bacteria, fungi, protozoa, metazoal parasites, and ectoparasites.

Viruses are the smallest pathogens and in one respect the most successful form of parasite. They consist of a template chemical that borrows from the living cell the enzymatic and nutritional elements necessary to reproduce. In doing so they deleteriously deplete or destroy the cells, which ultimately leads to organic dysfunction. As obligate intracellular parasites they can only replicate (reproduce) inside a living cell, a phenomenon that characterizes viral infections as the most insidious. The cells, tissues, and organs of the host in essence protect the virus from chemotherapeutic attack, which is the conventional means for dealing with the other categories of etiologic agents. There is a greater variety of viruses than of any other category of microbial agents of disease.

Rickettsiae are also obligate intracellular parasites but are susceptible to antibiotic suppression of replication. They also differ from viruses in being visible under a conventional microscope by special staining techniques.

Bacteria can readily multiply outside of living cells. This makes them amenable to cultivation on artifical media. They are also readily visualized by appropriate staining techniques. The detection and identification of a bacterial cause of disease are therefore much simpler relative to the special facilities and techniques necessary to detect, isolate, and identify viruses and rickettsia.

Fungi are the lowest form of infectious agent that bridge the gap between free-living and host-dependent parasites. Being of unicellular or multicellular form, they are rather easily characterized visually under the microscope and can be grown on selective artifical media.

Protozoa, as the term implies, are single-celled organisms. They are large enough to fix and stain for definitive microscopic identification according to nuclear and cytoplasmic structure. Although as living cells their nutritional and physiologic requirements are complex, some can be readily cultivated, which aids in their detection and identification. Forms vary from intracellular (malaria) to hematogenous (trypanosomes).

Metazoal parasites, because they are multicellular, occur in widely varied form that reflects the special adaptation characteristic of their parasitic cycles, which are reflected by the categorical terms trematodes, nematodes, and filaria.

Ectoparasites range from those that superficially affect the host, like lice and scabies mites, to those that invade the integument, such as larvae of dipterous flies.

RESERVOIRS OF CAUSATIVE AGENTS

Infecting organisms must have places where they can live and multiply. Such places are known as reservoirs of infection and are found mainly in human beings and in animals.

Human reservoirs include persons who are obviously ill with the disease (overt cases) as well as abortive and walking cases of the disease (subclinical cases). In addition, health workers have long been concerned with human carriers as a significant source of communicable disease. These are the "Typhoid Marys," for example, who are unaware of their condition and circulate freely in their communities until detected and diagnosed. All such cases—overt, subclinical, and carrier—serve as reservoirs from which disease may be communicated to other persons.

Animal reservoirs are mainly (although not exclusively) domestic animals and rodents. An animal disease that is transmissible to man is called a *zoonosis*. Usually, if an infection occurs, it is derived directly from the animal and is not further transmitted from man to man.

MEANS OF ESCAPE FROM RESERVOIRS

The causative agent or pathogenic organism must have a means of escape from its reservoir in order to bring about infection in another body. Sometimes an organism is unable to escape from its reservoir and therefore is of less public health significance than one that has a ready means of escape. Thus, a person who is infected with trichinosis is not a menace to others because the trichinae have no avenue of exit from his body or of transfer to someone else.

Principal avenues for escape (or *portals of exit*) of pathogenic organisms from reservoirs are the respiratory tract, through secretions from the nose, nasal sinuses, nasopharynx, larynx, trachea, bronchial tree, and lungs; the intestinal tract, through discharge with the feces; the urinary tract; and open lesions or discharges on the surface of the body.

The period during which the pathogen can escape from its reservoir is the *period of infectivity or communicability*. It is the time during which means for isolation and control against further transmission can be applied.

MEANS OF TRANSMISSION FROM RESERVOIRS

Once a pathogenic organism has escaped from its reservoir (human or animal) it must have either a direct or indirect mode of transmission to a new victim (host). In *direct transmission* the organism goes from one body to another without the aid of intermediate objects. In *indirect transmission* there is some vehicle which transmits the organism, and as a consequence the organism must be able to survive for a period of time outside the body. The inability of certain organisms to do this greatly reduces the likelihood of spread of the diseases for which they are responsible.

There are animate and inanimate vehicles for the transmission of pathogenic organisms. *Animate vehicles* are called *vectors* and include the various insects that can convey infection from one body to another. Thus, an insect is a vector which bridges the gap from reservoir to new victim. *Inanimate vehicles* are nonliving substances or objects and include water, milk and other foods, air, soil, and fomites (articles such as clothing, bed linen, utensils).

MEANS OF ENTRY INTO NEW, SUSCEPTIBLE HOSTS

Having achieved transmission from a reservoir, a pathogenic organism must next gain entry into a new victim or host. The principal entrance routes (or *portals of entry*) are the respiratory tract, the gastrointestinal tract, the skin, and the mucous membranes.

The interval of time between the entry of the pathogen into the host and the onset of symptoms of disease is known as the *incubation period*. It may be more or less precisely defined for certain diseases such as measles, for which the incubation period is normally ten days. Other diseases have variable incubation periods which may reflect the initial mass of infectious material introduced into the host, longer if in small amount, shorter if from a large infectious dose.

Even though a pathogen gains entry to the body it does not necessarily result in infection or disease. In order to fall victim to the disease, the new host must be *susceptible* to it. However, the body has certain defense mechanisms which help protect against invading pathogens and may aid in the latter's destruction. Such mechanisms are called *resistance*, and if sufficiently great, they constitute *immunity*.

Principal Prevention and Control Measures

IMMUNIZATION

Immunization is a process by which susceptible hosts are artifically prepared to resist infection by a specific disease agent. Immunization of a community to a calculable extent is a means for preventing establishment of a communicable disease. There are two types of immunization: active and passive.

Passive immunization is accomplished by the introduction of specific immune substances that act directly against exposure to an infectious agent within a reasonable period of time. For example, infectious hepatitis is sufficiently endemic and widespread in the human population to have produced specific antibodies in a large number of human beings. Immune globulin, extracted from blood plasma pooled from many people, contains in concentrated form specific antibodies against the virus of infectious hepatitis. Therefore, a sufficiently large dose of pooled human immune globulin inoculated into a person likely to be exposed to infectious hepatitis virus infection while traveling or living abroad (as with Peace Corps volunteers and servicemen in Southeast Asia) will provide protection for up to six months, by which time the antibodies in the immune globulin will no longer persist in sufficient strength. Prolonged exposure requires periodic reinoculation with passively immune substances such as gamma globulin.

Active immunization is the introduction of a specific antigenic substance to produce a specific immune reaction in the form of antibodies. The antibodies formed will oppose or combine with a specific infectious agent, preventing its invasion and multiplication in the tissues of the host or will prevent the effect of a toxin. Antigens (i.e., antibody generators) may be living, attenuated forms of the virulent agent, as in 17 D yellow fever vaccination, or they may be substances in which the infectivity is inactivated without destroying the antigenicity that stimulates the specific immune response. Examples of the latter are typhoid and cholera vaccines in which the virulent organisms have been chemically killed.

The Vaccination Assistance Act of 1963 put at the disposal of state and local health authorities the means for immunizing large sections of the population against such diseases as smallpox, diphtheria, pertussis, and measles. In mid-1971, the Public Health Service adopted a policy change involving discontinuance of routine smallpox vaccination in this country in favor of a selective vaccination program for those population groups who may be exposed to the disease. Circumstances influencing the new policy included the absence of smallpox from the United States for the past 22 years; the success of a global smallpox control program sponsored by the World Health Organization beginning in 1967; and the decreasing probability of smallpox importation into the United States.

QUARANTINE

Quarantine is the process of detecting infectious agents, infected persons, or other implicated hosts and vectors and preventing their introduction into a susceptible locality or population. Quarantine can be applied at the geographic source, which in the world at present is possible only under sanctions of the World Health Organization. It is usually applied at points of entry into a susceptible locality which is free of the agent in question. Thus, quarantine is one of the most effective measures for prevention of communicable disease occurrence in various parts of the world, particularly in the United States. Quarantine measures have prevented outbreaks of smallpox and possibly the introduction of yellow fever. They have slowed and sometimes stopped the movement of cholera and often work in concert with other preventive measures, such as immunization, to prevent geographic expansion of a variety of infectious diseases.

ENVIRONMENTAL CONTROL MEASURES

Preventive measures of a more permanent nature evolve from environmental control. Accomplishments of sanitary engineering such as pure water supply and proper disposal of sewage and other potentially infectious material have been legislated into building codes, city planning, state laws, and federal regulations to the point where they are almost an automatic, routine procedure in the physical development of the environment occupied by the growing population of the United States.

Associated with this, however, are biologic phenomena that so far have frustrated engineering design for exclusion. These are the zoonotic sources of infectious agents, i.e., vertebrate reservoirs and arthropod vectors. It is therefore necessary to maintain surveillance for the implicated vectors and reservoir animals. For instance, *Culex tarsalis* and *Culex pipiens quinquefasciatus* mosquitoes are vectors of arbovirus encephalitis. It has not been possible to engineer them out of existence, so continuous monitoring of their breeding and activity in previously affected or potentially susceptible localities is necessary. In the same way, dairy cattle reservoirs for Q fever and domestic canine and wild vertebrate hosts for rabies must be continually watched for the appearance of infected animals that could become a source of transmission of disease to man.

It is obvious that resources must also be developed, maintained, and continually changed in order to provide effective vector and vertebrate reservoir control. Every health authority responsible for a population in a mosquito-infested environment should have not only pest mosquito control but also means for dealing specifically with mosquito vectors of disease. The important role of the public health veterinarian pertains not only to the surveillance, but also to the control, of zoonotic sources of infectious agents.

In the realm of environmental control is the capability of disinfecting potentially infectious materials and premises, procedures that may well be within the capacity of a sanitary organization that effectively deals with vectors and animal reservoirs. Such a capacity would range from the rodenticidal control of rats to the fumigation and decontamination of rooms bacterially contaminated with such agents as staphylococcus or anthrax.

CONTROL OF HUMAN CARRIERS

Human carriers of such diseases as typhoid, amebiasis, and infectious hepatitis must, as vertebrate reservoirs, be kept under surveillance, detected, and controlled in a manner similar to other vector-reservoir species. It is often necessary physically to control human carriers by varying degrees of isolation. These may range from enforcement of rules segregating infected food handlers from eating establishments, to hospitalization of actual or suspected carriers for surgery or chemoprophylaxis. Examples are the extirpation of the *Salmonella typhii*-infected gallbladder, the chemotherapy of staphylococcus-infected nasopharynx or other lesions, and the suppression of *Neisseria meningococcus* by sulfa drugs. These means, which are often used on an individual basis, may on occasion be extended to a population such as the military personnel of a unit in which meningococcic meningitis exposure or epidemic has occurred, recognizing that one result may be the development of resistant strains, as has occurred in hospital infections with staphylococcus.

Public Health Roles in Communicable Disease Control

OBJECTIVES OF COMMUNICABLE DISEASE CONTROL PROGRAMS

A public health program in the area of communicable disease has several objectives. One is the detection of disease occurrence and the pinpointing of causes of disease outbreaks. Another is to keep track of the course of disease by assembling incidence and prevalence data on numerous specific communicable diseases. A third objective is the provision of adequate resources — material and technical — for application of control methods. Fourth is the utilization of methods for improving prevention of communicable diseases.

The eradication of communicable disease is frequently assumed to be the ultimate goal of communicable disease control programs. If eradication is interpreted to mean extirpation, the ultimate objective must necessarily be the elimination of the last viable representative of a specific pathogen from the earth. The enormity of such an accomplishment challenges imagination and does not seem practical. In other contexts, eradication simply means removal of a pathogen from a geographic region or population group. Or it may mean suppression of an infection or disease below an apparent or detectable level in a community or other definable situation. It is obvious that pursuit of any one of these latter goals of eradication can bring about effective disease control and actually accomplish widespread prevention of disease. Thus, the objective of disease eradication is a constructive public health concept provided there is a clear understanding of what is really meant.

Potential and actual deleterious effects of eradication campaigns are important considerations. Pressures on survival of biologic forms can cause genetic mutation, as has been observed in the development of antibiotic-resistant bacteria and insecticide-resistant mosquito vectors. Such developments have produced more perplexing communicable disease problems than existed before means were applied to eliminate these species. Another consideration is that removal of the immunizing prevalence of endemic infections such as malaria or poliomyelitis may result in intrusion of other parasitic forms that have, until now, not reached the human population. Finally, unsuccessful attempts to immunize a juvenile population by active immunization for a disease like measles may delay infection in sufficient numbers of persons who will then suffer more severe and more frequently fatal complications of the adult disease.

RESPONSIBILITIES FOR CONTROL PROGRAMS

Like other spheres of public health concern in the United States, communicable disease control is the responsibility of each sovereign state. The state health officer customarily delegates this full-time activity to a division of communicable diseases. A staff of physicians, public health nurses, and veterinarians works closely with the public health laboratory and state epidemiologist in detection, diagnosis, assessment, and control of communicable diseases. Because of their separate magnitude, tuberculosis and venereal diseases are often handled by associated divisions, specially designated for those diseases.

On the recommendation of the infectious disease experts, legislation is promulgated requiring every physician, practitioner, veterinarian, dentist, coroner, and responsible director of dispensaries, clinics, and hospitals to notify local health authorities (city or county) of the occurrence of cases of specified reportable diseases. This information is relayed to the state health department, where it is tabulated. The information may be of such type or extent to require further investigation or outside support and augmentation of local measures for control.

Such further investigation can be requested by the local authority or suggested by the state experts. An epidemiologist or other qualified person may be sent to investigate the reports and circumstances to determine whether it is a sporadic case or a component of an impending or current epidemic. Field and laboratory methodology and resources are utilized expeditiously to obtain a clear assessment of the situation. Where these are limited, the state health officer may request assistance from the Center for Disease Control

(Health Services and Mental Health Administration, Public Health Service).

The Center for Disease Control is located in Atlanta, Georgia, and until mid-1970 was known as the National Communicable Disease Center. The center is responsible for national programs for the prevention and control of communicable and other preventable diseases. Its epidemiology and laboratory programs provide skilled investigators and laboratory techniques of a type and quantity that may not otherwise be obtainable within state resources. The center also enforces quarantine regulations; conducts foreign quarantine activities; administers international activities for the control of malaria, smallpox, and measles; and provides consultation to other nations in the control of preventable diseases.

States are further assisted by the federal government through appropriation of funds to support communicable disease programs. Amendments to the Public Health Service Act in 1966 and again in 1970 provided for grants to states and communities to help meet the costs of a wide variety of specific control programs.

THE ROLE OF EPIDEMIOLOGY IN CONTROL PROGRAMS

The response of the epidemiologist to a reported disease is to determine in time, numbers, and geographic range the extent of the communicable disease process. The basic approach is *case-finding*. Starting with inquiry of the person who detected the earliest or first suspected case, called the index case, other suspected cases are located by telephone, house calls, hospital visits, and a variety of other means encompassed by the term "shoeleather epidemiology." On the basis of clinical suspicion and epidemiologic clues as to the etiology, appropriate specimens—blood, urine, feces, sputum, throat washings, skin scrapings, or purulent substances—are collected from cases and contacts. These are submitted to the public health laboratory for isolation, characterization, and identification of the causative agent or for serologic determination of the etiology.

As case-finding locates additional suspect patients, information is obtained that focuses on the time and location of exposure, possible source of infection, incubation period, clinical course, status of outcome (recovery, sequelae, or death), and pattern of dissemination. On receipt of laboratory characterization of the etiology, the fundamental basis for confirmation of suspect cases is established. Definition of the disease as to origin, time, evolution, and dissemination can be accurately assessed on the basis of epidemiologic data. Intelligent means for control and possibly prevention of other infections can then be applied.

Epidemiologic definition of a communicable disease in a human population is dependent on quantitative determination of incidence and prevalence of either infection or disease. Incidence is the occurrence at a point or within a unit of time. Prevalence may be considered the amount within a particular population. The more acute the process, the closer incidence approximates prevalence, as with measles. The more insidious, the greater variance between the two. For example, the incidence of active tuberculosis at any time in a community is distinctly less than the prevalence of persons showing past infection by x-ray or tuberculin test. Another example is the relationship of the annual incidence of overt cases of St. Louis encephalitis as compared with the prevalence of accumulated immunes owing to previous, usually inapparent infections as manifest by presence of specific antibody in serum detected by serologic tests.

NATIONWIDE SURVEILLANCE

The increased rapidity and frequency of human mobility have brought increasing need for recognition of communicable diseases beyond the confines of states and local communities. This has evolved into a collective communication of state information to the Public Health Service, which tabulates and assesses the data on a national scale. The resulting information is produced as the *Morbidity and Mortality Weekly Report* of the Center for Disease Control. The reports list the communicable diseases which are reportable in most states. Often, only on a national scale can current or evolving problems requiring urgent attention be visualized. An example of this is the cumulative reporting of hundreds of malaria cases in American servicemen returning from Southeast Asia to a nation where malaria as an indigenous problem was eliminated 25 years ago. Person-to-person-transmitted viral diseases such as influenza and poliomyelitis emerge from the national picture as a completely different order of importance for the attention of local and state public health personnel than if the status of these diseases was available only at the state level. The national reporting has not supplanted the basic state provision of information for its own localities, but it has given an additional and very useful perspective which is at the disposal of those who must detect and combat communicable diseases.

It must be emphasized, however, that without local observers such as the physician and nurse and other health personnel, who see or suspect a patient with an infectious disease, the higher echelons of information gathering, collation, and action would be impossible. The corollary is that without the individual professionals in various medical and health pursuits, measures of prevention and control derived from the regional and national assessments would be impossible. The local practitioners and health institutions are therefore the beginning and the end, initiator and recipient, of the essential chain of events that leads to control and prevention of communicable disease.

RESEARCH

There are those who suggest that research for further knowledge about infectious disease and its prevention not be stressed relative to the need for similar knowledge in other fields (i.e., cancer, heart disease, mental disease). However, being biologic phenomena, infectious diseases are continually shifting in nature to adapt to the changing patterns and circumstances of human behavior. It is therefore important to recognize the basic value of a vigorous, well-oriented research program in any continuing campaign to lessen the impact of infectious disease on individual and community health. Only through such continued study can appropriate means be applied for disease control. Such research ranges from basic laboratory studies to field investigations leading to detection, diagnosis, surveillance, and application of control.

Knowledgeable professionals, scientifically trained and provided with adequate facilities and appropriate equipment, are continually applying these resources to detection and definition of natural occurrence of infectious diseases in sporadic and epidemic form, systematically deriving data that can be formulated into new knowledge, interpretable in terms of new concepts and as a basis for application of new methods of disease control. While the definition of a communicable disease situation is often attempted by observational and statistical epidemiology, the use of the public health laboratory as an investigative and etiologically confirmatory instrument is inseparable. In fact, the public health laboratory is essential as the spearhead of the epidemiologic investigation.

PREVENTION

As means for control of communicable diseases have become more effective and widely applied, there has been a shift in emphasis from control to prevention. Laws and regulations enforcing reporting, investigation, rectification of sanitary and environmental deficiencies, isolation of cases, and disinfection are now infrequently applied and only under exceptional circumstances, because the conditions they were written to improve have now been virtually eliminated.

On the other hand, as preventive and curative medical services have become more universally available through prenatal, well-baby, school, and outpatient clinics, new types and more effective vaccines have been given to a much larger segment of the population. The widespread use of Sabin oral polio vaccine is an example. Regulations for commercially distributed foods in regard to absence of bacterial contamination are becoming more rigid. Animal inspections and meat product-processing standards are being used to prevent disease by enforcing sanitary practices consistently. This is far more effective than using such methods merely for the detection and prosecution of offenders after a disease outbreak has occurred.

The widely held misconception of a decade or so ago that infectious diseases were passé because of antibiotics, chemotherapy, new vaccines, and sanitation is no longer assumed by knowledgeable professionals in the health field. However, not enough medically oriented young people are selecting infectious diseases as a career as will be necessary to maintain vigilance in the United States and effectively deal with the exotic diseases abroad. Education of qualified professionals in the clinical, laboratory, epidemiologic, and preventive aspects of communicable diseases is one of the most important objectives to be pursued by those engaged in the health sciences. As a challenge, these diseases persist. They will continue to lurk, sporadically threatening—with some new ones developing—as far as can be seen into the medical future of mankind.

Principal Classes of Communicable Diseases

Many of the communicable diseases fall into definite groups which are similar in some important characteristic such as susceptibility or immunity. The following categorization of communicable diseases into nine classes is based on this principle of commonality of characteristics:[2]

1. Diseases to which susceptibility is general, against which there is yet no procedure for active immunization, an attack of which confers lasting immunity, and which nearly all persons acquire at some time, usually in childhood (for example, chickenpox)
2. Diseases to which susceptibility is general, against which effective active immunization is available and should be generally applied to young children throughout the community—for example, diphtheria, whooping cough (pertussis), poliomyelitis, measles, rubella (German measles), and tetanus

3. Diseases of gastrointestinal origin, closely associated with poor sanitation (for example, the dysenteries, bacterial food poisoning, and typhoid)
4. Diseases spread by arthropod vectors (for example, malaria, encephalitis, and Rocky Mountain spotted fever)
5. Diseases spread to persons from animal reservoirs (for example, rabies, brucellosis, and Q fever)
6. Diseases spread by close or intimate contact (for example, venereal diseases and tuberculosis)
7. Diseases of international importance, the so-called "international quarantinable diseases" (for example, yellow fever, smallpox, cholera, plague, and louseborne typhus)
8. Other diseases not belonging to any one of the categories above (for example, streptococcal infections, epidemic influenza, the pneumonias, and meningococcal infections)
9. Illnesses of unknown cause, occurring in outbreaks (nonrecognizable or ill-defined disease entities)

Selected Communicable Diseases

The remainder of this chapter provides accounts of selected communicable diseases—the venereal diseases and tuberculosis as well as several others of current interest. Descriptions of the etiologic, epidemiologic, and clinical manifestations of some 117 communicable diseases appear in a publication of the American Public Health Association entitled *Control of Communicable Diseases in Man.*[3] Information is also available in numerous textbooks of infectious disease, medicine, and preventive medicine.[1,4-8]

VENEREAL DISEASES

The venereal diseases are communicable, but unlike most of the other communicable diseases, only human beings serve as reservoirs and vectors, and the mode of transmission is almost exclusively sexual intercourse. If untreated, the venereal diseases become chronic, requiring more comprehensive treatment and management for rehabilitation or restoration and, therefore, are related to the kinds of conditions discussed in the next chapter.

The stigma of having such diseases, the tendency to chronicity if untreated, the remote sequelae of some of them, the length and cost of treatment, and the resulting personal inconvenience complicate the problem both for the individual and for public control. The individual who contracts a venereal disease comes into conflict with society's mores—which are changing, to be sure—and, in addition, public law requires that his case be reported to the health department. He may, therefore, be reluctant to seek diagnosis and treatment for fear that public identification of himself and his contacts may result in social ostracism and legal harassment. The confidentiality of official venereal disease records and epidemiologic follow-up is well protected by law and practice, but this fact is not fully recognized by the public or the medical profession.

The public attaches little significance to early signs and symptoms of venereal disease and sometimes is opposed to public education on the subject, yet the risk of chronic disease is great and costly. Complications of untreated or inadequately treated syphilis may lead to heart disease, blindness, paralysis, infected newborns, psychoses, and pathologic changes in many tissues and organs of the human body. Gonorrhea is still considered by many persons as nothing worse than a common cold, but there are, in fact, serious potential complications of sterility and urinary obstruction, especially for women and girls.

Types of Venereal Diseases. There are five separate and distinctly different venereal diseases. Syphilis and gonorrhea are the most common in this country; the three others, which are of lower incidence, are chancroid, lymphogranuloma venereum, and granuloma inguinale. There are a number of other diseases that are transmitted by sexual contact, such as venereal warts; monilial infections; trichomonal, crab, and lice infestations; and a few others. However, these diseases are not considered to be classic examples of venereal disease and are not serious social problems.

There are two major categories of *syphilis*, which reflect the stage of development of the disease. The first category is subdivided into primary syphilis, which indicates the initial point of contact and infection (usually the genitalia), and secondary syphilis, which indicates the early systemic involvement (usually skin lesions are present and are indicators of bodywide infection of all other organs). The second category consists of latent and late syphilis, which are the chronic stages of the disease and include the involvement and destruction of selected tissues and organs remote from the usual sexual point of initial contact and infection. Manifestations of this stage of development of the disease may be delayed for months or even years.

The causative organism of venereal syphilis is *Treponema pallidum*. It is a spirochete and is classified with the bacteria for lack of a better category in which to place it. The incubation period in syphilis is about three to six weeks. In order to acquire the disease, it is necessary to have warm, moist, prolonged contact (essentially sexual intercourse) with another human being who has accessible syphilis lesions containing the causative organism. The organism is capable of invading several kinds of tissues. A lesion will usually develop at the site where original entry of the causative organism occurred after the incubation period. This is primary syphilis and the lesion is referred to as a chancre. The lesion is usually single, elevated, ulcerated, indurated, and painless. The commonest site in the male is the glans penis, and in the female frequently on the cervix, where it may go unnoticed. This lesion vanishes spontaneously in around two weeks as *Treponema pallidum,* which have proliferated at this site, leave to enter the circulatory and lymphatic systems. At this time, syphilis is no longer a local disease, but becomes systemic; the entire body is now infected and the manifestations of secondary syphilis begin to appear.

Congenital syphilis represents asexual transmission of the disease from an untreated or inadequately treated, infected mother to the unborn fetus. After the seventeenth week of pregnancy, it is considered possible for live *Treponema pallidum* circulating in maternal blood to cross the placental barrier and infect the fetus. The father need not have syphilis. Congenital syphilis is amenable to prevention through premarital and prenatal examinations.

The most significant development in finding a cure for syphilis came in 1943 when Mahoney found that penicillin (first discovered in 1926) seemed to cure several male volunteers. Penicillin is now the drug of choice and is successful in almost 100 per cent of cases under proper management. Penicillin G in various forms is relatively innocuous and can cure syphilis with as little as one injection. Patients who are allergic to penicillin can be successfully treated with tetracycline or erythromycin.

The most pressing venereal disease problem at present is *gonorrhea* because of its incidence, complications, and lack of good diagnostic techniques. The causative organism, *Neisseria gonorrhoeae,* is found primarily in the urinary tract (especially in males), the reproductive system (especially in females), rectum, pharynx, and conjuctiva. In a few cases, it mimics its close relative, the meningococcus, and becomes invasive producing septicemia, meningitis, endocarditis, and arthritis.

The incubation period for gonorrhea is short, from three to ten days. Usually the male is symptomatic and communicable three days after exposure. Therefore, case-finding must be immediate in gonorrhea. The male who waits until he has been symptomatic for five days before seeking treatment can have had contacts who, in turn, have been capable of spreading the disease for two days. Gonorrhea is communicable as long as the patient remains infected; in the female particularly, this may last for years. She will by no means infect every sex partner but only an occasional one. It is not unusual for males to acquire several infections in one year.

The primary complication of gonorrhea in the male is urinary obstruction, which is seldom recognized early. Healing in the urethra results in scar tissue formation, which, over many years, results in scar proliferation and ultimate urinary obstruction. The prime site of female infection is in the deep secretory glands of the cervical os, i.e., the opening to the uterus. A problem of early recognition is that the cervix is insensitive to pain, and the physiologic manifestations, such as discharge produced, are minimal.

A fetus leaving an infected mother on delivery will obviously subject its eyes to infection. Gonorrheal conjunctivitis at one time was the leading cause of blindness of the newborn but may be prevented by instillation of silver nitrate solution or penicillin ointment directly into the infant's conjunctiva at time of birth.

Treatment of gonorrhea has varied as the organism has become resistant to each newly available chemotherapeutic agent. Local therapy with potassium and silver salts was at one time effective. The organism has become relatively resistant to sulfa drugs, and resistance to penicillin is increasing. However, penicillin given in large amounts is still the drug of choice because of its low cost and its availability as an intramuscular injection with prolonged absorption. As resistance to penicillin increases, tetracyclines may become the drugs of choice in spite of their cost and the requirement of patient responsibility to take medication as prescribed.

Incidence of Syphilis and Gonorrhea.   It is generally agreed that incidence figures (the number of new cases per year) and prevalence figures (the total number of cases in various stages of diagnosis, treatment, and rehabilitation at any given time) underestimate the magnitude of both syphilis and gonorrhea. The figures are influenced by the stage of the disease, the number of persons who seek diagnosis, and the number who are treated in public clinics versus by private physicians. Thus, the venereal disease problem reveals itself like an iceberg showing only a small part of its total mass; the bulk of the problem hides unreported in the community. Many of the individuals with undetected venereal disease may be unaware that they are infected because they have only minor symptoms or none at all. However, in spite of the problems resulting from the various kinds of gaps in reporting, available data probably do indicate at least the general direction of actual trends and differences, even if not the precise amount.

Table 10-2, which shows incidence for the period 1950–1970, reveals a downward trend in syphilis (total, all stages), from 154 cases per 100,000 population in 1950 to 44 cases per 100,000 in 1970. Gonorrhea rates, on the other hand, have shown a different pattern. Thus, from a rate of 204 cases per 100,000 population in 1950, the

TABLE 10-2. Cases of Syphilis and Gonorrhea and Rates per 100,000 Population Reported by State Health Departments, Fiscal Years, 1950–1970

Fiscal Year	Total Syphilis*		Gonorrhea		Total VD† (Syphilis All Stages & Gonorrhea)	
	Cases	Rate	Cases	Rate	Cases	Rate
1950	229,723	154.2	303,922	204.0	533,645	358.2
1951	198,640	131.8	270,459	179.5	469,099	311.3
1952	168,734	110.8	245,633	161.3	414,367	272.1
1953	156,099	100.8	243,857	157.4	399,956	258.2
1954	137,876	87.5	239,661	152.0	377,537	239.5
1955	122,075	76.0	239,787	149.2	361,862	225.2
1956	126,219	77.1	233,333	142.4	359,552	219.5
1957	130,552	78.3	216,476	129.8	347,028	208.1
1958	116,630	68.5	220,191	129.3	336,821	197.8
1959	119,981	69.3	237,318	137.0	357,299	206.3
1960	120,249	68.0	246,697	139.6	366,946	207.6
1961	125,262	69.7	265,685	147.8	390,947	217.5
1962	124,188	68.1	260,468	142.8	384,656	210.9
1963	128,450	69.3	270,076	145.7	398,526	215.0
1964	118,247	62.9	290,603	154.5	408,850	217.4
1965	113,018	59.7	310,155	163.8	423,173	223.5
1966	110,128	57.1	334,949	173.6	445,077	230.7
1967	103,546	53.2	375,606	193.0	479,152	246.2
1968	98,195	49.9	431,380	219.2	529,575	269.1
1969	96,679	48.1	494,227	245.9	590,906	294.0
1970	87,934	43.8	573,200	285.2	661,134	329.0

* Includes congenital and other syphilis.
† Excludes chancroid, granuloma inguinale, and lymphogranuloma venereum.
Source: Adapted from American Social Health Association, American Public Health Association, and American Venereal Disease Association: A Joint Statement. *Today's VD Control Problem—1971.* American Social Health Association, New York.

TABLE 10-3. Gonorrhea and Syphilis Infection by Age Groups, Calendar Year 1969 (Reported Cases Only)

Age (years)	Gonorrhea		Syphilis (Primary and Secondary)	
	Number of Cases	Rate Per 100,000	Number of Cases	Rate Per 100,000
0–9	1,928	5.0	35	.1
10–14	4,325	21.1	223	1.1
15–19	129,071	712.5	3,423	18.9
20–24	207,221	1,412.2	5,295	36.1
25–29	102,257	794.1	3,758	29.2
0–24	342,545	372.0	8,976	9.7
25 and older	192,327	178.8	10,154	9.4

Source: Adapted from American Social Health Association, American Public Health Association, and American Venereal Disease Association: A Joint Statement. *Today's VD Control Problem—1971.* American Social Health Association, New York.

trend was downward until 1957 and 1958, when the gonorrhea case rates were about 129. Since then they have been climbing steadily, reaching a new, 20-year high of over one-half million cases, or 285 per 100,000 population, in 1970. Gonorrhea rates have been consistently higher than syphilis rates during the past 20 years.

The highest rates of venereal diseases are found in the age group of 20–24 years, as shown in Table 10-3. Gonorrhea, as well as syphilis to a somewhat lesser extent, is more likely to be reported among males than females. Venereal disease reporting for males is probably more complete than for females because of the greater visibility of symptoms among males and because males may be less reluctant to seek treatment. Taking into account what is known and suspected about differential reporting generally, health workers are of the opinion that the present increase in venereal disease crosses both sexes and all age groups as well as all socioeconomic levels.[9]

Pattern of Spread of Venereal Diseases.   Every person infected with venereal disease (the primary case) has acquired his infection from another individual (his source case) and probably has infected others (his spread cases). Failure to seek immediate treatment for the primary case, the source, and spread cases increases the community reservoir and therefore increases the risk of infection spread. The identification of each source of infection and of all those exposed is a responsibility of the infected patient and his personal physician. It becomes the responsibility of public health agencies to protect the public by case-finding—that is, identifying the source and spread cases and treating them to prevent further spread of infection.

Figure 10-2 shows graphically how a case of venereal disease can spread if not treated promptly. Thus, one male student in a U.S. high school became infected with syphilis and initiated a chain of exposure of a large number of other students. Sixty-six of these students were examined, and among them, 14 were found to be infected, 27 were treated preventively, and 25 were found to be not infected.

Venereal Disease Control Measures.   Health officials view the venereal disease situation as a matter of serious concern. Gonorrhea, in particular, is classed as pandemic—"totally out of control" in the United States. Early in 1972, a $16 million national campaign was organized by the Center for Disease Control to fight gonorrhea. Most of the funds go to state and local health departments to administer the program under the center's supervision. The aim is to augment treatment facilities in hospitals and to encourage the involvement of private clinics operated by family planning groups and other organizations.

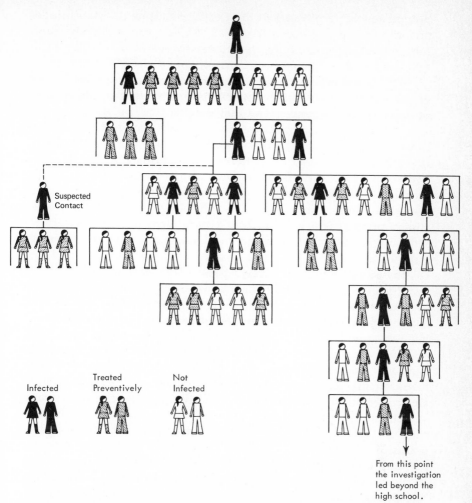

Suspected
Contact

Infected | Treated
Preventively | Not
Infected

From this point
the investigation
led beyond the
high school.

FIGURE 10-2. *Syphilis outbreak at a U.S. high school, 1969–1970.* [SOURCE: Adapted from American Social Health Association, American Public Health Association, and American Venereal Disease Association: A Joint Statement. *Today's VD Control Problem—1971.* American Social Health Association, New York.]

Conscientious case reporting, effective epidemiologic investigation and follow-up, and early treatment are principal public health methods for coping with venereal disease. These activities require cooperation between private physicians and health officials. In some areas, the apparent rise in venereal disease rates is merely the result of systematic reporting of source cases by physicians and diligent follow-up by the local health department.

Venereal disease prevention and control cannot be carried out effectively without public health laws and regulations requiring the prompt reporting of cases to the health department. This includes not only the newly discovered cases but also cases in the communicable stage who discontinue treatment without notifying the physician or clinic that treatment is being obtained elsewhere.

The single greatest need in the control of venereal diseases is, of course, the development of means to ensure that all infected persons receive treatment, and that they receive it early. Treatment is an effective control measure for infectious venereal disease because modern therapy can promise a cure to all, and once treatment is instituted, it renders the patient noncommunicable within a few hours. Therefore, clinical services must be freely available to anyone with actual or suspected venereal diseases. These services must be provided either through private physicians or through public clinics for those who cannot afford private medical care. The various kinds of inhibitions to seeking such treatment must be systematically identified and removed. Toward this end, 29 states and the District of Columbia had by 1971 passed laws permitting minors to give their own consent for venereal disease treatment; enactment of such laws was being sought in 9 more states and in Puerto Rico; and 8 other states had attorney general's opinions which allowed treatment of minors for venereal disease without parental consent.

Follow-up investigative services are important parts of a health agency's program, requiring well-trained investigators who can maintain the physician's cooperation and acquire the confidence and cooperation of the patient. In addition to the venereal disease investigator, the public health nurse, social worker, and health educator all have a role in community venereal disease control programs.

Public understanding of the natural, social, and biologic course of these diseases as they occur in population groups is essential. The public is generally ignorant of the cause, the mechanisms of spread, the effects, and the incidence of venereal disease in the populace. Therefore, education, beginning in high school with planned curricula, and carefully designed health education programs directed toward the general public, must be stimulated and promoted. The individual who is denied knowledge regarding the existence of venereal diseases and their causes, methods of transmission, symptoms, and effects is at a distinct disadvantage. The subject can best be handled in the classroom where the trained teacher can impart accurate, objective knowledge and can serve as a continuous resource to young people whose questions require definite, factual answers free of evasiveness and mythology.

Sex education too frequently has been equated with venereal disease education. However, sex education involves much broader issues than just the risks of venereal diseases. Physiology, anatomy, psychology, and moral issues are basic elements in sex education, and the range of sexual behavior as influenced by cultural backgrounds, family attitudes, and changing environmental stresses are other factors to be considered. It is reasonable to expect that free and open discussion of human biology and sexual behavior would have a favorable influence on community programs for the prevention of sex-related diseases. Venereal disease education probably will neither prevent nor stimulate promiscuous sexual activity. However, it may result in more selectivity in sexual behavior, and it certainly will result in infected persons seeking early treatment and cooperating with physicians or health departments in bringing source and spread cases under treatment.

Community programs in venereal disease education have lagged because of the point of view that the problem is individual and not social, that contracting a disease merely reflects irresponsible social behavior, and that good moral practice prevents risk of exposure. However, such views do not take into account the tendency toward more casual and informal sexual relationships that has developed as social mores change. Social taboos and related attitudes influence the individual in practicing prophylaxis, seeking medical care, and providing cooperation in the identification of sources and potential cases of venereal diseases. Prevailing attitudes toward promiscuity and discrepancies between society's mores and behavior also confuse the efforts to prevent these diseases. These are all problems of social ideology and behavior, and they cannot be ignored in efforts of public and professional education, prevention, and control.

TUBERCULOSIS

The causative organism or infectious agent in tuberculosis is *Mycobacterium tuberculosis* (tubercle bacillus). Man is primarily the reservoir, although in some areas diseased cattle are reservoirs. The source of infection is the respiratory secretions of persons with bacillary-positive pulmonary tuberculosis. The airborne route may be a frequent mode of spread; indirect contact through contaminated articles or dust is less important. The disease is communicable as long as tubercle bacilli are discharged. Prolonged household exposure to an active case usually leads to infection of contacts and frequently to active disease. What constitutes susceptibility, in terms of genetic mechanisms and specific environmental elements, remains an enigma. Certain age groups have increased tendency for infection, and others for progression of the disease following infection. Moreover, silicosis and diabetes are accepted as predisposing independent diseases.

Current Status of the Tuberculosis Problem. Mortality from tuberculosis in the United States is given in Table 10-4, which shows a marked regular decline from about 194 deaths per 100,000 population in 1900 to a rate of about 3 per 100,000 in 1969. Many factors have undoubtedly contributed to the decline in tuberculosis mortality in the United States since 1900. These include (1) a rise in the standard of living, including improved housing (lessened crowding and improvement in general household cleanliness), shorter working hours and lessened physical exhaustion, and better and more wholesome nutrition; (2) social legislation and social services affecting residents of urban and rural slums; (3) general improvements in community sanitation; (4) dissemination of public information regarding cause and control of tuberculosis; and (5) improvement in scientific knowledge regarding treatment of the disease.

Although the tuberculosis mortality picture has improved significantly in the United States, it still persists as a public health problem in urban areas, especially among the poor and among certain other high-risk groups. Mortality rates increase with age, are higher among males than females, and are much higher in nonwhite than white groups. Although females generally have lower mortality rates from tuberculosis, they die earlier.

The number of active, new cases of tuberculosis reported each year has also been declining, from about 76,000 cases in 1955 to about 39,000 cases in 1969 (Table 10-4). Youth and early adult life are the periods when *infection* is most likely to occur; adult life is the age at which the more common forms of the *disease* manifest themselves; and old age is the period in which the *death rate* is highest.

Prevention and Control of Tuberculosis. Adequate machinery for the control of tuberculosis consists of systems for early case detection and reporting; thorough examination of contacts and follow-up of suspects; provision of prompt, effective, and continuous medical treatment and other needed care; supervision of relapse and reinfection cases at risk; reduction of environmental and social factors that contribute to and complicate the disease; maintenance of records and data-retrieval apparatus for sequential effectiveness rating; and finally, coordination of community resources and regulatory agencies in order to ascertain responsibilities and to channel resources toward defined goals. Such goals could include the targeting of the community toward a 10 per cent decline in new active case rates over a succeeding decade.

Principal methods for the detection of tuberculosis are the tuberculin test and chest x-ray. The purpose of the *tuberculin test* is

TABLE 10-4. Tuberculosis: Deaths and New Cases, United States, Selected Years

	Death Rate Per 100,000 Population*	Number of Active Cases Newly Reported
1900	194.4	. . .
1905	179.9	. . .
1910	153.8	. . .
1915	140.1	. . .
1920	113.1	. . .
1925	84.8	. . .
1930	71.1	. . .
1935	55.1	. . .
1940	45.9	. . .
1945	39.9	. . .
1950	22.5	. . .
1955	9.1	76,245
1960	6.1	55,494
1965	4.1	49,016
1969	2.6	39,120

* All forms of tuberculosis.
Sources: Adapted from U.S. Bureau of the Census. *Historical Statistics of the United States, Colonial Times to 1957*. Washington, D.C., 1960, p. 26. Also, *Statistical Abstr. t of the United States, 1971*, pp. 58, 77.

to identify individuals who have been infected with the tubercle bacillus at some time in the immediate or distant past, and the testing procedure can be easily adapted to mass screening. In many communities, a 1 per cent tuberculin-positive rate among 14-year-olds is a long-term goal to be established by periodic cross-sectional tuberculin surveys of children at various school ages. The *chest x-ray* has been discarded for most screening purposes because of its high false-positive rate and low yield of new active cases. However, it does have utility in the screening of adult populations in communities where the prevalence of tuberculosis is excessive and in the examination of certain groups at special risk of infection. Contacts of active cases, both familial and otherwise, deserve consideration as part of a community detection program.

Among the measures designed for the prevention of tuberculosis infection, *BCG vaccination* (a living culture of bovine tubercle bacilli) is to some extent effective in providing resistance. Mass vaccination has little role in areas where the risk of infection is low, but it may be used for household contacts of active cases or for special-risk groups. *Chemoprophylaxis,* consisting of the administration of isoniazid, has also been tried with promising results as a preventive measure for contacts and special-risk groups and under certain other circumstances. The most general method of prevention consists of *health education* of the public regarding the importance, mode of spread, and methods of control of tuberculosis.

Advances in the treatment of tuberculosis have occurred in connection with new drug therapy and surgical techniques. Whereas in 1900, the sanitaria were used for protracted confinement of tuberculosis patients, today the hospital stay serves as a useful introduction to drug therapy and rehabilitation. Surgical intervention is reserved principally for cases of advanced cavitation. With drug treatment, the sputum test can be expected to become negative within a period of a few months, and a chemotherapy surveillance program maintained over the next few years averts relapse. The antimicrobial drugs used in the treatment of tuberculosis are isoniazid, para-aminosalicylic acid, and streptomycin, administered for one or more years.

Certain patterns in the control and treatment of tuberculosis are now generally accepted. For the *active cases* of tuberculosis, in addition to the x-ray and sputum examinations at monthly intervals, hospitalization is advisable to initiate uninterrupted chemotherapy. Reporting of active cases to the local health authority is required in most states, and it is recommended that health departments maintain a current register of such cases. *Probable active cases* should also be hospitalized and have a complete medical work-up. For *inactive cases,* the periodic sputum examination should be done as long as chemotherapy is given, or for at least one year. For those individuals who are only *quiescent cases,* chemotherapy should be continued indefinitely and sputum examinations repeated at quarterly intervals. *Casual contacts of active cases* should be examined at least once.

RUBELLA (GERMAN MEASLES)

Rubella is a viral infection that is highly infectious by person-to-person contact with nasopharyngeal secretions. It may be aerosol-transmitted after a 14-to-21-day (average 18 days) incubation period; fever, catarrhal symptoms, and maculopapular rash with cervical lymphadenopathy and leukopenia develop. It is an epidemic disease usually seen in spring and summer. Infectivity lasts up to four days following onset. While it is a disease of childhood, it has often occurred in young adults, military recruits, and pregnant women. If it occurs in the first trimester of pregnancy, it causes congenital defects in the fetus frequently enough that termination of pregnancy is considered. The epidemic of 1964–1965 produced congenital defects in thousands in the United States. The erythematous-to-maculopapular rash often causes diagnostic confusion of single or sporadic cases with other erythematous and exanthemic diseases such as measles, erythema infectiosum, exanthem subitum, Boston exanthum (ECHO virus infection), and Coxsackie A virus infection.

Treatment is symptomatic. An effective attenuated virus vaccine is currently under evaluation which promises to give lifelong protection and will be most useful prior to marriage. Since it is a mild disease, voluntary exposure of female children to epidemic cases has often been practiced as means for early infection and immunization.

The control of rubella was made possible when the rubella virus was first isolated in 1962. In a short time, live attenuated virus vaccines were developed, which produce an antibody response in over 90 per cent of recipients. The vaccines were first licensed for use in the United States in mid-1969. The principal objective of rubella control is to prevent infection of the fetus. This can best be done by eliminating the transmission of virus among children, since they are the major source of infection for susceptible pregnant women. Furthermore, the live attenuated rubella virus vaccine is safe and protective for children, but not for pregnant women because of an undetermined risk of the vaccine virus for the fetus.

INFECTIOUS HEPATITIS
(EPIDEMIC OR CATARRHAL JAUNDICE)

Infectious hepatitis is an acute febrile infection with a heat-resistant gastrointestinal virus transmitted by finger to mouth, person-to-person contact, food handler-contaminated food, or fecal- or sewage-contaminated water. Incubation period is weeks to two months, resulting in onset of fever, marked anorexia, nausea, malaise, gastrointestinal discomfort, and often jaundice. Leukopenia is frequent. Anicteric cases of mild nature are frequent. Fatalities due to liver damage are rare but occur more frequently in adults, pregnant women in particular.

Infectivity occurs prior to onset and continues for at least a week. Carriers may be infectious for many months. Sporadic cases may occur, but the disease is often seen in epidemics. While it is thought to be caused by a single virus type, providing lifelong immunity, there is a possibility that there are several types.

Best protection is by personal hygiene and good sanitation, with emphasis on feces disposal and pure or treated water supply, and by preemployment examination, history, and surveillance of food handlers with isolation of suspects or cases from contact with food. Patients should be isolated during the first week of jaundice.

Effective prophylaxis for persons exposed or at high risk (e.g., personnel assigned to overseas occupations, Peace Corps workers, missionaries, or military personnel) in poorly sanitated areas is by pooled human gamma globulin (5 ml) every six months. The virus has not been isolated in other-than-human volunteers; so no active immunization is yet available.

SERUM HEPATITIS
(HOMOLOGOUS SERUM JAUNDICE)

Serum hepatitis is an acute infection by heat-resistant virus causing a disease indistinguishable from infectious hepatitis. It has a distinctly longer incubation period of two to six months, usually 60 to 120 days. Transmission has long been considered possible only by inoculation, as in vaccination with contaminated needles or by blood and plasma transfusion. Recent evidence suggests occasional transmission by the oral route. There is no cross-protection with infectious hepatitis virus; so repeated attacks of clinical jaundice are possible.

Prophylaxis is also by pooled human gamma globulin, although it is not so certain. Prevention is by use of disposable single-use needles and transfusion equipment. Where necessary, disinfection by heat-penetrating steam (autoclave or pressure cooker) and nacent halogen disinfectants (Clorox) is the only reliable means. Even *prolonged boiling* cannot be relied on to inactivate heat-resistant serum hepatitis virus. No vaccine is available.

STAPHYLOCOCCAL INFECTIONS

Staphylococcal infections include a variety of disease manifestations resulting from infection, growth, and contamination by a group of selectively cultivable, antigenically closely related bacteria, morphologically identifiable as staphylococcus.

Impetigo (Impetigo Contagiosa). Impetigo is a dermal infection and purulence that produces dermatitis with vesicular and crusted seropurulent lesions that are highly infectious by person-to-person contact. Control is by maintenance of cleanliness, isolation of lesions and affected persons, and treatment of the infection.

Focalized and Systemic Staphylococcal Disease. Impetigo and systemic infections, including those of the eye (conjunctivitis) and nasopharynx, may be a source of more serious staphylococcal infections. These are furuncles and carbuncles seen most often in the young; deep-seated tissue infections such as tonsillitis and pneumonia; and suppuration as in emphysema and osteomyelitis, leading to organic abscesses and septicemia in the debilitated and elderly. These more serious complications may result in death, particularly with antibiotic-resistant strains.

The widespread use of antibiotics, which were initially almost universally effective in the control of staphylococcal infections, has resulted in the evolution of antibiotic-resistant strains of these bacteria. They are particularly hardy, often escape even diligent attempts at disinfection, and cause widespread postsurgical and contact infections that are not amenable to antibiotic therapy. Because clinical facilities, particularly hospitals, focalize diseased people, the problem of hospital, antibiotic-resistant staphylococcal infections has become a major communicable disease problem. It results in serious complications of intractable postsurgery infections and epidemics among newborn babies.

Only through careful disinfection, application of sanitary and isolation measures, and selective use and testing of antibiotics can safety and intelligent control be accomplished.

Staphylococcal Food Poisoning.   Certain strains of staphylococcus grow well in artificial media as provided by prepared foods, such as those made with milk, eggs, and chopped meats. Unrefrigerated, at room temperature, the bacteria grow rapidly and produce an enterotoxin which results in severe gastrointestinal reactions. These reactions include abrupt and often violent nausea, vomiting, diarrhea, and prostration which, although serious, are rarely fatal because of expulsion of the toxic material. Staphylococcal food poisoning occurs soon (one-half to four hours) after consumption of prepared foods that have been held unrefrigerated for a substantial period of time, often being initially contaminated by a food handler shedding staphylococcus from a dermal or nasopharyngeal infection.

Staphylococcal food poisoning is most frequently manifest as a common food source epidemic of short incubation period. It follows consumption of a food contaminated by enterotoxin-producing bacteria, usually easily identifiable by case history and by culture.

Prevention is by surveillance of food handlers for infection or lesions and sanitary preparation and refrigeration of food. Treatment is symptomatic. Cases are not directly infectious to others.

MALARIA

Malaria is caused by a protozoal parasite which invades, multiplies in, and destroys red blood cells in a cyclic rhythm varying from 48 to 72 hours. The sporozoites of any of four species of *Plasmodium* (*vivax, falciparum, malariae,* and *ovale*) which develop by sexual reproduction in the definitive *Anopheles* mosquito host are injected into the intermediate human host during the process of taking blood. After invasion of the parenchymal cells of the liver, mesozoites form, which are released into the blood to invade red cells to form schizonts. It is the schizogony that produces cell destruction resulting in febrile paroxysms.

The incubation period may be as short as 11 or 12 days, but may take months or even years. The sudden onset of fever and shaking chills, called a paroxysm, is characteristic but of limited duration, and occurs intermittently. During the interim, the patient is usually afebrile, apparently normal, but may feel weak.

Control of malaria has been by protection from the bite of anopheline vectors and by destruction of vectors through use of residual insecticides such as DDT, dieldrin, and malathion. While this is directed at breaking the transmission chain, elimination of the parasite from the blood and liver is attempted by chemotherapy with drugs such as chloroquine, Daraprim, primaquine, and quinacrine. Development of drug-resistant strains of plasmodia has led to use of natural quinine for treatment, intravenously in the case of cerebral malaria. The drugs are also used prophylactically for prevention of malaria attacks.

References

1. Anderson, G. W., Arnstein, M. G., and Lester, M. R. *Communicable Disease Control*, 4th ed. The Macmillan Company, New York, 1962.
2. California State Department of Public Health. *A Manual for the Control of Communicable Diseases in California*. The Department, Berkeley, 1966.
3. Benenson, Abram S. (ed.). *Control of Communicable Diseases in Man*, 11th ed. American Public Health Association, New York, 1970.
4. Sartwell, Philip E. (ed.). *Maxcy-Rosenau Preventive Medicine and Public Health*, 9th ed. Appleton-Century-Crofts, New York, 1965.
5. Dauer, Carl C., Korns, Robert F., and Schuman, Leonard M. *Infectious Diseases*. American Public Health Association, Vital and Health Statistics Monographs. Harvard University Press, Cambridge, 1968.
6. Top, Franklin H. *Communicable and Infectious Diseases: Diagnosis, Prevention, Treatment*, 6th ed. The C. V. Mosby Company, St. Louis, 1968.
7. Hunter, G. W., III, Frye, W. W., and Swartzwelder, J. C. *A Manual of Tropical Medicine*, 4th ed. W. B. Saunders Company, Philadelphia, 1966.
8. Beeson, P. B., and McDermott, W. (eds.). *Cecil-Loeb Textbook of Medicine*, 13th ed. W. B. Saunders Company, Philadelphia, 1971.
9. American Social Health Association, American Public Health Association, and American Venereal Disease Association: A Joint Statement. *Today's VD Control Problem—1971*. American Social Health Association, New York.

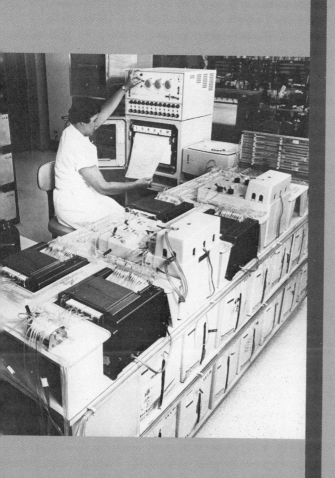

11
CHRONIC
DISEASES

CHAPTER OUTLINE

Courtesy of City of Milwaukee Health Department. Staff photo.

Perspective Concerning the Major Chronic Diseases

Chronic diseases, viewed from the standpoint of either the provision of care for long-term illness or the sequelae of disability, have emerged as major scientific, medical, public health, and socioeconomic problems to be faced throughout the world.[1,2] Particularly in the United States, these problems have stimulated governmental concern as well as a significant amount of legislative, professional, voluntary organization, and community debate.

Concern over mounting chronic disease and disability has been expressed periodically since the early 1920's. However, recognition of a need for a national program to reduce the cost of these diseases is of more recent origin. Initially, it was the economic depression of the 1930's and, subsequently, World War II that stimulated chronic disease rehabilitation on a mass scale. Industry found ways to use many handicapped persons in providing essential services during the war effort. Beginning in the 1940's, many persons returning from military service with service-connected impairment received the benefit of modern methods of rehabilitation.

In 1947, a joint committee of the American Hospital Association, the American Medical Association, the American Public Health Association, and the American Public Welfare Association issued a statement urging that prevention be considered a basic approach to chronic illness. The joint statement also focused on the need for diagnostic and treatment facilities for chronic illness and set as an objective the availability of high-quality services to all income groups. When the statement was written, it was recognized that home care, care in nursing homes, rehabilitation teamwork, and the coordinated efforts of many groups in the community would be required in order to make a chronic disease control program effective.

As a result of the joint committee statement, the National Commission on Chronic Illness was organized in 1949. The commission conducted studies, served as a clearinghouse for information, and prepared a four-volume series of reports to establish guidelines for program planning. The commission defined chronic illnesses as comprising all health impairments or deviations from normal that have one or more of the following characteristics: permanency of residual disability caused by nonreversible pathologic alterations; a requirement of special patient training for rehabilitation; and a long period of medical supervision, observation, or care.

Long-term care is a sensitive topic in the United States today and a matter of national concern because of the demands that it makes on the economy. Long-term illnesses occur in all age groups and in all ethnic and socioeconomic groups, and demand a strenuous application of the principles of prevention, diagnosis, treatment, and rehabilitation. Even though the young in the population are affected to some extent, it is the older population that incurs the bulk of suffering from chronic conditions.

Chronic illness cannot be viewed in isolation; rather, it must be considered as part of the problem of general medical care. In planning for the care of the chronically ill, consideration must be given to the entire spectrum of illnesses and to the appropriate care provided for all gradations of patient need, from the acute exacerbation, or flare-up, to the stable chronic condition. The concept of comprehensive care is of particular importance in relation to chronic illness, and includes inpatient care, home care, and outpatient care.

Changing Mortality and Chronic Diseases

Chronic diseases are not new in occurrence, but there has been an improvement in diagnostic methods and a recognition of the social importance of these diseases. Environmental factors have influenced the etiology, early detection, and management of chronic conditions. Changing infectious disease patterns, a shifting age distribution of the population and longevity, and a rising standard of living generally are considered interrelative factors which have affected the trend toward chronic disease as a major cause of death and disability.

The overall downward trend in the mortality rate in the United States no doubt began during the early nineteenth century and accelerated during the latter half of that period. A consistent mortality rate decline occurred between 1900 and 1954, and the rate has exhibited a slower, uneven decline since then. By the turn of the century, control over certain of the infectious diseases was under way; and as early as 1900, the deaths from chronic diseases were already proportionately higher than those from acute diseases. By 1955, the chronic diseases accounted for more than 80 per cent of all deaths.

The three leading causes of death in 1900 (pneumonia and acute respiratory diseases, tuberculosis, and gastrointestinal conditions) amounted to only one twentieth of all deaths by 1960. The diseases that could be influenced through environmental control, such as water, food, general sanitation, hygienic practices, and medical care, demonstrated the greatest decline. Table 11-1, which shows the ten leading causes of death in 1968, reveals that three categories of chronic diseases head the list. Diseases of the heart have the highest death rate—about 373 deaths per 100,000 population—followed by malignant neoplasms and cerebrovascular diseases.

A reduction in death rates has occurred in the younger age groups, which permits a higher percentage of the population to reach the age of greater risk from chronic diseases. More than 60 per cent of all deaths are among persons 65 years of age and over. The mortality rate for the broad category of major cardiovascular diseases is about seven times as great for persons over age 65 as it is for those between the ages of 45 and 64. In contrast to this, deaths from malignant neoplasms are only about three times as great in the older age group. Deaths due to other chronic diseases have become relatively more important in younger age groups, so that although

TABLE 11-1. The Ten Leading Causes of Death, United States, 1968*

	Death Rate per 100,000 Population
Diseases of heart	372.6
Malignant neoplasms†	159.4
Cerebrovascular diseases	105.8
Accidents	57.5
Influenza and pneumonia	36.8
Certain diseases of early infancy	21.9
Diabetes mellitus	19.2
Arteriosclerosis	16.8
Bronchitis, emphysema, and asthma	16.6
Cirrhosis of liver	14.6

* For method of selecting the leading causes of death, see U.S. Department of Health, Education, and Welfare, Public Health Service, *Vital Statistics of the United States, 1968,* Technical Appendix, Part A.

† Includes neoplasms of lymphatic and hematopoietic tissues.

SOURCE: Adapted from U.S. Bureau of the Census. *Statistical Abstract of the United States, 1971,* p. 59.

they are the most frequent causes of deaths from middle age on-ward, these diseases are also not insignificant at earlier ages.

Marked alterations in life expectancy have accompanied these changes in mortality and causes of death. In 1900, the expectation of life at birth was about 50 years. By 1968, it was more than 70 years. The rate of this gain, however, appears now to be decreasing. In 1900, the expectation of life at birth for females was greater than that of males, and the trend has been a continuing spread in this differential. Thus, longevity was 2 years greater for females at the turn of the century and is more than 6 years greater at the present time. On the other hand, the life expectancy of ethnic groups has been converging over time. In 1900, the average expectancy was al-most 15 years greater for whites compared with nonwhites, whereas recently this difference diminished to less than 6 years.

The increased impact of chronic diseases is not attributable, however, solely to the aging of the population. Only until 1940 was the proportion of the total population in the older age groups increasing. Past, as well as current, levels of fertility are responsible for this recent reversal of the general aging trend in the United States population. In the past two decades, there has been an *increase* in the relative proportion of persons under 20 years of age, with a corresponding *decrease* in the major wage-earning groups of 20 to 44 years. Thus, rather than observing an increase in prevalence or mortality *rates* owing to the chronic diseases, it is more likely that with the population growth, little change will occur. However, the *absolute numbers* of persons affected and disabled by chronic diseases and the numbers of deaths from these diseases will be ob-served to increase over the next 25 years.

Morbidity Attributed to Chronic Diseases

The chronic diseases, with the exception of a few that are infec-tious (e.g., tuberculosis), are not reportable conditions as are the communicable diseases. Therefore, it has been difficult to establish reliable trends of incidence and prevalence. Nevertheless, several methods have been used to establish rough estimates of the in-cidence and prevalence rates of some chronic diseases in recent years. There seems to be no question of general increase in these rates, with some identification of risks for specific age, sex, ethnic, occupational, and other groups.

Incidence rates are conjectures in many instances and have limited usefulness because they require data related to onset, early signs, and initial symptoms of disease, whereas most of the chronic diseases have an indeterminable "incubation" period, variable biologic and psychologic manifestations, and a delayed diagnosis. These factors also influence the validity of prevalence rates. The prevalence of the major chronic diseases, derived from many reports, parallels the rank order of mortality. However, there are also other chronic disorders of frequent occurrence which primarily interfere with normal function and social adjustment. Such conditions include peptic ulcer, arthritis and rheumatism, hernia, allergies, chronic bronchitis and sinusitis, blindness, deafness, neurologic and sensory diseases, and mental disorders.

Information on chronic disease morbidity can come from several sources. One consists of *case registries,* which serve as repositories of information—usually accumulated over an extended period of time—about a limited number of specific chronic diseases. Other sources include chronic disease reporting by physicians, chronic disease surveys involving household interviews of a probability sample of the population, chronic disease examination surveys, industrial periodic examinations, health record surveys, and data derived from the conduct of various chronic disease screening procedures.

Periodic *household interviews,* which have been used over the past 40 years as a means of obtaining information on chronic disease morbidity, usually involve drawing a representative sample of a large number of families in a given area. One member or more of each household is interviewed about social characteristics, illnesses, and disability of a specified severity and occurrence, and within a specified period of time. The interview is structured by the use of a detailed questionnaire, and provisions are made for minimizing both respondent and interviewer reporting errors. The Health Interview Survey, which is one of the three activities of the National Health Survey, is an outstanding example of the household interview method and has been in operation since 1957. Annual modifications of the questionnaire permit collection of data on a large number of topics, more topics than could be included in a single-visit interview. As shown in Table 11-2, the National Health Survey found in 1968–1969 that about 11 per cent of the population (an estimated 22 million persons) reported they were limited in their activities as a result of a chronic condition. About two out of every five persons 65 years and older had some activity limitation caused by chronic conditions, and over half of these were limited in the amount or kind of major activity they could do (Table 11-2).

A *health examination morbidity survey* is a clinical examination of a well-defined sample of a population. This examination includes a physician-administered interview, physical examination, and review of all available laboratory results. In many situations, a physician-administered examination is repeated on the same popula-

TABLE 11-2. Degree of Limitation of Activity Due to Chronic Conditions, by Age, United States, 1968–1969

	Age (Years)				
	All Ages	Under 17	17– 44	45– 64	65 and Older
	Per Cent				
Persons with no limitation of activity	88.8	97.6	92.8	81.3	57.6
Persons limited because of chronic conditions	11.2	2.4	7.3	18.7	42.4
But not in major activity*	2.1	1.2	2.0	3.0	4.1
In amount or kind of major activity*	6.3	1.0	4.3	11.4	22.4
Unable to carry on major activity*	2.8	0.2	1.0	4.3	15.9

* Major activity refers to ability to work, keep house, or engage in school or pre-school activities.
Source: Adapted from U.S. Department of Health, Education, and Welfare, Public Health Service, National Center for Health Statistics. *Age Patterns in Medical Care, Illness, and Disability, United States, 1968–1969* (data from the National Health Survey). HEW Publication No. (HSM) 72-1026, Series 10, No. 70, April 1972, p. 44.

tion, thereby providing information as to the number of new cases of chronic disease that have occurred during the intervening period of time.

Control of Chronic Diseases

PREVENTION

There are two basic approaches to the prevention of chronic diseases: (1) the application of communitywide health measures and (2) the utilization by the individual of knowledge and methods of personal health promotion and maintenance. Both approaches would be greatly facilitated and more effective if the cause of each chronic disease was known and if each had a specific preventive available, as is the case with many communicable diseases. Unfortunately, the causes of chronic diseases are generally not known. What is known is something of the circumstances associated with their development (incidence), and it is on this knowledge that preventive activity must be based until further research sheds more light not only on causes but on the entire natural history of chronic diseases.

The prevention of certain infectious or communicable diseases and their sequelae can in turn prevent a few chronic diseases. Thus, rheumatic heart disease can be the aftermath of rheumatic fever, and syphilitic heart disease may result from untreated syphilis. Prenatal care for mothers guards against premature birth which increases the risk of congenital defects, and medical care at child-birth decreases the possibility of birth injuries which may cause permanent damage. Regular health appraisals for preschool and school children can reveal conditions that, if uncorrected, could result in chronic impairment as the child grows older. Adequate nutrition and diet appear to be related to forestalling certain chronic diseases, and controlling obesity may help prevent diabetes, hypertension, and arthritis. Accidents, which can be the source of severe chronic disability, can be reduced or avoided by safety measures in the workplace, at home, and on streets and highways. The control of environmental pollution removes, if not the cause, at least the source of aggravation of several chronic conditions.

Social habits and attitudes may have major influence on chronic disease, such as the use of tobacco, alcohol, and drugs, as well as the stressful accompaniments of the competition for excellence, economic status, or superiority. The stresses of the urban environment, of increasing population density, noise, tightly scheduled living, 60-to-80-hour "portal-to-portal" workweeks for many persons, reduced physical and mental recreation, and the increasing pressures of conformity are among the many sociophysical stresses believed to have some influence on chronic disorders.[3]

Prevention of chronic disease often requires the development by the *individual* of responsibility in matters such as diet or the alteration of smoking habits. *Society's* role in prevention includes the responsibility for broad programs such as improvement of the standard of living, slum clearance, and occupational hygiene. The task confronting behavioral scientists is to establish a framework through which personal habits can be influenced, but until this level of competence is reached, case-finding and early detection are the best hope for reduction of disability and premature death from chronic diseases.

DETECTION

The two principal methods currently in use for the detection of chronic diseases are periodic health appraisals or examinations and mass screening tests. The purpose of both methods is to detect and diagnose a disease at the earliest possible stage so that treatment can be initiated promptly. "Well" people are the targets of both methods, which means they must seek the examination or testing without being prodded by symptoms of illness.

Although *periodic health examinations* are strongly recommended by health professionals, they are not usual except in pediatric, obstetric, and industrial medical practice. There are various obstacles to more extensive use of periodic examinations by well persons, including insufficient physician time, financial cost to the individual, and lack of personal motivation. Most people wait until they are bothered by symptoms of illness, and even then they are likely to put off going to the doctor as long as possible. The physician, in turn, usually becomes preoccupied with diagnosing and treating the acute illness and does not use the opportunity to look for asymptomatic chronic conditions.

There are a number of possible *screening tests* that can be used in a variety of circumstances.[4] A screening program may consist of administering a single test, such as the traditional (and now less used) chest x-ray, or it may consist of a battery of tests that screen for a number of diseases in the same person. The latter is known as multiple screening, and this technique is usually more economical than testing for single diseases on separate occasions. Screening programs are generally administered by official or voluntary health agencies and institutions and may be offered to an entire community or to one or more segments of the population considered to be at high risk of disease. The specific tests are given by health and medical personnel, and the results are evaluated for signs of disease in the individual. The tests provide information specifying the probability that a follow-up physician examination would validate a given diagnostic condition. For example, a positive test finding on tonometry (the measurement of intraocular tension) should properly be the basis for a referral for follow-up diagnostic procedures which would lead to the final step of a physician diagnosis of, for instance, wide-angle glaucoma.[5] Physician services are often utilized in the interpretation of suspicious findings obtained by screening procedures and for performing follow-up diagnostic studies of suspects.

An important consideration in screening tests is that of screening level. Whether one is dealing with a biochemical analysis of serum or an interpretation of an x-ray, there should be a definition of what concentration of a given metabolite or what type of observation on the film will be considered as having an acceptable probability of leading to diagnostic confirmation. This defines the level of "abnormality" that is appropriate to the screening procedure and is to be considered a *"positive test."* Consideration in assigning this "positive" screening level must be based on a composite formula which estimates the overall health value to the community of screening at each given level. This formula is composed of balancing the value of true-positives and true-negatives, as opposed to the detriment of false-positives and false-negatives. The potential for improving the health of those screened as "positive" must be considered in terms of the cost to patients' families and to the community, as well as from the standpoint of facilities existing for treatment (following the necessary diagnostic follow-up) and the physicians available for such services.

TREATMENT

Chronic disease treatment is a highly individual matter and there are, therefore, countless possible patterns of therapy. Medication, diet, and exercise—singly or in combination—may provide the basis for a fairly uncomplicated treatment regimen in some cases. Other cases of chronic illness may require the use of one or more organized community health facilities as described in Chapter 4: outpatient clinics, hospitals (both general and those designed specifically for chronic diseases), and nursing homes.

Follow-up care after hospital or nursing home stays is an important part of the treatment pattern and may include the use of home health services (see Chapter 4). There are several home health services that are particularly appropriate for chronic disease patients, such as home nursing, homemakers and home health aides, equipment rental and lending, various specialized therapies (physical, speech, occupational), and friendly visitors.[6] If the patient has financial or adjustment problems associated with his chronic condition, counseling or social work services become significant aspects of the treatment process.

REHABILITATION

The goal of rehabilitation is to restore the patient to the maximum function that his chronic condition permits. The rehabilitation effort involves assessing the individual's abilities, disabilities, and needs as well as canvassing the community for the facilities and skills that are available and appropriate for the particular case. Rehabilitation may consist of restoring the patient to the activities of daily living, of teaching him to live within his limitations, or of retraining him for another type of occupation (vocational rehabilitation). Special living and work arrangements may be an appropriate part of the rehabilitation of some patients and may be found in cooperative living centers, sheltered workshops, and selective placement in industry.

Maximizing the restoration of function depends substantially on the motivation and attitude of the patient and those around him. Lack of knowledge about available resources for rehabilitation or a defeatist attitude about their utility can seriously interfere with an individual's realizing his full potential. Counseling and social work services, therefore, again have an important role in this stage of chronic disease control.

Chronic Disease Programs

CONCEPTS OF CARE AND PROVISION OF COMMUNITY SERVICES

Programs directed toward the control of chronic disease and the provision of treatment facilities require special attention to the unique characteristics of each of the diseases in this heterogeneous group. For example, a program of prevention, early detection, and treatment aimed at cerebrovascular disease must take into account whatever is known about causes as well as means for restoration and improvement of function. Community services, such as a rehabilitation center, home care, visiting nurse service, or long-term hospital care, can be organized to serve persons with all types of chronic disease, but each specific program is normally tailored to the individual patient with suitable recognition of the unique characteristics of his disease.[7] Pessimistic attitudes about many of the chronic diseases, such as cerebrovascular disease, are now giving way to more realistic expectations that many individuals with this condition can recover a substantial amount of function through intensive diagnostic and therapeutic efforts, coupled with the utilization of recent developments in physical medicine and other aspects of rehabilitation. It is now recommended that many such patients live at home rather than in hospitals or nursing homes. Rehabilitative services have been directed toward job reemployment of such impaired adults.

There is a gradual assumption of responsibility for the care of the chronically ill in general hospitals and a deceleration in the growth of separate chronic disease institutions. In many instances, the large public hospital has served as a focus for organized medical home care programs, utilizing extensive outpatient facilities and a carefully developed visiting nurse service. Many community agencies, including health departments, have participated in the development of chronic disease home care programs. In view of the relatively large proportion of the population in this country that is afflicted with chronic disease conditions, it is easily seen that one cannot isolate care of patients with long-term illnesses from the general medical care of the community. A dream, as yet unachieved, is true continuity of care wherein the general hospital conducts community-based programs which are integrated with nursing home-care programs and community agency activities to provide comprehensive care.

Comprehensive care can be viewed as a galaxy of services that can be called upon when needed. The first step in effecting such a service is the periodic reevaluation of a patient's physical status, his psychosocial state, and the economic resources available to him and his family. A setting wherein comprehensive care is given has a full spectrum of organizational patterns. Outpatient care includes not only an outpatient department of a hospital but also programs such as the ambulatory service of a rehabilitation center and visits of chronic disease patients to their family physician in their own community.

Probably one of the most significant developments in long-term care has been the interest in the area of *continuity of care.* Many hospitals have developed services in which the follow-up care plan was made during the course of confinement as an inpatient and extended well beyond discharge. Frequently, a public health nurse in the patient's community and a medical social worker play important roles in linking the hospital staff and resources to the patient in his home. A very carefully planned discharge and periodic reevaluation of the individual's rehabilitation status form the nucleus for this type of service.

One obstacle to full rehabilitation is the lack of continuity in providing social and vocational service at the time and place of need. It does little good to restore a person with medical services and subsequently fail to provide him with the vocational training or the social work counseling which he needs to prepare himself for work or for a life situation suitable to his impairment. The programs of public and voluntary agencies in the health or welfare fields have benefited from the work of rehabilitation coordinators, who provide an understanding of the importance of sequence and continuity in all types of services. Medical services only form the platform from which the other rehabilitative services are launched. Significant aspects of the activities of the public health and social welfare fields are aimed at preventing the progress of disease, evaluating disability, and restoring the handicapped to optimum usefulness. A lesson learned long ago in the care and treatment of tuberculosis was the need for community planning in order to complete the rehabilitation process.

ROLE OF HEALTH DEPARTMENTS AND OTHER AGENCIES

Despite a considerable growth of activity in the area of public health concern with chronic disease control, many state and local public health departments have not undertaken an extensive program such as that recommended by the American Public Health Association.[8] Reasons for the lag include shortages of funds and personnel, opposition of local medical societies, interagency conflicts, and many others. Usually, the health officer with a direct interest in chronic diseases will find ways to circumvent these difficulties. To most informed local health officers, the chronic disease field will represent a constellation of activities which extend from community surveys to early detection of disease, rehabilitation, planning for patient care (particularly for the indigent and other special groups), nursing home supervision, and activities in mental hygiene.

The health department usually cannot provide the totality of chronic disease services, but it can make its resources available in developing a comprehensive community plan. The health officer can provide tools and equipment within his own organization or persuade other agencies to do so. The health department can administer regulations which support programs of other groups and agencies — for example, the establishment of standards of care in various types of facilities such as nursing homes, convalescent homes, hospitals, and homes for the aged. Even a small health department can undertake many types of services for chronic conditions that might be integrated with the general community health programs.[6]

Welfare agencies have an important role in serving the social and economic needs of the person with a chronic condition by aiding him to plan, pay for, and obtain maximum benefit from the health services available. Official vocational rehabilitation services help individuals achieve independence and satisfaction through suitable jobs. Other educational services, which are often provided by the school system, are of value in the prevention of chronic illness as well as in the care and rehabilitation of patients. Voluntary agencies of a vast variety participate in the fight against chronic disease by assisting in direct patient care, providing financial support to patients, coordinating community health efforts, and conducting public or professional education programs.[6]

PROGRAMS OF THE FEDERAL GOVERNMENT

National Institutes of Health.   Several institutes of the National Institutes of Health (Public Health Service, U.S. Department of Health, Education, and Welfare) have responsibilities for research and training activities in a broad array of chronic diseases. The National Cancer Institute conducts research relating to the cause, prevention, and methods of diagnosis and treatment of cancer. It also supports such research, as well as training programs, in universities, hospitals, laboratories, and other public or private nonprofit institutions. The institute cooperates with many state and local agencies, organizations, and institutions engaged in cancer activities and collects information on cancer for dissemination through publications and other media. The National Heart and Lung Institute has a similar series of responsibilities with regard to diseases of the heart, lungs (including emphysema), and blood vessels, as does the National Institute of Neurological Diseases and Stroke in connection with neurologic and sensory diseases. The National Institute of Allergy and Infectious Diseases has responsibilities pertaining to chronic diseases with an allergic or infectious component. The National Institute of Arthritis and Metabolic Diseases is concerned with arthritis, rheumatism, and metabolic diseases and conducts and supports research in these and related fields. Among its activities, the institute conducts a research and development program in the improvement of artificial kidneys and related treatment modalities for the maintenance of patients with chronic kidney failures. The National Eye Institute is responsible for training and research programs in vision, and conducts studies in areas such as retinal degeneration and cataract management.

Social and Rehabilitation Service (SRS). The administration of programs for handicapped persons, including those disabled by chronic disorders, is the responsibility of the Social and Rehabilitation Service (U.S. Department of Health, Education, and Welfare).

Within SRS, the Community Services Administration promotes the development of social services for handicapped adults and others by assisting the states in establishing a comprehensive range of such services at the community level. It provides technical assistance and guidelines and is responsible for extending and strengthening the social service delivery system.

The SRS Rehabilitation Services Administration has responsibility for programs aimed at achieving productive employment for persons with disabilities. It also administers a training grant program for professionals in various rehabilitation specialties, and it provides grants for construction and expansion of rehabilitation facilities as well as for extension and improvement of existing services and programs for the disabled. The basic program of vocational rehabilitation services is carried out cooperatively between the states and the federal government. Under this program, disabled persons apply or are referred to the state vocational rehabilitation agency to receive whatever combination of services they require. Provision is made for medical, surgical, hospital, and psychologic services, as well as vocational and other educational training, job placement, follow-up in employment, and several other related services. While some services may be provided directly by the state agency, most are obtained by purchase from physicians, hospitals, rehabilitation centers, clinics, schools, sheltered workshops, and other sources. Federal funds are allotted by a formula involving the state's population and fiscal capacity as measured by its per capita income.

Regional Medical Programs Service. Within the Health Services and Mental Health Administration (Public Health Service, U.S. Department of Health, Education, and Welfare), programs dealing with the chronic diseases reside in the Regional Medical Programs Service. This agency is responsible for the Regional Medical Programs (described in Chapter 4) as well as a chronic renal disease program (which includes a home dialysis aspect) and the National Clearinghouse for Smoking and Health (with the purpose of reducing disability and death associated with cigarette smoking).

The Regional Medical Programs are an outgrowth of recommendations made in 1964 by the President's Commission on Heart Disease, Cancer and Stroke.[9] The programs are intended to increase the availability and quality of care for patients with heart disease, cancer, stroke, or related diseases. About half of the component activities of the programs are involved in training and continuing education for health professionals; one third are related to demonstrations of patient care; and the remainder are devoted to research and development. Within a designated geographic region, all the component activities are interrelated as part of a total program effort.

Cardiovascular Diseases

The cardiovascular diseases consist of a broad heterogeneous grouping of conditions primarily involving the heart and blood vessels. Table 11-3 shows the principal subdivisions of disease categories within this grouping (according to the International Statistical Classification of Diseases, Injuries and Causes of Death, eighth revision), and provides an indication of the relative importance of the categories in terms of death rates. The table indicates that, as a cause of death, the cardiovascular diseases as a whole accounted for 512 deaths per 100,000 population in 1968. By far the largest contribution came from diseases of the heart (about 373 deaths per 100,000 population) followed by cerebrovascular diseases (about 106 deaths per 100,000 population) and arteriosclerosis (with a much lower rate, 17 deaths per 100,000). It will be recalled from Table 11-1 that diseases of the heart and cerebrovascular diseases were the first and third leading causes of death, respectively, in 1968. Among diseases of the heart, ischemic heart disease was responsible for most of the deaths in that category (Table 11-3).

In older age groups, *death rates* for diseases of the heart or for

TABLE 11-3. Classification of Major Cardiovascular Diseases and Deaths Due to These Diseases, United States, 1968

	Death Rate per 100,000 Population
Major cardiovascular diseases	512.1
Diseases of heart	372.6
Active rheumatic fever and chronic rheumatic heart disease	8.2
Hypertensive heart disease*	8.9
Ischemic heart disease	337.6
Chronic disease of endocardium and other myocardial insufficiency	3.9
All other forms of heart disease	14.0
Hypertension	4.5
Cerebrovascular diseases	105.8
Arteriosclerosis	16.8
Other diseases of arteries, arterioles, and capillaries	12.4

* With or without renal disease.

Source: Adapted from U.S. Bureau of the Census. *Statistical Abstract of the United States, 1971,* p. 58.

cerebrovascular diseases were higher for men than for women in 1968, as shown in Table 11-4. For both sexes the death rates for these diseases were far greater for persons aged 65 and over than for those 45 to 64 years of age. Thus, elderly men were the group at greater risk for either disease, but particularly for diseases of the heart, with 3,393 deaths per 100,000 population.

The *prevalence* of heart disease in older age groups is strikingly

TABLE 11-4. Deaths Due to Diseases of the Heart and to Cerebrovascular Diseases in Older Age Groups, by Sex, United States, 1968

	Diseases of the Heart	Cerebrovascular Diseases
	Rate per 100,000 Population in Specified Group	
Men		
45–64 years of age	677.7	90.3
65 years and over	3,392.6	927.7
Women		
45–64 years of age	231.4	68.4
65 years and over	2,410.1	886.8

Source: Adapted from U.S. Department of Health, Education, and Welfare, Health Services and Mental Health Administration, National Center for Health Statistics. *Health in the Later Years of Life,* October 1971, pp. 8–9.

TABLE 11-5. Prevalence of Heart Disease in Older Age Groups, by Sex and Race, United States, 1960–1962

	45–64 Years of Age	65–79 Years of Age
	Per Cent in Specified Group	
MEN		
White	16.1	33.0
Negro	36.9	51.8
WOMEN		
White	15.2	43.7
Negro	41.7	70.0

SOURCE: Adapted from U.S. Department of Health, Education, and Welfare, Health Services and Mental Health Administration, National Center for Health Statistics. *Health in the Later Years of Life,* October 1971, p. 18.

different between whites and Negroes. As shown in Table 11-5, nearly one sixth of white men and women have definite heart disease at ages 45 to 64. However, among Negro men and women of that age group, over one third have a heart disorder. After age 64, the proportion of persons — both sexes, both races — who have heart disease increases markedly.

Prevalence and incidence studies have identified several factors associated with an increased risk of developing heart disease, although (as has been pointed out in Chapter 9) such associations do not necessarily mean that the factors cause the disease. The risk factors that have been found to be associated with heart disease include an elevated serum cholesterol level, elevated blood pressure levels, cigarette smoking, and obesity. Investigations of possible social influences have shown some indication that incidence of heart disease among males is related to factors such as urban background and frequent changes of residence or occupation, but such findings provide only inklings, and the role of social, psychologic, personality, and stress factors still remains to be more completely determined. The same is true for genetic and environmental factors, although evidence regarding the influence of the environment on heart disease is beginning to grow.

Prevention is a particularly urgent need in heart disease because the mortality from an acute heart attack is so high (one third of those who suffer an attack die within three weeks, a large percentage of these within 48 hours), and even survivors have a shortened life expectancy. Greater emphasis on provision for emergency treatment with minimum delay has begun to save lives that formerly would have been lost to heart attacks. Since optimal prevention and control measures depend on knowledge of the etiology of disease, expanded research efforts in many different aspects of cardiovascular diseases are of primary importance. In order to provide a program for preventing disability and premature death, it is recommended that physicians assist in the early recognition of the disease and educate their patients on the risk factors. Screening efforts frequently include chest x-ray to detect enlargement of the heart, pulse check for regularity of rhythm, measurement of the blood pressure, review of symptoms referrable to cardiorespiratory function, and examination of the electrocardiographic tracing. Unfortunately, as a screening effort, these tests are not very specific. In one screening project, only 32 per cent of the persons subsequently diagnosed as normal were screened as negative. The sensitivity of any one of the tests is generally of the order of only 50 per cent.

Cancer

The term *cancer,* or malignant neoplasms, includes a group of diseases characterized by the transformation of normal body cells into abnormally growing parasitic cells. From the standpoint of both treatment and research, cancer presents one of the most complex and difficult medical problems because of the nature of the biologic change involved and the fact that it can occur in any part of the body. Malignant neoplasms have certain biologic features in common, but they differ widely with respect to known etiology, diagnostic and treatment methods, clinical course, and curability.

As the second leading cause of death (Table 11-1), malignant neoplasms claim victims at increasing rates as age advances. There are also differences in mortality from cancer according to sex and race as shown in Table 11-6 for the period 1945–1967. The table shows—over time—an increase in death rates for males, both white and nonwhite; a slight tendency toward decreasing death rates for white females; and a somewhat variable pattern for nonwhite females. In 1967, mortality rates per 100,000 population from highest to lowest for these groups were as follows: nonwhite males (218), white males (181), nonwhite females (143), and white females (125).

The more common kinds of cancer involving various biologic systems and sites include (1) gastrointestinal malignancy—colon, stomach, pancreas, rectum, liver, and biliary tract; (2) respiratory malignancy—lung, larynx, nasopharynx; (3) breast malignancy; (4) genital malignancy—prostate, uterus, ovary; and (5) leukemia and lymphomas. There are also many types of skin cancer, thyroid cancer, and the more uncommon malignancies of various organs in

TABLE 11-6. Deaths Due to Malignant Neoplasms, by Race and Sex (Age-Adjusted Rates), United States, Selected Years*

| | White | | Nonwhite | |
	Male	Female	Male	Female
	Death Rate per 100,000 Population			
1945	142	139	104	127
1950	148	132	138	141
1955	157	128	160	140
1960	159	121	174	136
1965	164	119	192	137
1967	181	125	218	143

* Rates are 3-year averages around the base years 1945, 1950, 1955, 1960, 1965, and 1967.

SOURCES: Adapted from U.S. Department of Health, Education, and Welfare, National Cancer Institute. *Patterns in Cancer Mortality in the United States: 1950–1967,* Monograph 33, May 1971, p. 587; and *1972 Fact Book,* January 1972, p. 12.

the body. The sexes differ according to the site of the malignancy that causes death. Among males, the most frequent single site is the lung (accounting for at least one quarter of all cancer deaths), followed by the prostate (about one tenth of all cancer mortality). Among females, the most common site of malignancy is the breast, followed by the colon (about 20 per cent and 12 per cent, respectively, of all deaths from cancer).

Morbidity methods have yielded certain information about the number of new cases of cancer in this country during a given year. One estimate is that more than one-half million new cases occur each year, and the prevalence of cases treated in one year is close to one million. This kind of information comes from a special type of cancer morbidity survey performed by the Public Health Service, plus the cancer case registry data provided by several state health departments and by many large hospitals. Information may also be obtained from physician and hospital records. Thorough canvassing of these records has yielded information about the number of new cases occurring in a given area over a specified period of time. Registry data are generally considered better for providing survival information but are more liable to underreporting problems. Another drawback is that registry information which is collected in a valid and useful fashion is expensive and is not feasible for all state and local health departments.

It has been thought that cancer may be caused by genetic or hereditary factors, but studies of recent years suggest interrelated influences of physical environment and the functioning of the body's immune system. Familial factors have been found particularly with respect to breast cancer, where an incidence twice that expected occurred in members of families with breast cancer histories. The same kind of association, but to a lesser extent, has been observed with respect to stomach, colon, and cervical cancers. However, the only form of cancer with a recognized hereditary etiology is retinoblastoma, a relatively rare childhood malignancy of the retina of the eye. In general, the search for cancer causation at present is in terms of a specific virus, a specific carcinogenic chemical, or exposure to some physical agent, such as ionizing radiation.

Viruses of many kinds have been found to cause cancers in animals, and research investigators are trying to determine whether or not there is also a cancer-causing virus in humans. The production of cancer by chemicals is part of a larger problem of the hazards confronting man in today's environment. The chemical agents that are receiving particular attention include agricultural chemicals, such as pesticides, which may contaminate foods; artifical sweeteners, such as cyclamates; hormonal compounds widely used as oral contraceptives; and "natural" products of various molds and fungi, which occur on improperly harvested or stored food crops. Chemical inhalants from cigarette smoke have been implicated not only in cancer of the lung but also in cancer of the larynx, bladder, and oral cavity. There is some epidemiologic evidence that not only cigarette smoke but also air pollution should be considered as a factor in lung cancer. For more than half a century the increased risk of cancer from radiant energy has been known. Energy from ultraviolet rays of sunlight and ionizing radiations from x-ray, radium, and other radioactive materials under some conditions may cause cancer, such as skin cancer, leukemia, and bone cancer.

Prevention of most cancers is obscure and in many cases impossible. Early diagnosis and treatment seem to influence disability and longevity for some types of cancer, whereas in many others little effect can be expected; the reasons for these differences are not understood. Various screening centers or cancer detection centers have been established throughout the United States, and the effectiveness of screening procedure varies considerably among the types of cancer. Several surveys have been performed to establish the prevalence of "cancer-suspect" abnormalities of cells examined under the microscope. These usually relate to examination of tissue from the cervix of the female. A related detection study is that of sputum cytology, which has suggested that even with a negative x-ray, positive or suspicious cells can be indicative of a marked increase in lung cancer risk. Chest x-ray programs are another method of cancer detection. Analysis of the results of such programs has led to the conclusion that a chest x-ray every six months would be the absolute minimum necessary for adequacy and that probably for most of the population such a program would not be suitable as a method for early detection. A development that points toward some possibility of success in detection of breast cancer is that of *mammography*, or diagnostic x-ray of the breast, as an early screening procedure for nodules that are not palpable.

Chronic Metabolic Diseases

DIABETES

Diabetes is a hereditary, metabolic disease resulting from malfunction of the pancreas, pituitary, or other endocrine glands. These glands are interrelated in their hormonal influence on carbohydrate metabolism. Imbalance of glandular function and metabolism contributes not only to the development of diabetes but also to the long-term complicating diseases of the neurologic, cardiovascular, and other biologic systems.

One form of diabetes, diabetes mellitus, ranked seventh among the ten leading causes of death in 1968 (as shown earlier in Table 11-1). In that same year, diabetes mellitus caused more than 38,000 deaths. Nonwhite female mortality due to diabetes was considerably higher than the white female death rate, which in turn exceeded the male rate for both races.

It is estimated that over 3 million people in the United States have diabetes, and that approximately half of them are not aware of it. Diabetes is rarely reported for young people; in fact, the disease is about 10 times more prevalent after age 65. At every age level, individuals who receive treatment shortly after the onset of their disease improve their chances of survival. Even so, the life expectancy is still only about two thirds that of the general population.

Since diabetes is a metabolic disease characterized by a high blood sugar level and excretion of sugar in the urine, its etiology is clearly more hereditary than environmental. For identical twins, where one has diabetes, the frequency of diabetes in the paired sibling is about 50 per cent, whereas a fraternal twin or a nontwin sibling has a risk of about 5 to 10 per cent. However, this does not imply that factors other than heredity are unimportant. Thus, although heredity determines diabetes susceptibility in most cases, the occurrence of the disease among adults is closely correlated with obesity. It has been estimated that more than half of all diabetics sometime during their life are 20 per cent or more above average weight. If one considers that diabetes involves genetic recessive type of heredity, the occurrence of this disease in succeeding generations could at least be reduced by family counseling. The usefulness of this method, however, is mitigated by the fact that diabetes generally is not detected until the adult years.

In most instances, the control of diabetes consists of early detection, which is important because diabetics with minimal complications at the time of diagnosis have a lower death rate than patients who are not diagnosed before they have serious complications. Short-term complications are diabetic coma and various types of infections. The long-term complications are cataract, neuritis, retinitis, and glomerulonephritis, as well as risk for coronary heart disease, cardiovascular disease, and peripheral arteriosclerosis.

The principal means for the detection of diabetes are urine tests and blood tests. Screening programs frequently concentrate on members of families where a diabetic has been identified, persons who are overweight, or persons over 40 years of age. This will yield the greatest return in screening tests. Once diabetes is established by diagnosis, it becomes important that both diet and drugs be regulated. This often requires a long period of time.

The discovery and almost universal use of insulin, oral hypoglycemic agents, and nutritional management all have contributed to a significant control of diabetes during the past several decades. In many cases, medical control can be achieved without insulin. For example, weight reduction and weight control are effective in almost half of adult-onset diabetics. In many cases, the oral hypoglycemic agents can be used rather than the injection of insulin. Another item of considerable importance is the reeducation of the individual to control his physical and psychosocial stress. Special emphasis must be placed on long-term avoidance of infection with its associated complications. Giving detailed instructions in hygiene and diet for diabetics can be very time-consuming, and efforts have been made to organize such teachings in group classes.

Despite substantial progress, diabetes remains a major health problem in the United States, particularly for the middle- and old-age groups. The focal point of the attack must be on early detection, because management of the disease from its incipiency not only reduces disability but also offers the hope of some restoration of pancreatic function and the obviation of long-term complications of the disease.

OBESITY

Obesity is a condition marked by excessive deposition and storage of fat in the body. No scientific quantitative definition exists for this condition, either in terms of a specific method of measuring the fat or in terms of the pathogenesis of the condition. It has been demonstrated that weight and height alone are not good indicators of "fatness," and that as a practical matter one must view obesity with a composite picture of the sex, weight, age, body type, state of health, and specific measurements such as skinfold thickness.

Almost all prevalence data relative to obesity are based on the height-adjusted weight, or the deviation of observed weight from a "desirable" weight estimate. Despite the inadequacy of this incomplete measure, the figures suggest that a high proportion of the population of the United States weighs more than is "desirable." A considerable increase in overweight occurs with advancing years.

Since a large proportion of overweight is due to excessive fat, one could presume to associate this prevalent condition with an increased risk to disease and increased mortality. However, an unequivocal answer to the question of obesity as a health hazard is not easily attained. There have been many large-scale studies conducted by insurance companies which seem to support the contention that obesity carries with it a high risk of heart and circulatory disease and shortened longevity, with mortality experience being apparently most unfavorable for the young, obese adult. Another study reported not only an association with mortality from all causes but also an increase in death attributable specifically to diabetes, heart and circulatory diseases, and digestive diseases. This, of course, does not mean that obesity was the cause of the increased mortality, and in addition, one can question what might have been observed in an uninsured population in this regard. Moreover, there was no standardization in the method of measuring the overweight or in the reporting of causes of death in the insured population.

A study conducted by the Public Health Service in Framingham, Massachusetts, suggested that relative weight did not appear to be associated with an increased risk of developing heart disease unless both hypertension and elevated serum lipids were present. Whether or not obesity is causal relative to adult-onset diabetes is controversial; however, many obese diabetics appear to benefit by a weight-reduction program.

The many psychologic disturbances frequently found in obese patients pose a special health problem. It has been suggested that psychologic processes are responsible for overeating and play a role in maintaining the individual in his obese state. It is difficult to describe and measure this disturbance and document its implications from an epidemiologic point of view.

The past decade has witnessed a research interest in the neurophysiologic and biochemical basis for obesity. Recent twin studies have strongly suggested the existence of a hereditary factor. Also, the prevalence of obesity in children has been shown to be four times higher if one parent is obese, and eight times higher if both parents are obese. However, the fact that the nature of the diet in the United States tends to be high in calories and that there is limited exercise expenditure of these calories raises a question regarding the importance of genetic influence and highlights the difficulty of segregating hereditary factors from the environmental milieu.

It is apparent that the mechanism for regulating food intake is vulnerable to many neurologic, metabolic, and psychologic disturbances. The relative importance of each of these etiologic factors in the various types of obesity is not clear, and hence the question of disease risk remains obscure. One study seems to show clearly that obesity in childhood tends to persist into adulthood, and that the degree of overweight is directly proportional to the adult attainment. Obese children in adolescence constitute a major reservoir for obesity in adult life. As a consequence, the importance of controlling obesity in childhood has gained a significant amount of recognition.

In spite of the lack of knowledge as to the causes of obesity, prevention and treatment can be undertaken and can be strongly recommended. Obese persons have been observed to have a higher prevalence of serum lipids, fasting blood sugar, and blood pressure, all of which can be more or less reversed by a weight-reduction program. These changes accompany the psychologic benefits often reported by patients undergoing weight reduction. Until more is known about the mechanism of the early development of obesity, preventive measures will be based essentially on action to curtail food intake and increase energy expenditure. The evidence relative to the health problems and treatment failures in this method of control clearly points toward a need for early obesity prevention. Health education, particularly as part of a school health program, should include information about the caloric value of food and the caloric cost of exercise.

Chronic Obstructive Lung Diseases

As the ninth leading cause of death (1968; see Table 11-1), bronchitis, emphysema, and asthma are often referred to as "chronic obstructive lung diseases," which comprise one of several categories of the chronic respiratory diseases. Other categories are chronic lung diseases in which an infectious agent plays a prominent role (tuberculosis and several other infectious diseases affecting the lungs, such as histoplasmosis and brucellosis); sensitivity diseases including recurrent acute asthma and chronic granulomatous diseases associated with sensitivity to inhalants; predominantly occupational diseases in which the agent is a pneumoconiosis-producing dust or a chemical irritant; and various other conditions, including diseases of the pulmonary vascular tissue and neoplasms of the lung.

Principal *agent factors* in chronic respiratory diseases are dust and chemicals. Larger dust particles in inspired air tend to be deposited in the bronchi and bronchioles, while the smaller-sized particles affect the alveoli. A similar pattern tends to occur for other particulate matter such as organic material, including infectious agents. Chemical agents have unique effects when absorbed onto particles which are capable of reaching the bronchioles and alveoli. There may be acute exposure to high levels of dust, chemicals, and other particulate matter which may produce an immediate reaction, or there may be long-term exposure to low concentrations of chemicals or other airborne materials which may produce insidious disease and disability. Some of the airborne materials may produce an allergic reaction, which may be acute or anaphylactic owing to hypersensitivity of the host; other reactions may be insidious, arising from long-term exposure and less positive sensitivity.

In addition to the agent factors that can produce chronic lung disease, there are host and environmental factors which determine susceptibility and modify the exposure to specific agents in the population. Examples of *host factors* are age, sex, race, genetic endowment, nutritional state, and immunologic experience. The *environmental factors* which impinge on certain individuals of the population and increase or decrease risk include crowding, place of residence, occupation, climate, and many undefined psychosocial elements. The interaction of each of these primary or accessory factors in determining the prevalence of emphysema or chronic bronchitis has not been well studied. For example, it is well known to clinicians that atopic conditions, such as asthma, are familial, but the genetic mechanism is not clear.

There were about 33,000 deaths from "chronic obstructive lung diseases" in 1968. The mortality ascribed to emphysema, chronic bronchitis, and chronic asthma has had its impact primarily in individuals over 45 years of age. It may also be noted that the increase largely occurred in the adult male population where it became a frequent cause of disability and sickness absence.[10] The Social Security Administration reported that 7 per cent (21,000) of its total cases of disability were due to chronic obstructive pulmonary diseases. The bulk of these cases during 1967 occurred in the age group 50 to 64. It is difficult to estimate the incidence or prevalence of chronic bronchitis, chronic asthma, and emphysema in the general population at this time. Part of the difficulty in this estimate is the lack of a definition of early disease and a suitable yardstick to measure stages of disease.

Since the "chronic obstructive lung diseases" are the prevalent chronic respiratory diseases, a major national effort is taking shape to define their incidence, identify areas vulnerable to control, and provide for early treatment and/or rehabilitation. In some sense this challenge is shared by organizations oriented toward combating the parallel menace, lung cancer. Moreover, clinicians are making inroads in defining preventive programs for special-risk groups. Programs to detect early "chronic obstructive lung disease" generally have utilized a questionnaire to elicit symptomatology referable to one of the diseases and/or a spirometry test to assess the probability of obstructive or restrictive abnormality.

References

1. Lilienfeld, Abraham M., and Gifford, Alice J. (eds.). *Chronic Diseases and Public Health.* The Johns Hopkins Press, Baltimore, 1966.
2. Myers, Julian S. (ed.). *An Orientation to Chronic Disease and Disability.* The Macmillan Company, New York, 1965.
3. Dodge, David L. and Martin, Walter T. *Social Stress and Chronic Illness.* University of Notre Dame Press, Notre Dame, Indiana, 1970.
4. Wilson, J. M. G. and Junger, G. *Principles and Practice of Screening for Disease.* World Health Organization, Geneva, 1968.
5. Thorner, R. M., and Remein, Q. R. *Principles and Procedures in the Evaluation of Screening for Disease.* Public Health Monograph No. 67 (Public Health Service Publication No. 846). U.S. Government Printing Office, Washington, D.C., 1961.
6. The American Public Health Association. *Control of Chronic Diseases in Man.* The Association, New York, 1966.
7. American Hospital Association. *Care of Chronically Ill Adults.* The Association, Chicago, 1971.
8. Program Area Committee on Chronic Disease and Rehabilitation. *Chronic Disease and Rehabilitation—A Program Guide for State and Local Health Agencies.* The American Public Health Association, New York, 1960 (also, Breslow, Lester, ed., 2nd edition, 1971).
9. The President's Commission on Heart Disease, Cancer and Stroke. *A National Program to Conquer Heart Disease, Cancer and Stroke: Report to the President,* Vol. I and Vol. II. U.S. Government Printing Office, Washington, D.C., December 1964.
10. Breslow, Lester. Chronic disease and disability in adults. In: Sartwell, P. E. (ed.). *Maxcy-Rosenau Preventive Medicine and Public Health,* 9th ed. Appleton-Century-Crofts, New York, 1965.

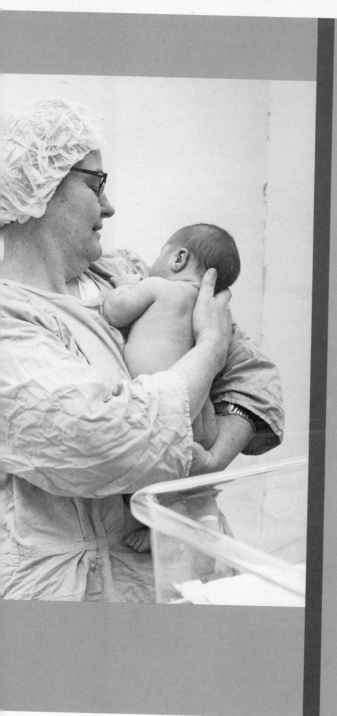

12

HEALTH OF MOTHERS AND CHILDREN

CHAPTER OUTLINE

Courtesy of California's Health, *California Department of Public Health. Staff photo.*

The Health of Mothers, Infants, and Preschool Children

PUBLIC HEALTH CONCERNS IN MATERNAL AND CHILD HEALTH

Efforts to promote health and prevent illness in mothers and their children include all aspects of physical, mental, and social well-being. The goal of these efforts is a healthy child, delivered and cared for by a healthy mother. There are several factors in this process which have played a role in making maternal and child health a matter of public health concern.

First, childbearing women and growing infants and children are, in general, the more dependent members of a society. As a society evolves, there is a trend toward greater concern for these dependent members, and public efforts develop in their behalf.

Second, there is the economic significance of childbearing and rearing to the future of any civilization. Some community activity to ensure healthy arrival in the production of its members is essential to the maintenance of the society's future.

A third reason stems from the fact that at the turn of the century, deaths of mothers and children were major contributors to mortality in every community in the United States. Approximately 60 mothers died for every 10,000 pregnancies that produced liveborn infants. Out of every 1,000 of these liveborn infants, 100 babies did not survive their first year of life. Improving community health, which is the primary purpose of public health, meant preventing the diseases that led to maternal and infant deaths.

The fourth reason for the role of public health in maternal and child health is the ever-increasing complexity of organizing and meeting the high cost of the services necessary to provide the best solution for many of the health problems of mothers and their children. Only through organized community efforts can the necessary services be made available to all citizens who are in need.

PRINCIPAL MATERNAL AND CHILD DEVELOPMENTAL PERIODS

For descriptive purposes, the development of mothers, infants, and young children may be divided into several periods. These developmental periods are enumerated and defined as follows and are presented schematically in Figure 12-1.

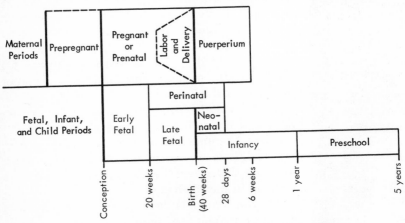

FIGURE 12-1. *Principal developmental periods of the maternal, infant, and preschool years.*

The maternal periods include the following:

Prepregnant: all nonpregnant time during the mother's reproductive years

Pregnant or Prenatal: from conception until the delivery of all products of conception, including the placenta

Labor and Delivery: that portion of the prenatal period from the beginning of true labor until the delivery of all products of conception including the placenta

Puerperium: the six weeks following delivery

The periods related to infants and children include:

Fetal: from conception until delivery—
   Early: from conception through the twentieth week
   Late: from the twentieth week to delivery
Neonatal: from birth through 28 days of life—
   Early: from birth through the first seven days of life
   Late: from the eighth day of life through the twenty-eighth day

Perinatal: from the twentieth week after conception through the first 28 days after birth, thus combining the late fetal and neonatal periods

Infancy: from birth to the first birthday

Preschool: from the first birthday to the fifth birthday

It is important to keep in mind that while developmental periods are convenient descriptive devices, they are artificial. Growth and development are continuous processes which proceed at all times, rather than in a series of arbitrary periods.

MATERNAL HEALTH

Maternal Mortality. The primary vital statistic which public health has traditionally used to follow the degree of health of pregnant women has been the maternal mortality rate. This rate is defined as follows:

$$\frac{\text{All mothers dying while pregnant} + \text{All women dying within 90 days of having delivered an infant}}{\text{All live births}} \times 10,000$$

The numerator is considered to include all women who die from causes related to the pregnant state. While the denominator is actually a measure of birth, it will, at least in theory, include most women who have been pregnant. The resulting fraction is multiplied by 10,000 because in recent years in the United States, the maternal mortality rate has fallen to less than 1 per 1,000 and it is desirable to have the statistic expressed in a whole number.

From Figure 12-2 it is apparent that between 1922 and 1935 the maternal mortality rate in the United States was fairly stable at about 60 per 10,000 live births among white mothers and 100 per 10,000 in the nonwhite group. By 1968, this figure had dropped to 1.7 per 10,000 in the white group and 6.4 per 10,000 in the nonwhite group. In addition to this racial variation, there is also considerable variation from state to state and from urban to rural areas. It is now felt by many that a maternal mortality of two deaths per 10,000 live births is not an unreasonable goal for all groups throughout the nation.

The most direct causes of maternal deaths include toxemia of pregnancy (a poorly understood condition which includes swelling, elevated blood pressure, and protein in the urine), as well as hemorrhage, abortion, death due to anesthesia, and sepsis (infection of the bloodstream). Approximately three quarters of these deaths are judged to have been avoidable and thus can be considered to be the

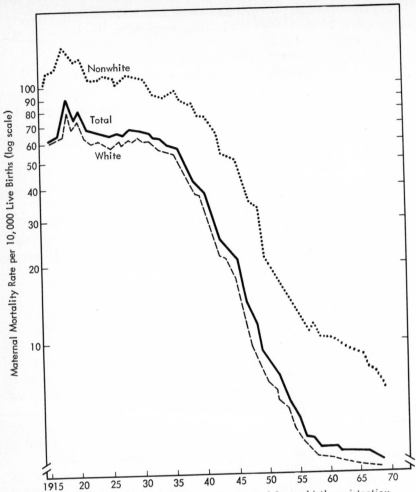

FIGURE 12-2. *Maternal mortality by color, United States birth registration area, 1915–1968.* [Source: Adapted from National Center for Health Statistics. *Vital Statistics of the United States, 1965,* and from U.S. Bureau of the Census, *Statistical Abstract of the United States, 1971.*]

result of inadequate quality or quantity of maternal care. In the various states in this country, maternal mortality committees investigate the causes of maternal deaths. These committees (experts in all fields germane to maternal health) investigate the details of events surrounding each maternal death reported and submit a report summarizing the events of the death, including a judgment as to whether or not it was avoidable.

Prepregnancy Period. Whether or not a woman will survive a pregnancy and provide an adequate physiologic environment for the growing child depends to an enormous extent on her health prior to and at the time of conception. Any chronic disease in the mother that alters her normal physiologic homeostasis can profoundly affect both the mother's health and that of the developing child.

Pregnancy may be a time of stress for the mother, both psychologically and physiologically. If the mother enters pregnancy with any serious emotional problems, these may become exaggerated. Sometimes, however, the opposite may occur: on occasion, an emotionally unstable woman will have fewer adjustment problems during pregnancy.

Closely intertwined with the mental health of the mother is the quality of her social environment. While a marriage certificate prior to the onset of pregnancy does not in any way guarantee a better pregnancy, a stable social environment for the mother is very important during pregnancy. The value of emotional support during this period cannot be overestimated. The important consideration is that the mother be comfortable and happy with her social environment and receive support from others during the pregnancy.

Because all the preceding factors have become increasingly recognized as being important to the outcome of pregnancy, a new field known as preventive obstetrics is developing. The purpose of preventive obstetrics is to ensure that physical, emotional, and social factors are as satisfactory as possible prior to the onset of pregnancy. Family planning is, of course, an important part of preventive obstetrics so that the children will be wanted and the pregnancy will occur when desired and when personal and family conditions are optimal for the outcome.

Pregnancy Period and Prenatal Care.   Pregnancy involves profound physiologic and biochemical changes in the mother. Therefore, it is essential to diagnose pregnancy as soon as possible in order that supervision can be provided which will assure maintenance of good maternal health and will help to minimize the chance of pregnancy wastage. The phrase "pregnancy wastage" has been coined in recent years to refer to unfavorable results of pregnancy with regard to the fetus or infant. This includes the entire spectrum from fetal and infant death through all degrees of sublethal damage which can cause lifelong handicapping conditions such as cerebral palsy, mental retardation, or congenital malformations.

Proper health supervision during pregnancy, or prenatal care, is now accepted as an important part of public health. In most parts of the United States, prenatal care is provided by private physicians. Nearly all counties, however, also provide public prenatal clinics for those who cannot afford this service privately. These public clinics may be administered through a county hospital or through the county or city health department. The quality of medical care provided by the professional staff in public clinics is in general quite high.

In spite of the availability of good prenatal care, large numbers of women are known to go through all or much of their pregnancy without such care. There are a number of reasons for this. Since prenatal care is primarily preventive in nature, the pregnant mother must present herself for this care when she may not feel ill in any way. While the value of preventive health care is understood by many people in the United States, there are still large groups of individuals who would never consider going to a doctor unless they felt sick. Hence, for a number of women, even in the present day, going for a checkup during pregnancy when they feel fine is unthought of. While health education would help overcome this negligence, it is difficult to locate these women so that the health education may be applied. There is no system in the United States, as there is in many countries, for ensuring the case-finding of new pregnancies in the population. At the present time, a valuable resource is for public health nurses to be observant while working in the districts they serve. Maternal and infant care centers and neighborhood health centers are also now playing significant roles. When an expectant mother is discovered, the nurse (or other health worker) can explain the value of care and make an appropriate referral.

The shortage of trained personnel in the United States is a significant problem in providing prenatal health care. Even if all pregnant women should present themselves early in pregnancy for prenatal care either to private physicians or to public clinics, it would be impossible for these women to be cared for adequately. At present, there are not enough obstetricians, general practitioners, or clinics; and even with the rapidly growing number of medical schools it will be a long time before there are enough physicians to provide a sufficient quantity of prenatal care.

Other nations, such as England and the Scandinavian countries, have at least partly solved the problem of the personnel shortage through the use of nurse obstetric assistants (nurse midwives). After the prenatal patient has been examined on the first visit by the physician, she is placed in a high-risk or low-risk category depending on her medical history. If she is unlikely to have any complications, she is considered low risk and may be followed on subsequent visits by a nurse midwife and subsequently may even be delivered by the nurse midwife. The high-risk pregnancy and any mother followed by nurse midwives who develops complications are referred to the physicians for follow-up and delivery.

Lay midwives have traditionally played a significant role in maternal care, although in the United States their numbers have reduced from approximately 21,000 in 1948 to about 4,100 in 1970. There were approximately 1,200 qualified *nurse midwives* in the United States in 1970. Nurse midwives function as members of the obstetric team and provide prenatal, intrapartal, and postpartal care. There are at least 10 nurse midwife training programs in the United States and Puerto Rico, leading to either the certificate of qualification (6 to 8 months) or the master's degree plus certificate (12 to 24 months).

There has been resistance in the United States to the use of nurse midwives in spite of the fact that several of the major medical centers in the country, including Johns Hopkins University and Columbia University, train such specialists. The fear is that these individuals may not be able to cope with some of the unanticipated complications of pregnancy and delivery, but such fears appear unfounded in view of their thorough training and experience.

Labor and Delivery Period.   Whereas pregnancy lasts nine months, labor and delivery usually last less than 24 hours. This 24-hour period is, however, by far the most critical time for the health and survival of both the mother and the infant. The physiologic stresses on both these individuals are high.

The risks for the mother at this time include hemorrhage, complications of anesthesia, and the introduction of infectious agents into her uterus. Because of such risks there has been a trend in the United States over the past 50 years toward more and more deliveries to be performed in hospitals, so that now about 98 per cent of the deliveries occur in a hospital. Hospital delivery has the advantage of having all facilities to handle sudden problems as they arise during these critical hours. It has the disadvantage of having the mother out of the familiar surroundings of her home and the familiar comforts of her family. In England, where there is a serious shortage of hospital beds, a system has been devised whereby all low-risk mothers with uncomplicated pregnancies may be delivered at home by nurse obstetric assistants. There is always available, on immediate call, an ambulance from the nearest hospital which contains all the necessary equipment for any obstetric emergencies.

Obviously the fact of being in the hospital does not in itself guarantee good supervision of labor and delivery. In order to correct and forestall unsatisfactory procedures, many cities, counties, and states have developed standards of hospital practice of obstetrics. In New York City, for example, hospital licensure rests in part on thorough study by the health department of the practices in the labor rooms, delivery rooms, and newborn nurseries. Many private hospitals have their own appointed committees to conduct a similar surveillance of practices. It is difficult, however, for one physician in a private hospital to criticize a fellow physician in the same hospital. For this reason, there are distinct advantages in having an independent, outside agency such as the health department provide such surveillance. It is also beneficial to be able to use licensing as a means of ensuring good practices.

Puerperal Period.   The puerperium is a period of important physiologic and psychologic readjustment for the mother. Because of the shortage of hospital beds and because of the importance of early ambulation, most mothers are now discharged from the hospital within three days of delivery. In some busy county hospitals they may be discharged within 24 hours of delivery. A subsequent checkup by a physician (postpartum checkup) thus becomes a very important procedure. Again, however, this is primarily a preventive measure, and unfortunately, large groups of women will not return for such checkups. Public health nurse follow-up of recently discharged new mothers is of considerable help in getting these women back to their doctors.

FETAL AND PERINATAL HEALTH

In addition to having effects on the mother, pregnancy, of course, also has effects on the developing child. The normal nine-month pregnancy is actually 40 weeks long. For research and statistical purposes, these 40 weeks are usually divided into two equal periods. The first 20 weeks is the period of early fetal development and takes place before the developing child is capable of survival outside the uterine environment. The second 20 weeks, the late fetal period, is the time when a child is, at least theoretically, capable of surviving in the outside world.

The problems of the late fetal period and those of the first 28 days after birth (the neonatal period) are intertwined inexorably. Any attempt to study these problems must include both periods in order to be meaningful. It is for this reason that the concept of the perinatal period has been developed, which, it will be recalled from an earlier section, combines the late fetal and the neonatal periods.

Early Fetal Period.   Information about the health needs and problems of the fetus during the first 20 weeks of gestation is still very limited. Even the number of deaths that occur during this period can only be estimated. Only a few states require the reporting of a fetal death prior to 20 weeks of gestation, and even in these states the reporting of such deaths is very poor. Many pregnant women will miss one or two menstrual periods and then spontaneously abort ("miscarry") a very small fetus without even realizing they have been pregnant. Many early fetal deaths may be the result of induced interruption of pregnancy and sometimes will not be reported. It is estimated that more than 10 per cent of all human pregnancies spontaneously abort prior to 20 weeks of gestation. Many investigators feel spontaneous abortion represents nature's way of taking care of imperfectly formed fetuses. Others, however, believe that a significant proportion of the women are aborting unnecessarily.[1] This group includes mothers who have a characteristic tendency to lose their pregnancy spontaneously in the early weeks.

Factors that influence early fetal growth are very poorly understood, but it is known that the first 20 weeks is the critical period in the development of all major organ systems of the body. This is the period when insults such as infections, drugs, or an adverse environment may cause congenital malformations or even fetal death. The discovery of the relationship between an undesirable outcome of pregnancy and German measles infection in early pregnancy, or thalidomide taken in these early weeks, has brought widespread attention to such problems. There has also been a great deal of discovery recently in the area of the genetic causes of congenital abnormalities, but it is still not possible to state whether the genetic components of the developing fetus or the intrauterine environmental factors are more important in the production of defects. It is perhaps most likely that there is an interaction between the environment (including infectious agents and drugs) and the genetic components which determines the development of many congenital abnormalities. As more is learned about genetics, the fetus, and the intrauterine environment, it will be possible to prevent some of this pregnancy wastage.

Perinatal Period. The perinatal period is one of great importance with respect to the survival and future well-being of the child. During the last weeks of pregnancy, the fetus becomes capable of independent existence outside the uterus, and during the first weeks after birth numerous complex changes necessary for physiologic independence take place.

The risk of death is greater during the perinatal period than at any other time until after age 60. Perinatal mortality is defined as death after 20 weeks of gestation but prior to delivery ("stillbirth"), plus death in the first 28 days of life. To determine a perinatal mortality rate, deaths during this period are used as the numerator; the denominator consists of all infants at risk and therefore includes all live births plus all stillbirths. Thus, the perinatal mortality rate is computed as follows:

$$\frac{\text{Deaths after 20 weeks' gestation} + \text{deaths in the first 28 days of life}}{\text{Stillbirths} + \text{live births}} \times 1,000$$

There were 32 deaths per 1,000 live and stillbirths in 1968, with a perinatal mortality rate of 29 and 49 deaths in white and nonwhite groups, respectively. The single most common cause of death before birth is anoxia, or lack of oxygen. The most common cause of death during the first seven days after birth is "prematurity," which accounts for somewhere between one quarter and one third of these deaths. The next most common cause is asphyxia, or suffocation, which accounts for approximately one quarter of the deaths.

Many authorities agree that little headway will be made in the reduction of perinatal mortality until something can be done about prematurity. The problem with prematurity is that it is a phenomenon and not a specific disease. It is also difficult to define. Since body weight in general increases with increasing length of pregnancy, and since this measurement is easily obtained internationally, the World Health Assembly defined prematurity in 1948 as an infant weighing less than 2,500 g (5 lb, 8 oz), and later changed the term from "premature" to infants of "low birth weight."

More recent investigation has suggested that there may be at least two separate subgroups among infants under 2,500 g. Infants with birth weights between 1,500 and 2,500 g in general have a much lower mortality rate and seem to have much less difficulty in later life. On the other hand, infants weighing less than 1,500 g at birth may represent a different phenomenon. Seventy-five to 80 per cent of these infants die in the first week of life, while only 10 to 15 per cent of the larger babies succumb. In addition, longitudinal follow-up studies have demonstrated conclusively that even if the smaller infants survive the neonatal period, they carry a definitely increased risk of mental retardation, neurologic handicaps, eye defects, and other medical problems.

The incidence of low birth weight in a given population varies with a wide number of factors. One of the most important factors is socioeconomic status. As socioeconomic status declines, the rate of low birth weight rises and, secondarily of course, the perinatal mortality rate also rises. In addition, the incidence of low birth weight increases with the following factors: multiple birth, young mothers (under 16), older mothers (over 35), first pregnancy, fifth or greater pregnancy, smoking by the mother, illegitimacy, history of previous premature delivery by the mother, and poor prenatal care.

INFANT AND PRESCHOOL HEALTH

Infancy, it will be recalled from an earlier section of this chapter, is defined as the period of life from birth to the first birthday; the preschool period extends from the first to the fifth birthday. Infancy is a time of particularly rapid rate of growth and development. At birth, many organs have yet to reach their maximum efficiency in carrying out their essential physiologic and biochemical functions. By the end of the first year, these organ functions have matured considerably. In addition, numerous outwardly visible evidences of physical and psychologic growth and development occur in infancy and continue throughout the preschool period.

Infant and Preschool Mortality. The infant mortality rate is the number of liveborn babies under one year of age who die during a calendar year, per 1,000 live births during the same time period. The method of computation and the general utility of this rate have been described in Chapter 9. Figure 12-3 shows a reasonably steady decline in the infant mortality rate in the United States over a 54-year period, from about 100 infant deaths for every 1,000 live births in 1915 to 22 in 1968.

As has been suggested in earlier chapters, most of the long-range decline in the infant mortality rate has been due to the control of infectious diseases through a combination of improved environmental control, immunization, and antibiotics. In view of these accomplishments and the generally high standard of living in the United States, it might appear that the infant mortality rates which have prevailed over the past several years reflect a biologic lower limit precluding further significant improvement. However, when comparisons are made with other nations of similar economic and social development, the error of this conclusion is apparent. Thus, as shown by Table 12-1, the United States had the *highest* infant mortality rate among a list of 15 nations in 1968–1969.

Excessive deaths among the nonwhite infants in the United States are a major source of the higher overall infant mortality rate. Figure 12-3 indicates that, although nonwhite infant mortality has dropped over the years, it still remains at about 34 deaths per 1,000 live births. White infant mortality fell below that point about 25 years ago. Health workers believe this racial differential to be the result of socioeconomic factors rather than biologic differences. Poverty is no doubt one of the nation's major maternal and child health problems. It should not be assumed, however, that infant mortality in the United States is entirely the result of the unfortunate socioeconomic status of the nonwhite population. By 1968 only five states

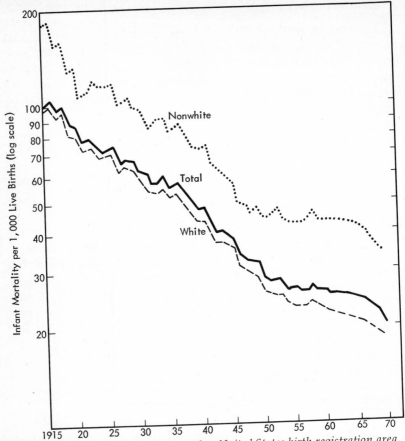

FIGURE 12-3. *Infant mortality by color, United States birth registration area, 1915–1968.* [SOURCE: Adapted from National Center for Health Statistics. *Infant and Perinatal Mortality in the United States,* Series 3, No. 4, 1965, and from U.S. Bureau of the Census, *Statistical Abstract of the United States, 1971.*]

and the District of Columbia had reported white infant mortality rates of less than 17 per 1,000 live births: North Dakota with 16.9, Delaware with 16.0, Utah with 16.6, Alaska with 16.6, Hawaii with 15.6, and the District of Columbia with 16.6. Thus, even if the status of the nonwhite population were on a par with that of the white population, further improvement in conditions affecting all mothers and children, white and nonwhite alike, would still be needed in order to match the accomplishments of several other nations in the world.

Risk of death among infants declines with age, the most critical period being the first month of life. After a child has reached his first birthday, the risk of death drops sharply to about 4 per cent of

TABLE 12-1. Infant Mortality, Selected Countries, 1968–1969

	Infant Mortality per 1,000 Live Births
Iceland	11.7
Sweden	12.9
Netherlands	13.2
Norway	13.7
Finland	14.0
Denmark	14.8
Japan	15.3
Switzerland	15.4
France	16.4
Luxembourg	16.7
New Zealand	16.9
Taiwan	17.5
Australia	17.9
United Kingdom	18.6
United States	20.8

SOURCE: Adapted from United Nations. *1970 Demographic Yearbook,* 22nd ed., 1971, pp. 646–52.

what it was in the first year. At present, 1 child out of every 1,000 in the preschool age group dies each year in the United States. The mortality rate of nonwhite children during the preschool years continues to be about twice that of white children, or nearly 2 deaths per 1,000 nonwhite children of preschool age. Accidents are the number-one enemy of today's preschooler, accounting for more than one third of the deaths between one and four years of age.

Health Needs of the Infant and Preschool Child.   Infant and preschool years are a time of building foundations which will provide good support for a long, productive, and enjoyable life. Because of the very rapid rate of physical and psychologic growth and development, insults that might be minor at a later stage in life may cause lifetime deviations from normal when they occur in these early years. Basic health needs can be divided into three groups: environmental, physical, and emotional.

The child's *environment* should be comfortable, clean, and safe. The water, milk, and food supply must be free of harmful toxins or infectious agents. Disease-carrying insects must be excluded. Accident hazards need to be removed or controlled in accord with the ability of the infant and child, in order to prevent the much too frequent tragedy of accidental death or permanent disability. This is of major importance for preschoolers.

Physical needs include being kept reasonably clean and appropriately dressed. Nutrition must be adequate for good physical growth. Children's teeth should have attention during preschool years. Immunization should be started as early as the infant's immune mechanism can respond, currently considered to be about two months of age. Regular physical examinations to detect any deviations from normal as soon as possible are also among the physical health needs of infants and preschool children.

The *emotional* needs of the developing child are of major importance to his future well-being. Parental love of an unselfish and undemanding nature will help develop trust and confidence in the world and its people. Some regularity of surroundings and responses is necessary in order that security can be created through predictability, yet there must be enough variation to meet the need for diversity and thus help to avoid the development of an excessively rigid personality. Inadequate human contact and stimulation may result in disturbed behavior, a failure to thrive, and even death. It is not necessarily the presence of the infant's biologic mother that is important, but rather the fact that he receives "mothering" kinds of attention such as cuddling, being played with, and being talked to.

Well-Child Supervision. Physical evaluations including an assessment of development, immunizations, dietary advice, and anticipatory guidance are best provided together in programs of well-child supervision. Such supervision begins in the hospital during the newborn period. It is recommended that an infant be seen at monthly intervals thereafter for the first six months, bimonthly for the next six months, every three or four months in the second year of life, and every six months until school age.[2]

Well-child supervision is most frequently provided by a private physician, commonly a general practitioner. Unfortunately, many families cannot afford to have their children cared for privately. For such children, the community usually provides well-child clinics. At the present time, health departments are the main, though not exclusive, provider of public, well-child supervision, augmented by maternal and infant care centers and neighborhood health centers. In some communities, clinics are sponsored by voluntary organizations such as service clubs or churches, which provide funds for equipment and salaries and a convenient place for holding a clinic at regular intervals. The Visiting Nurses Association is another organization that is very active in providing well-child clinics.

The emphasis of the clinics is prevention, and clinic personnel are usually quite enthusiastic about this aspect of child health care. The clinic facility is also usually staffed by a physician, one or two public health nurses, a registered nurse, a social worker, and one or more volunteers. Some arrangement for consultation with various medical specialists is also provided. Through the public health nurse and other allied health personnel, the service may even extend into the home. This team approach offers a broad kind of service which is sometimes difficult to provide in private practice.

Public well-child supervision is, however, far from ideal. There are problems of financial eligibility of children for program support. Public agencies are always short of funds, but even if there were unlimited financial resources for establishing more clinics, the shortage of medical personnel would still be a problem. These financial and personnel problems have resulted in many clinics across the nation limiting their service to infants and children under two years of age in spite of the recommended visit every six months thereafter throughout the preschool years.

A number of suggestions regarding better use of available funds and personnel in public well-child clinics have been made in the past few years. In a demonstration clinic where public health nurses had been given considerably more responsibility, infants and mothers were seen by the nurse, only, for four out of seven visits during their first year and five out of ten visits during their preschool years. A physician saw the baby at 1, 6, and 12 months, and at every other visit thereafter unless the nurse felt consultation was necessary.[3] Another solution to relieve some of the patient load problem has been to develop high-risk infant clinics, which many of the newer maternal and infant care centers are, in reality. Infants with suspicious factors in their early fetal, perinatal, or family history receive special, more intensive well-child supervision. Such an approach enables the more skilled but scarce personnel to focus on a smaller group which has a relatively greater need for health surveillance.

The artificial separation of well-child care from sick-child care is probably the major weakness of clinic supervision. If an abnormality is found, the child must be referred elsewhere for treatment. Obtaining health services from a variety of resources is unsatisfying for both the provider and the recipient. In order to improve the continuity of care, several solutions have been proposed. Some clinics have affiliated with approved hospital pediatric services in order to provide a more direct referral system. Community health centers, which have been developed in low-income areas, offer a full range of outpatient services. In other approaches, a public health nurse is assigned to the families and works with the private physician (paid for service by the health department) just as she would with a clinic physician. A social worker may also be utilized. At present each community must take stock of its own needs and resources and develop a design for comprehensive care within its own limits.

HIGH-RISK MOTHERS AND CHILDREN

There are several groups of mothers and children who are at especially great risk for having health problems. High-risk mothers also include those with an increased risk of pregnancy wastage.

Mothers with Age, Parity, or Medical History Problems. Women under 16 and over 35, women having their first child, and women having their sixth child or more have been shown definitely to have an increased risk for their own health and for the health of the developing child during pregnancy. All such women should receive special attention and careful supervision of the progress of their pregnancy. Furthermore, any mother who has a history of previous pregnancy failure is at higher risk of having a succeeding pregnancy failure. A woman with such a history needs to be identified early in pregnancy and followed closely.

Mothers and Children of Low Socioeconomic Status. There is no doubt that women in the lowest socioeconomic groups are at high risk both for death and for having complications that lead to pregnancy wastage. Earlier in this chapter it was noted that maternal mortality in the United States was considerably higher among non-white mothers than among white mothers. Low socioeconomic status offers many obstacles to the healthy development of the infant and the young child. Both mortality and morbidity are higher among children of lower-income families. Some means must be found for providing more comprehensive and well-coordinated health care for mothers and children from low-income families.

Unwed Mothers and Their Children. In 1968, there were 339,200 babies born in the United States who were reportedly born out of wedlock. Of these babies, 165,700 were born to mothers younger than 20 years of age, with 7,700 under 15 years of age. The total represents a marked increase over 20 years ago, when about 150,000 infants were reported to be born out of wedlock. These unwed and frequently very young mothers have more health problems but receive less prenatal care. Social customs and sometimes regulations in prenatal clinics discourage unwed mothers from seeking health care during pregnancy. For example, some prenatal clinics require that any girl under 18 years attending the clinic must be accompanied by her mother. On the other hand, some health departments are developing new and imaginative programs to provide for the special needs of unwed mothers. Thus, the health department and the school district may jointly sponsor a program for pregnant teenage girls, which provides instruction in child care and other aspects of health, in addition to the regular school curriculum. There are also many homes run by voluntary agencies and religious groups throughout the country where unmarried mothers may live during their pregnancy and receive both regular prenatal care and health education. There is still, however, an urgent need for many more thoughtfully initiated programs, if the problems of this high-risk group are to be met.

Working Mothers and Their Children. There is still some question as to whether or not a woman who must work during pregnancy is a high-risk mother. Everyone agrees, however, that if a woman is working during pregnancy and has an additional health problem, she should be relieved from work. In the United States, there are frequently many factors to discourage such a woman from seeking relief from employment. Foremost, of course, is the loss of income for the family. In addition, she may risk loss of seniority or even loss of the job itself. These considerations may deter an employed woman from seeking prenatal care for fear that a problem will be discovered and the doctor will insist that she stop working. Such fears are unfortunate because there is general agreement that working mothers urgently need prenatal care to determine whether or not they have a health problem for which work may be detrimental.

In 1971, there were 25.7 million children under 18 years of age who had working mothers. About 5.6 million of these children were under 6 years of age. The mere fact that a mother works is not necessarily harmful to a child. What is of vital concern is the arrangement made for child care while the mother is away. There is a real need for more and better arrangements. Most states have laws governing standards, inspection, and licensing of larger child care facilities. However, a great many children are cared for in situations that do not come under public jurisdiction. For example, there may be a neighbor who takes five or six local infants or children into her home every day. The environment may be crowded, unsanitary, unsafe, and inadequately supervised, but the enterprise is not large enough to be subject to existing laws.

Mothers and Children in Migrant Families. In 1960, the United States census indicated that there were 400,000 to 500,000 domestic migrant workers. These people are one of the most underprivileged groups in the nation. They have all the problems of low socioeconomic status plus the very significant added difficulties of separation from relatives, isolation from community life and resources, lack of legal residence status, and no protection by minimum wage laws and unemployment insurance.

Mothers in the migrant labor group are an extremely high-risk group. Even though they have low incomes, they are often ineligible for prenatal care because they do not live in one place long enough to establish residency. They also frequently work throughout their entire pregnancy whether or not they have additional health problems.

Approximately 300,000 children belong to migrant families. They are often malnourished and anemic, have severe dental problems, are plagued with intestinal parasites, and have frequent skin, respiratory, and gastrointestinal infections. Also, because father, mother, and older siblings may all work, young children and even infants may be left unsupervised for many hours of the day. Newer federal legislation is focusing some health care attention on the need of migrant families, but a great deal more is required.

Children with Congenital Abnormalities.   Children with known congenital abnormalities suffer from three major groups of problems. The first group of problems consists of the handicaps, impairments, or limitations that arise from the particular abnormality. The second results from the difficulties which parents and others responsible for day-to-day care have in providing for the child's normal emotional needs. Thus, the child with a known abnormality may not receive enough essential loving care or may be so excessively responded to that he is never allowed to develop any independence. The third problem area is that of medical care. While the particular malformation may be well treated, the care is often so highly specialized that the overall needs of the child are totally neglected. All too frequently such children progress through their entire first year without well-child supervision and reach their first birthday or even later with no immunization, with nutritional deficiencies, and with a firm start toward lifetime behavior problems.

The Child of Abusive Parents.   The child of abusive parents has come to be known as the battered child. This problem has recently been brought to public attention as a significant cause of disability and death in children. The child is commonly under three years of age and too young to give any explanations for his multiple bruises, swellings, and recent and old fractures. Frequently, though not always, there is also evidence of general neglect, malnutrition, and poor hygiene.

Laws against child abuse exist in all states, but the situation must come to the attention of proper authorities before any legal action can be taken. Since most of the battering episodes do not occur in public, they are seldom reported. It is not uncommon, however, for the child to be brought to a clinic or hospital for treatment of the most recent injury. Parents usually attribute the injuries to accidents or place the blame on baby-sitters or siblings. Many medical personnel have found it difficult to believe that a parent could be responsible for the injuries to his own child and have tended to accept whatever story was provided. Others, who may have been suspicious, have been afraid of becoming liable in some way if they interfere.

Public concern for the abused child increased so greatly that in 1963 the Children's Bureau and the American Humane Association prepared model laws which would make reporting of suspect cases by a physician mandatory, but would at the same time protect against civil or criminal liability. By the first part of 1966, all except three states had passed such laws. Reporting of a case does not mean immediate court action will be taken, but only that a careful investigation by trained child welfare workers will be carried out. If the suspicions are found to be true, steps are taken to protect the child and to help the family, if possible.

The Health of Schoolchildren

BACKGROUND AND COMPONENTS OF SCHOOL HEALTH PROGRAMS

When laws regulating child labor and making school attendance compulsory were enacted, new responsibilities were imposed on local government as well as on parents. If a child is required to attend school, then government must provide the school, and, in addition, if there are any health hazards peculiar to school attendance, it becomes the responsibility of government to exert every reasonable effort to offset these hazards. It is in the discharge of this obligation that school health services were first developed. Gradually it became recognized that the school setting provides an opportunity to improve as well as protect the health of children.

School health programs began in the United States in the late nineteenth century and were directed principally toward the control of communicable diseases and minor infections which were rampant in the school population. With improved methods of communicable disease control, this aspect, although still important, is not the major emphasis in the modern school health program.

Contemporary school health programs have been broadened to include three primary components: medical, educational, and environmental. The *medical* component of school health services involves the prevention of disease, the detection of physical or mental conditions which might handicap the schoolchild, and the provision of procedures for the correction of such defects. The *educational* aspect pertains to basic instruction in health for the child and to some extent for the school staff and the parents. The *environmental* component includes the provision and maintenance of sanitary, safe, and comfortable conditions in the school.

In the past, the greatest concentration of school health work has been with children in the first eight grades. The children in these grades are usually from 6 to 14 years of age and constitute approximately 65 per cent of the total school population. However, the age distribution is changing, and state and federal programs are providing for schooling for younger children, particularly those with working mothers or in one-parent families. There are increasing numbers of children in public and private schools, preschools, and nursery schools. Furthermore, with the increasing emphasis on higher education, an unprecedented number of young people are attending high schools, junior colleges, colleges, and universities. Table 12-2 illustrates the increase in all categories of school enrollment that has occurred from 1960 to 1970.

TABLE 12-2. School Enrollment, United States, 1960 and 1970

	1960	1970
	Number of Persons (in Thousands)	
Kindergarten	2,092	2,726
Elementary (grades 1–8)	30,349	33,950
High school	10,249	14,715
College	3,570	7,413
TOTAL	46,259	58,804

SOURCE: Adapted from U.S. Bureau of the Census. *Statistical Abstract of the United States, 1971,* p. 103.

Significant physical, mental, emotional, and social changes characterize the growth of the school-age child. Although certain norms may be used to describe the various stages of development, it should be kept in mind that deviation from the average does not necessarily constitute abnormality. Individual differences in the rates of growth must always be recognized. During childhood, growth rates also vary in the different body systems. For example, the child of six to ten years of age shows increasingly slow growth in height and increasing rapid gain in weight; this trend continues until the onset of puberty, when an accelerated gain in height and a still more accelerated gain in weight normally occur. During this period, the child is exposed to common communicable diseases, malnutrition may be seen because of faulty or inadequate diet, and postural deviations may develop. During the adolescent period profound physical, emotional, mental, and social changes occur because of endocrine functioning, resulting in sexual growth and maturity. With growth, needs differ and the pattern of health care should be adjusted to meet the needs. The health program in the primary grades cannot be the same as that in a secondary school or college. Staff should be selected according to their ability and training to serve pupils at various school levels.

It is generally acknowledged that dental defects are the most common health problems found among school-age children. It has been estimated that dental caries are found in 50 to 70 per cent of all schoolchildren examined. Health problems of lesser frequency include defective vision, defective hearing, obesity, orthopedic and posture defects, diseases of the nose and throat, and nervous, emotional, and neurologic problems.

Implicit in the school health program is the development of health awareness, specifically as it relates to the needs of pupils and staff. This awareness is promoted through health examinations done at predetermined intervals and through health inspections and classroom instruction. Examinations and inspections enable the identification of pupils who are in need of special school programs, remedial measures, and referral for care. A valuable role school physicians and nurses perform is that of consultant to the teachers or the administration about pupils who are having physical or emotional problems.

In conducting a program, it is important to coordinate the school health activities with other health activities in the community in order to avoid duplication and waste of efforts. A major responsibility of the school is discovering health problems that may interfere with the child's ability to benefit to the maximum from the educational experience; it is also a responsibility to see that these problems are corrected whenever possible. The case-finding activities of the school health worker gain in meaning when correction of defects is accomplished.

ORGANIZATION OF SCHOOL HEALTH SERVICES

Throughout the United States, there is a wide variety of school health services ranging from comprehensive to minimal; in some communities there are no school health programs at all. There is also considerable variation from state to state and among communities with respect to the agency that is responsible for school health programs. Thus, school health services may be provided by a local, county, or state health department, or they may be provided by a department or board of education. In a number of instances, the services are administered jointly by the health department and the educational agency. Occasionally, still other kinds of administrative patterns occur, such as the provision of school health services by local medical groups.

Within the school system, patterns of administration and organization of health programs vary with the jurisdiction responsible for the program. In larger school systems, the health services may be a branch of a pupil personnel division, or they may constitute a special or auxiliary services division, usually the same division as for other pupil services such as child welfare and attendance, or vocational guidance and counseling services. Most health services are headed by a medical director, with supervisors representing the major disciplines serving as chiefs of their respective sections.

In the more comprehensive school health programs, services are provided by a number of different persons representing various professional specialties. These include physicians, dentists, nurses, teachers, and, depending on the magnitude of the program, several other categories of specialists.

Physicians perform physical examinations of school pupils; almost all corrective work, however, is done in private offices, clinics, or hospitals. In large school systems that have numerous children with special problems (vision, hearing, heart, chest, neurologic, psychiatric, etc.), medical specialists are employed by the school district to render diagnostic services. These services are largely designed to assist in pupil placement in school and referral for prompt correction of remediable defects.

Dentists perform periodic dental examinations and participate in dental health education programs in the school. The school dentist may also do certain limited corrective work, although most dental corrections are done by private dentists and dental clinics.

Nurses assist the physicians in physical examinations of the children, make inspections of children referred by the teacher and arrange follow-up, and give first aid in minor injuries. The school nurse may assist the teachers in providing health instruction in the classroom and serve as a resource person. She may also visit parents in connection with health problems of their children, such as the need for correction of defects, and matters of personal hygiene, health habits, and school adjustment. She may arrange for treatment in free clinics for children whose parents are unable to pay for private care. Assisting parent-teacher groups in their health programs and helping to promote community understanding and participation in the school health program may also be important aspects of the work of the school nurse.

Teachers in many school systems provide formal health instruction as part of the regular classroom work and stimulate an interest in health among the children and their parents. In secondary schools, special health teachers conduct classes in personal hygiene, nutrition, and physical education.

Depending on the size of the health program, other specialists may participate in school health work, including audiometrists (who perform audiometric examinations at stated grades and on pupils especially referred because of suspected hearing problems), dental hygienists, clinical psychologists, psychiatric social workers, and others.

The physicians, nurses, and dentists may be employed either by the department of education or by the department of health. Special teachers in health and physical education are usually employed by the schools. When the health program is divided between the department of health and the department of education, the health department is responsible for the medical, dental, and nursing elements of the program, leaving the health instruction largely to the schools. When the entire health program is under the jurisdiction of the school system, these programs may be divided among different divisions; for example, there may be a health service in one division and a health education program in another division where the teaching staff has the major responsibility.

There are differences of opinion regarding how the goals of school health programs can best be accomplished, one consideration being which of several possible administrative patterns, or jurisdictional arrangements, is preferable. There are both advantages and disadvantages if either the department (or board) of education or the department of health has *sole* responsibility for the administration of school health services. Even when the responsibility is *shared,* questions arise as to how the various components of school health service should be allocated between the two departments.

The jurisdictional arrangement which appears to some to be preferable places primary responsibility on the health department for planning and administering school health services, while the department of education is responsible for the approval of policies.[4] One advantage of this arrangement is that the health department remains the single agency responsible for all official community health programs, thus minimizing the possibility of fragmentation and duplication of services. Moreover, under this administrative pattern, the health department can endeavor to provide uniform services among all categories of schools — public, private, parochial, and special schools. Since the provision of health services is its customary activity, the health department may find it easier to develop a high-quality program and to attract better qualified personnel.

On the other hand, if the school system is responsible for the administration of school health services, there is the advantage that the services are an integral part of the educational program. Under this jurisdictional arrangement, school health workers are able to give their full attention to the conduct of the school health program and thus can engage in certain kinds of relevant activities that otherwise might not be possible. Within the school, this includes the design of special programs to meet the health needs of pupils with particular problems such as the physically handicapped, the emotionally disturbed, the teen-age pregnant girl, and others. Moreover, the school-based health worker frequently serves on policy-making committees, works closely with parent and pupil groups, participates in the development of the health curriculum, and is readily available as a resource person for the teaching and administrative staff. By maintaining a close working relationship with private physicians, the health department, and other health agencies, the school health worker can form a bridge between the school and the various health workers in the community.

Other administrative considerations in the school health program have to do with matters of policy, such as how much school health service should be provided for children whose families can afford private care, and how much should be provided for children from low-income families. In either case, certain problems arise from the fact that while the school health program offers preventive and some diagnostic and follow-up services, the child usually must go elsewhere for treatment regardless of his financial status. The principal problems in this arrangement pertain to where the child should go for such treatment, and how the goal of treating the "whole child" can be achieved when his care is divided among agencies.

There are also certain considerations regarding the optimal method of work for school health personnel, notably the physician and the nurse. Although the physician is able to perform many of his usual functions and some special ones in the school health program, his activities are limited largely to referral and follow-up of pupils with health problems. As a consequence, his customary role of providing treatment is markedly curtailed, which raises some question regarding whether his training and experience are being utilized sufficiently. With respect to the method of work of the nurse, some prefer that she be full time in the school program, while others consider that she can best carry out her responsibilities for the health of schoolchildren by functioning as a public health nurse in the community. Under the latter arrangement, she divides her time between the school, the health department clinic, and home visiting, thus serving not only the schoolchild but also his entire family. One work pattern of the nurse that appears to be emerging involves having public health nurses in elementary schools and full-time school nurses in secondary schools.[4] However, the pattern of having nurses assigned exclusively and full time to school health programs in both elementary and secondary schools is still considered to have numerous advantages.

Official and Voluntary Health Resources for Mothers and Children

COMMUNITY SERVICES

City or county health departments, as well as hospitals and neighborhood health centers of various types, provide many of the primary services for mothers and young children such as prenatal and well-child clinics. Crippled children's programs may fall within health department supervision or be administered by some other local agency such as a welfare department or an independent crippled children's agency. The quality and quantity of all services provided at present still vary considerably from place to place throughout the nation.

Community resources are used by the health worker in follow-up activities required for the correction of remediable defects among school-age children. The private physician, clinic, and parent-teacher association, as well as community service and church groups, are utilized to augment follow-up and corrective procedures.

Many communities have organized school health councils composed of representatives from official and voluntary agencies. School health representatives also work with civic and church representatives to coordinate school health activities. In large urban communities, the Welfare Planning Council has a school health committee. Local medical associations have school health committees, pediatric societies, or other relevant groups. Cooperation with these various organizations tends to maximize the school's efforts in the conduct of health programs.

STATE PROVISIONS

State health departments provide some direct service for mothers and children in the more rural areas, but for the most part their role is to administer funds, establish and maintain standards, consult with local agencies about current and future programs, provide professional educational activities and publications, and act as a central coordinating agency throughout the state and with neighboring states.

In many states, legislation has been enacted which requires health instruction in public schools on such subjects as accident and fire prevention and the effects of narcotics, alcohol, and tobacco; some states have statutes regarding teacher inspection of children for health problems.[5] Requirements for certification of teachers may include health qualifications and health education courses in pre-service training. The state health department establishes sanitation standards for school plants and for food services.

Crippled children's programs vary from state to state with respect to administrative methods, services, and eligibility requirements. Administration can be through any designated state agency. Health, welfare, education, universities, and specially created agencies are all represented among the programs. All programs, of course, have some kind of arrangement for diagnostic services, hospitalization, and the provision of required appliances and any special therapy recommended. While eligibility requirements are somewhat different in each state, in general they include the condition and its treatment outlook, the estimated length of care and cost, the family income and family size in relation to income, and family resources and obligations. Diagnostic services are offered regardless of financial status. Only after a diagnosis is made is it possible to determine whether the condition would be sufficiently aided by treatment, how long it would take, and what the cost would be. If a child is either medically or financially ineligible, the family will be referred to a private-care source.

FEDERAL PROGRAMS

Several agencies of the U.S. Department of Health, Education, and Welfare offer programs and services for mothers and children. The Office of Child Development (a unit of the Office of the Secretary) was established in 1970 to plan and organize special services for children and youth, working with private organizations and other federal agencies in these endeavors. Within the Health Services and Mental Health Administration (Public Health Service), the Maternal and Child Health Service is responsible for administering a national program of grants for services, research, and training to improve the health and well-being of mothers and children under authorization of the Social Security Act. The Social and Rehabilitation Service, through its Community Services Administration, has responsibility for programs in child and family services (aid to families with dependent children and child welfare services), group and day care of children, child abuse control, services to unwed mothers, adoption services, foster family care, and other services. Principal agencies engaged in a vast panorama of research studies on children and youth are the National Institute of Mental Health and the National Institute of Child Health and Human Development.

The U.S. Department of Agriculture in its Food and Nutrition Service administers four programs designed to improve the nutrition of schoolchildren, particularly those from low-income families: national school lunch program, school breakfast program, equipment program to initiate or expand school food service, and special milk program for children. In the national school lunch program, grants-in-aid to the states provide financial assistance to public and private schools, of high-school grade or under, operating nonprofit school lunch programs. The funds are provided to schools on the basis of their need for assistance and the number of meals served. Participating schools also receive foods bought specifically to help them meet meal standards and are eligible for food acquired under price support and surplus removal programs of the U.S. Department of Agriculture.

VOLUNTARY AGENCY ROLES

Local, state, and national voluntary agencies play a major role in improving the health of mothers and children. A variety of direct services, research, lay and professional educational activities, legislative promotion, and fund raising to support their particular activities are among the programs of these agencies. Maternal and child health in the United States benefits greatly from the cooperative interaction of voluntary and public agencies, which share the common goal of achieving a higher level of health for all mothers and children.

Many professional and voluntary organizations and associations also are concerned with school health. The National Congress of Parents and Teachers is an important force in the promotion and support of health of the school-age child. The National Education Association and the American Medical Association have established a joint committee on school health policies and practices.[6] The American Public Health Association has a section on school health, with an annual meeting for the consideration of school health programs and problems. The activities of the American School Health Association and the American College Health Association are devoted to the consideration and promotion of school health programs in the nation.

References

1. Hellman, L. M., and Pritchard, J. A. *William's Obstetrics,* 14th ed. Appleton-Century-Crofts, New York, 1971.
2. American Public Health Association, Committee on Child Health. *Health Supervision of Young Children.* The Association, New York, 1955.
3. Siegel, Earl, and Bryson, S. A redefinition of the role of the public health nurse in child health supervision. *Am J Public Health,* **53:**1015–24, July 1963.
4. Harper, Paul A., and Stine, Oscar C. Health services for children. In: Sartwell, P. E. (ed.). *Maxcy-Rosenau Preventive Medicine and Public Health,* 9th ed. Appleton-Century-Crofts, New York, 1965.
5. Nemir, Alma. *The School Health Program.* W. B. Saunders Company, Philadelphia, 1965.
6. Wilson, Charles C. (ed.). *School Health Services,* 2nd ed. National Education Association and American Medical Association, Washington, D.C., 1964.

Additional Reading

Eliot, Martha M. The Children's Bureau — fifty years of public responsibility for action in behalf of children. *Am J Public Health,* **52:**576–91, April 1962.

McLachlan, Gordon, and Shegog, Richard (eds.). *In the Beginning — Studies of Maternity Services.* Oxford University Press, London, 1970.

Randall, Harriett B. Mental health of teachers. *J Sch Health,* **34:**411–14, November 1964.

School Nursing Committee, American School Health Association. The nurse in the school health program — guidelines for school nursing. *J Sch Health,* **37:**entire issue, February 1967.

Shapiro, Sam, Schlesinger, Edward R., and Nesbitt, Robert E. L., Jr. *Infant, Perinatal, Maternal, and Childhood Mortality in the United States.* Harvard University Press, Cambridge, Mass., 1968.

Turner, C. E., Sellery, C. M., and Smith, S. L. *School Health and Health Education,* 6th ed. The C. V. Mosby Company, St. Louis, 1970.

U.S. Department of Health, Education, and Welfare, Maternal and Child Health Service. *Maternal and Child Health Service Programs.* U.S. Government Printing Office, Washington, D.C., 1971.

U.S. Department of Health, Education, and Welfare, Maternal and Child Health Service. *Services for Crippled Children.* HEW Publication No. (HSM) 72-5001. U.S. Government Printing Office, Washington, D.C., 1972.

World Health Organization, Regional Office for Europe. *Child Health.* The Organization, Copenhagen, 1970.

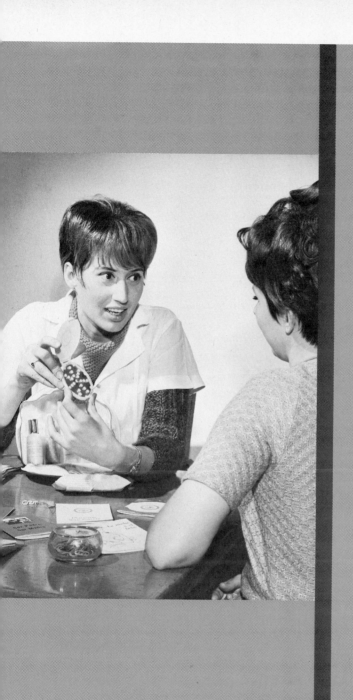

13

POPULATION
AND
FAMILY
PLANNING

CHAPTER OUTLINE

*Courtesy of Los Angeles County Health Department, Division of Public
Health Education.*

Population Dilemmas of the 1970's

There was a time in history—worldwide—when high birth rates were substantially offset by high death rates and a balance was achieved, characterized by a slowly increasing world population. Today there is a wide imbalance, in which high birth rates and declining death rates have resulted in more rapidly increasing world population. The social and economic consequences of this imbalance have become matters of worldwide concern.[1-3]

Biologists, demographers, economists, health experts, and biostatisticians have for several decades directed national and international attention to the implications and consequences of an accelerated rate of world population growth which ultimately may exceed the capacity to meet the needs for food, clothing, shelter, health care, education, and employment. There are two general options in coping with the situation: one is to concentrate on economic development; the other is to dwell on measures that seek to regain former population balances.

To some extent, the impending population crisis can be alleviated by international resource planning efforts. Such planning would involve devising the means to expand agricultural production, to utilize and share available natural and man-made resources, and to improve education. A common experience, however, of nation after nation, particularly in the developing world sector, is that population expansion in the short run outpaces the gains made in economic development and erodes the economic and social gains that might otherwise have been accomplished. Most nations of the world, therefore, have recognized that efforts in economic and resource development must also be accompanied by specific measures to limit population growth by *lowering the birth rate* if the threats inherent in "too many mouths to feed" are to be minimized.

PAST AND FUTURE GROWTH OF WORLD POPULATION

The world population doubled in about 1650 years from the beginning of the Christian era until the middle of the seventeenth century; it doubled again in about 200 years; doubled again in less than 100 years, and if the current rate of population increase were to remain constant, it would double every 35 years. Thus, it was not until 1850 that world population reached an estimated one billion persons, but it took only about 75 years for the second billion and 35 years more for the third billion, in about 1965. In 1971, world population stood at 3.7 billion, and it has been estimated that there will be more than 7 billion persons on earth in the year 2000. The changing nature of the world population scene requires close surveillance by demographers and others regarding birth rates and death rates, resulting in realistic population forecasts.

World population currently is increasing at the rate of about 2 per cent per year, and has an astonishing geometric quality. If this rate of increase had existed since early Christian times, there would be about 20 million individuals in place of each person now alive, or 100 people to each square foot of space. If the present world population should continue to increase at its present rate of 2 per cent each year, within two centuries there will be more than 150 billion people.

The increase in world population is occurring because 120 to 130 million infants are born each year, whereas only 50 to 60 million people die annually, resulting in a net gain of approximately 60 to 70 million. Such rapid population growth is clearly out of proportion to present and prospective rates of increase in socioeconomic development and the ability to advance human welfare. The long-term prognosis, according to the Committee on Science and Public Policy of the National Academy of Sciences, is that "either the birth rate of the world must come down or the death rate must go back up."[4]

POPULATION GROWTH IN VARIOUS PARTS OF THE WORLD

The rate of population growth varies among regions of the world and among nations. One notable difference occurs between the more developed and the less developed areas of the world. This is illustrated by Table 13-1, which shows that the less developed areas already have almost three quarters of the world's population and among the highest rates of population increase. Thus, it is estimated that Latin America, Africa, and Asia will double their populations in from 24 to 31 years. Latin America is one of the fastest

TABLE 13-1. Estimated Population in 1971, Annual Per Cent Increase, Number of Years for Population Doubling, Population Projections to 1985, Major World Areas

	Estimated Population, 1971		Estimated Annual Rate of Population Growth (%)	No. of Yr. for Population to Double at Indicated Rate	Population Projected to 1985 (Millions)
	Millions	*Per Cent of World Total*			
WORLD TOTAL	3,706	100.0	2.0	35	4,933
LESS DEVELOPED AREAS	2,748	74.1			
Africa	354	9.6	2.7	26	530
Asia	2,104	56.7	2.3	31	2,874
Latin America	291	7.8	2.9	24	435
MORE DEVELOPED AREAS	960	25.9			
North America	229	6.2	1.2	58	280
Europe	466	12.6	0.8	88	515
USSR	245	6.6	1.0	70	287
Oceania	20	0.5	2.0	35	27

SOURCE: Adapted from Population Reference Bureau, Inc. *1971 World Population Data Sheet*, August 1971 (with permission).

growing population regions in the world, increasing at the rate of almost 3 per cent per year, and the rate of increase is accelerating. The death rate dropped sharply following World War II, but the birth rates have remained high. Latin American countries, where excess of births over deaths is particularly high, include Honduras, Mexico, Colombia, Ecuador, Venezuela, and Paraguay. In these countries, unchecked growth will result in a doubling of the population in 21 years.

Birth rates are uniformly high in all of Africa (about 47 per 1,000 population). The highest population growth is, however, taking place in North Africa where the annual death rate is well below the rest of the continent.

Asia is, of course, the world's population colossus, with more than 2 billion persons. Population crisis spots, because of sheer size, include Pakistan and Indonesia (each in excess of 125 million) and India (almost 600 million). Among the Asian nations, India and Japan provide a marked contrast. India has more people than North and South America combined and more people than there are in Europe; the population of India will be over 1,200 million by the year 2000 if the present growth rate continues. Japan is unique among the Asian countries because it is the only nation of any size that is industrial, urban, and literate. Japan's birth and death rates are among the lowest in the world. Both rates have been declining since 1920, but the most significant change occurred during the ten years after World War II when there was a 50 per cent drop in the birth rate. The birth rate is now a little below long-term replacement of the population. Mainland China (population 773 million in 1971) has a birth rate of 33 per thousand and a death rate of 15 per thousand, with a doubling rate between that of Japan and India.

Among the more developed areas, Table 13-1 shows that the growth rate in Europe is the slowest of any region in the world, requiring 88 years to double the population. Among European countries, the lowest rate of increase is in Finland, Austria, and West and East Germany, and the highest is in the Netherlands, Switzerland, and Spain. Birth and death rates of the United States and the U.S.S.R. are low and the doubling periods are 58 and 70 years, respectively.

The United States has undergone a steady increase in population since the first census was taken in 1790. This is indicated by Table 13-2, which also shows, however, that the percentage of increase has fluctuated widely. The greatest increases occurred in the decades before the Civil War, after which there was a decline, the percentage decline reaching a low during the depression years

TABLE 13-2. Population and Increase over Preceding Census, United States, 1790–1970

	Number*	Per Cent Increase Over Preceding Census
1790	3,929,214	†
1800	5,308,483	35.1
1810	7,239,881	36.4
1820	9,638,453	33.1
1830	12,866,020	33.5
1840	17,069,453	32.7
1850	23,191,876	35.9
1860	31,443,321	35.6
1870	39,818,449	26.6
1880	50,155,783	26.0
1890	62,947,714	25.5
1900	75,944,575	20.7
1910	91,972,266	21.0
1920	105,710,620	14.9
1930	122,775,046	16.1
1940	131,669,275	7.2
1950	150,697,361	14.5
1960	178,464,236	18.4
1970	203,184,772	13.3

*Excludes Alaska and Hawaii, 1790–1960.
† Not applicable.
Source: Adapted from U.S. Bureau of the Census. *Statistical Abstract of the United States, 1971,* p. 5.

of the 1930's. The history of population growth in the United States has been affected by several factors, including immigration (which was stimulated by developments such as land expansion and the need for labor manpower) and the birth rate.

Between 1910 and 1935, United States birth rates dropped gradually from 30.1 per 1,000 population to a low of 18.7 in the middle of the depression. The birth rate began to climb during World War II, reaching a postwar high of 25.0 in 1955. Since then, there has been a steady decline, and in the first quarter of 1972 the rate dropped to 15.8 per 1,000 population, its historical low point. The present decline in the birth rate has been attributed to several factors, including economic uncertainty, rising contraceptive use, increased abortion, and current general feelings about population growth. Despite the decline, the present birth rate is still above the so-called replacement rate, and it is possible still to forecast a rise in United States population by 1985.

Influences on Population Increases

The major influences on population increase are those that contribute to increased longevity and a sustained high birth rate. A country with a birth rate of 20 per 1,000 population and a death rate of 10 or less per 1,000 population risks a doubling of its population in 40 to 50 years. Nations with birth rates of 40 to 50 and death rates of 8.5 to 15 (per 1,000 population) will have a much faster rate of population increase. Survival rates at birth, during the first year of life, and in early childhood have been spectacularly favorable in recent decades for most countries, although there are still 34 countries in which the rates exceed 100 infant deaths per 1,000 live births and 16 countries in which infant deaths exceed 150 per 1,000 live births.

As is well known, the basic significant contributions to survival and longevity came through knowledge about causes of epidemic illness and the adoption of control measures that had been perfected over time, including sanitation (water and waste), immunization, and so on. As discussed earlier, increased longevity has also resulted from the general advances in curative medicine, distribution of pharmaceuticals, and the greater availability of medical care and facilities. These advances improved the treatment of chronic and degenerative diseases as well as of acute illness. Better nutrition, rising standards of living, and improved working conditions, supported by increased educational opportunities, are a few of several other kinds of factors that have probably helped to enhance life expectancy over the past several decades. The more developed nations first began to experience the benefits of these advances almost a century ago. Although the less developed countries began to share in the benefits only fairly recently, the period of time has been sufficiently long to effect a noticeable reduction in mortality rates even in those countries.

Several significant factors affect infant survival (and thus indirectly longevity in the present epoch of relatively low adult mortality). The first is that because of low infant mortality more females survive into and through their childbearing period. Thus for a given generation of females, the possibility of having a maximum number of children is increased, and this possibility in turn is extended to their children and to their children's children, and so on.[5] In fact, at any one point in time the birth *rate* itself may be a less important factor in determining the actual number of infants born than is the number of females of childbearing age.

A second factor of extreme importance is the cultural ethos regarding childbearing. In most nations, there are a host of social forces and incentives that are promotive of childbearing and child rearing. These forces and incentives are differently expressed in different cultures. They have evolved over the centuries subtly and unconsciously to permit fertility to counteract the almost certain high mortality of past times. The result is the feeling of pride in children, the "machismo" or maleness in men, and the womanliness and "fulfillment" in women. These concepts are everywhere differently expressed and modulated by prevailing social custom and personal feelings and emotions. In Western society—although this situation is lessening as time goes by—childless adults are often penalized for deviation from childbearing norms, and sometimes undergo loneliness, ostracism, and ridicule. Thus, social customs and institutions, backed up by government policy, consciously and unconsciously promote policies that lead to population increase. Much of this will no doubt change as women in many societies and nations adapt to new opportunities for personal lifelong expression in significant occupations and careers, in addition to or instead of fulfilling maternal roles exclusively.[6]

Consequences of Population Increase

While there are many influences on population increase, as has been suggested, such growth in turn has important effects on social and economic outlook. Moderate population growth is acknowledged by most economists as a valuable stimulus for economic development. As population grows, there is an expanding market for goods produced—aside from export—as well as the opportunity for a larger labor force. As an economy develops toward self-sufficiency, education and technology go ahead together. This idealized scenario permits all components to fit into their place in "moderately" accelerating fashion.

When population grows too fast, for some of the reasons already mentioned, there is too great a drain on limited resources, depressing their availability, eroding their quality, and ensuring maldistribution and high costs. In addition, there is too great a demand on local natural resources, with further setback for technology, manpower, and finance.

There is grave concern about the possibility that the world's food-producing capacity may not be able to keep pace with the continued growth of world population. For a number of years, the world's food supply has fallen short of population growth by at least 1 to 2 per cent a year. In addition, the food supply is not distributed evenly throughout the world. The distribution of arable land also is very uneven, and the supply of readily reclaimable land is not endless and is nearing productive limits. Latin America can claim only 5 per cent of its area as arable, and India apparently has little additional land that can be brought into ready and productive cultivation. Widespread efforts to increase yields per acre on existing lands encounter obstacles because many changes in agricultural techniques would have to be achieved, including the use of fertilizer in amounts that would exceed current world production.

In the less developed countries which have a predominantly agrarian economy, the struggle to obtain the bare necessities of life is particularly severe, and a rapidly growing population only presses harder against the relatively fixed resources of food and other production. A country with a high birth rate and a declining death rate has many dependents to provide for; for example, in the less developed areas, children under 15 years of age constitute between 35 per cent and 50 per cent of the population. Such an age imbalance presents not only a severe problem of support, but also an enormous burden of education in a nation that probably already has a low educational level and a high rate of illiteracy. Furthermore, until the educational deficit is overcome, these nations have little hope of obtaining the skilled manpower needed to achieve a more advanced economy.

The vast majority of nations in Africa and Asia have a per capita gross national product of less than $300 per year (compared with more than $2,000 per annum, average, in western Europe and Canada and almost $4,000 in the United States). The average per capita income in less developed countries is estimated to be about $100 a year, and such marginal subsistence associated with high birth rates creates a trap from which neither families nor the nation can escape. When a rapidly expanding population is engaged largely in agriculture, the amount of cultivable land that can provide employment becomes insufficient, and there is not enough industry in urban areas to absorb the excess labor force. Thus in less developed areas, migration to urban centers often means only exchanging rural unemployment for urban unemployment.[7]

In more developed nations, the consequences of unchecked population growth are not related to marginal economic events in the same way as they are in developing regions. However, even in the United States there are certain economic effects of population—for example, the marked increase in the elderly population since 1900 that has placed an extraordinary pressure on the medical care system. The greatest concern is that unchecked population growth in developed countries has contributed its share to urban crowding, environmental pollution, transportation congestion, and dwindling open space and recreational areas. Thus, population has had its impact upon a deteriorating quality of life in the highly urbanized areas.

Alternative Methods of Population Control

INDIRECT OR INVOLUNTARY METHODS OF CONTROLLING POPULATION

In individual nations, inhibition of population growth is associated with certain economic factors. Thus, as population increases out of proportion to a country's gross national product, family limitation tends to occur, but only perhaps in the upper 10 to 30 per cent of the socioeconomic strata. There is also evidence in western Europe and in the United States of an inverse relationship between the labor force participation of married women and the size of their families. Historically, the birth rate has been observed to decline during an economic depression.

While the converse has prevailed on many occasions, *social policies* may be devised to limit population growth, such as the provision of incentives for later marriages and for smaller families. For example, a number of German states in the mid-nineteenth century restricted permission to marry to those couples who presumably would be able to support a family. The social and political climate in most nations today is, of course, not favorable to such methods for controlling population growth.

Methods of *involuntary fertility control* that have been proposed from time-to-time include (1) a "fertility control agent," with predictable fertility reduction capability (from 5 to 75 per cent), administerable in the water supply, etc.; (2) temporary "time capsule" sterilization which is reversible; and (3) compulsory sterilization of males with three or more living children. Not all of these methods are at present technically feasible, nor is there scientific readiness for their early development. The main obstacles would appear to be their low ethical acceptability and their lack of political and administrative viability.[8]

FAMILY PLANNING AS A METHOD OF POPULATION CONTROL

Family planning and family limitation programs constitute the most direct approach to the problem of accelerated population growth and, because they can be universally applied, are probably the only means that, in the long run, can be effective. The concept and methods of family planning are influenced by the social and cultural institutions of the various countries of the world. However, a growing appreciation of the small family and the practice of family limitation is found in both Western and Eastern countries, in industrial and agricultural societies, and among many social, economic, and religious groups.

In the ideal family-planning program, the children who are conceived and born are wanted, and the number of offspring are commensurate with family, community, and national resources, thus assuring a reasonable standard of living and the opportunity for personal development for all children. Furthermore, information on family planning is made available equally to all socioeconomic groups, and with a knowledge and understanding of the methods, the individual then has complete freedom to make a choice that is compatible with his cultural and religious background. Family planning programs operate on a systematic, organized basis and include appropriate educational and medical services.

Family planning methods and practices for the prevention of unwanted pregnancies have developed over the centuries and vary widely throughout the world. The oldest practices for family spacing are periodic or total abstinence and withdrawal, or coitus interruptus. One form of periodic abstinence is the *rhythm method* (approved by the Roman Catholic Church) which involves refraining from sexual intercourse while the woman is at highest risk of conception during ovulation. The principal problem in the rhythm method is that of reliability—establishing the true menstrual pattern and thus determining the exact period during which abstinence must be practiced (varying from 11 to 18 days). The failure rate of this method tends to be higher than with some other methods.

A variety of well-known contraceptive devices and methods are selectively in use today, but are of varying reliability. These include jellies, creams, and foams, as well as douches which are sometimes used after intercourse. The diaphragm and spermicidal jelly provide a method that has been popular and relatively effective as a mechanical form of contraception. Condoms go back to Biblical times and are still widely used by men.

In recent years, oral contraceptives and various intrauterine devices have become popular and well known. *Oral contraceptives* are synthetic progesteronelike steroid pills which prevent ovulation and permit the regular recurrence of uterine bleeding at about 28-day intervals. This method is very widely used and affords a high degree of protection once it is regulated and carefully practiced. It is satisfactory for some population groups, but the costs and use requirements are beyond the reach of much of the world population. Drawbacks include regularity of use (danger of "forgetting"), minor annoying and transient side effects in the very early periods of use, and more importantly, *possible* serious endocrine alterations and other possible serious effects (e.g., blood clots). Adaptations of the "basic" pill are in the process of development, including the "morning-after" pill, not yet fully tested.

There are many *intrauterine devices* (IUD) of various shapes, generally made of flexible plastic material. These plastic rings, coils, or other shapes are inserted through the cervical canal and return to their original form in the uterus. This method of contraception is believed to be both safe and very effective, requiring little action by the individual once the device is inserted. It has a low cost, is protective over a long period of time, requires only the decision to use it, and probably is the most effective contraception for the less educated, less motivated, and less self-controlled. Special intrauterine devices (small, flat, plastic shapes) are in wide use in family planning programs in developing nations. Several problems in their use include rejection by the body and spontaneous dislodgement after insertion as a result of bodily activity.

Sterilization is being used by an increasing percentage of selected population groups in the United States, Japan, and India. This method of birth control requires a safe, simple surgical technique in either the male or the female. The vasectomy for sterilization of the male is the surgical removal of a portion of the vas deferens, which is the excretory duct of the testicle. Female sterilization is also a safe procedure, requiring a small abdominal incision to tie and cut the fallopian tubes, which prevents the ovum, or female egg, from reaching the uterus and being united with the male sperm. Both male and female sterilization is widely used in Japan and to a lesser extent in India, and female sterilization is popular in Puerto Rico. The advantage of this method is the degree of permanency and the freedom from the need for continuous application that characterizes other methods of contraception. Owing to the permanency, use of this method is often delayed until the family has "enough" children. Thus, this procedure tends to be used by older age groups. There apparently is rarely any psychologic or related physiologic reaction following the sterilization and none in cases adequately evaluated and selected beforehand.

Induced abortion has been and is being used as a means of terminating pregnancy in many nations in the world, one estimate placing the world figure at 30 million abortions per year. Induced abortions are divided into legal and illegal. In Japan, where abortion is legal, more than one million abortions are performed annually by specially licensed technicians.

In the United States in past years, it is estimated that one million pregnancies were terminated annually by abortion, the vast majority illegally. As mentioned in Chapter 12, abortion has been one of the major causes of maternal mortality, and in almost every case, the abortion was illegally induced. The serious health problem associated with illegal abortions is that they are likely to be either self-induced or performed by a nonmedical person using techniques or agents that are extremely dangerous. Furthermore, a large but unknown number of attempted illegal abortions which fail undoubtedly damage the progress of the pregnancy and result in a deformed child. This is particularly likely when drugs or chemicals are used.

Because of these and other problems, there has been a strong pressure for broadening provisions for legal abortion in the United States. In general, state laws may be said to fall within three categories according to degree of restrictiveness. The *"more* restrictive" laws are those that allow abortion only to protect the life of the pregnant woman; about 33 states have such laws. The *"less* restrictive" category of laws permits abortion to preserve not only "life" but also "health" (i.e., for therapeutic reasons, including risk to life or "mental health" of the mother, rape, high probability of malformed infant, among other reasons). The *"least* restrictive" category has no legal restriction on reasons for which an abortion may be performed; the four states in 1971 in this group were Alaska, Hawaii, New York, and Washington. The laws in these states require that the abortion be performed by a physician, and generally in a hospital or approved facility.

Early in 1973, the most decisive step taken so far in the United States to liberalize abortion occurred when the U.S. Supreme Court ruled that women have a constitutional right to an abortion during the first six months of pregnancy, although the states can still exercise some controls in the interest of protecting the mother's health and the child's life. Thus, the ruling provided that within the *first three months* the decision about an abortion (and the conditions under which it is performed) must be left to the woman and her doctor. During the *second three months* of pregnancy certain state-imposed controls would be permissible in order to preserve and protect maternal health (e.g., requirements that the abortion be performed by a physician or in a licensed hospital). After the fetus becomes capable of surviving outside the uterus—generally between the *24th and 28th weeks* of pregnancy—even stiffer controls would be permissible and the states could outlaw abortion. However, even at this stage the states would be constrained to permit terminating pregnancy in order to preserve the mother's life or health.

There are arguments, supported somewhat by European (particularly Scandinavian) and American experience in the past, that population groups with higher standards of living and increased education will practice family planning, utilizing the methods that are available and acceptable. While improved socioeconomic conditions may have a favorable influence in reducing population increase, the goal of achieving population balance demands realistic world programs of control through voluntary individual family planning, irrespective of economic considerations. In general, for programs for voluntary control of family size to be effective, there need to be both a high degree of individual motivation *and* availability and knowledge of the utility of birth control procedures.

Research will undoubtedly in the long run lead the way to the most efficient, practical, and acceptable methods of birth control. Immunologists may someday develop a vaccine for the female against the spermatozoa or against the development of placental tissues. A vaccine for males may be discovered someday which would prevent the development of active sperm mobility or of sperm ability to fertilize the ovum. Vaccination is a procedure well accepted and would enhance fertility control. In the meantime, it will be necessary to continue to incorporate already available family planning methods into regular health and medical care practice as an essential part of comprehensive health care.

Family Planning in the United States

Until the 1960's, the American public, the various levels of government, and professional and religious groups were reluctant to recognize the potential effects of excessive population increases on future health and welfare. This had resulted in a lag in generating broad and systematic programs in family planning in the United States. The higher socioeconomic groups of the population were able to some extent to obtain advice and assistance through private medical care, but the poor, who rely on public tax-supported programs for much their medical care, were denied family planning services.[9]

In spite of general apathy and resistance, efforts were made during the past several decades to promote and provide programs in family planning. A number of local health departments for many years "bootlegged" family planning and counseling into their maternal and child health programs. The Population Council and the Planned Parenthood-World Population organization (the latter founded by Margaret Sanger 50 years ago) promoted family planning clinics, public education, and demonstrations. Policies and positions in support of family planning were developed by many state health and welfare agencies, the World Health Organization, the United Nations, the National Academy of Sciences, and several professional groups (e.g., the American Public Health Association, the American Social Welfare Association, and the American Medical Association).

More recently, attitudes have begun to change, so that a large majority of the public, in opinion polls, now expresses approval of making birth control information available to everyone who wants it. There is a growing recognition of the desirability of family planning as a means of permitting the American woman to make an independent contribution to society. Family planning allows her to be both a mother and a participant in the labor force if she wishes, to protect her own health and that of her children, and to assist in the maintenance of a more economically secure family unit.

INTERESTS OF THE UNITED STATES GOVERNMENT IN FAMILY PLANNING

There is increasing involvement of various agencies of the federal government in family planning services, stimulated by both the executive and the legislative branches. In 1966, in a special message to Congress, the President stated that, "We have a growing concern to foster the integrity of the family and the opportunity for each child. It is essential that all families have access to information and services that will allow freedom to choose the number and spacing of the children within the dictates of individual conscience." In 1968, the President appointed a Committee on Population and Family Planning, which subsequently issued a series of recommendations related to both domestic and international matters and covered areas of service, research, and training.[10] By congressional action in 1969, the Commission on Population Growth and the American Future was established, and undertook a two-year detailed assessment of the impact of population growth on the economy, government, and the quality of life. The commission stated that "no substantial benefits would result from continued growth of the nation's population," and proposed a national and deliberate population policy which could enable parents to avoid unwanted childbearing. In December 1970, the President signed into law the Family Planning Services and Population Research Act of 1970, which included authorization of funds for family planning services through project grants and funds for population research.

The federal government became actively involved in supporting family planning programs in 1964, when the Office of Economic Opportunity (OEO) made the first federal grant to a family planning program. Since then, the OEO and, to an even greater extent, the U.S. Department of Health, Education, and Welfare have rapidly expanded assistance to providers of family planning services and information. The Department's increased commitment is illustrated by the growth of fiscal appropriations: for its family planning program to bring services and information to persons without other access to such provisions, appropriations increased from $80.3 million in 1971 to $147.7 million in 1972; and funds for population research increased from $40.3 million in 1971 to $51.3 million in 1972.

The U.S. Department of Health, Education, and Welfare supports family planning through programs in several of its operating agencies; the Office of Population Affairs (within the Office of the Secretary) is responsible for coordinating all family planning activities of the Department. The National Center for Family Planning Services (within the Health Services and Mental Health Administration, Public Health Service) is the focal point in the Department for delivering family planning assistance to an estimated 5.4 million low-income women of childbearing age in this country who have not had access to such service but desire to obtain it. The center develops, funds, evaluates, and coordinates comprehensive family planning project grants under provisions of the Social Security Act. Through grants and contracts, the Center for Population Research (within the National Institute of Child Health and Human Development, National Institutes of Health) supports research and research training in several areas, including development of new contraceptives, medical effects of existing methods of fertility control, and social and behavioral aspects of population changes. The Social and Rehabilitation Service includes family planning in its public assistance reimbursement programs for social and medical services. The Food and Drug Administration is concerned with drug safety research of compounds used for contraceptives.

THE STATES AND COMMUNITIES IN
FAMILY PLANNING

Before 1960, publicly assisted family planning services were provided by only a few states. By the end of that decade nearly all states and about one half of the counties in the United States had family planning programs. Such services were available in large metropolitan areas, but less so in smaller ones, and they were almost nonexistent in rural areas.

In 1970, there were an estimated 3,000 to 3,500 discrete geographic sites where family planning services were in operation in the United States. Of these, approximately 1,000 were federally supported sites with over 400,000 patients. Out of almost 7,000 hospitals surveyed in 1970, about 9 per cent had an organized family planning service available through a hospital-based staff.

A basic function of a public health agency in family planning, whether on the state or community level, is to provide leadership within its area which will ensure that all families have ready access to information and services. Both the need and the potential for continued development of family planning services have been well documented. The women presently denied access to these services can be identified, and in general it is known how to design programs with respect to optimum location, auspices, budgeting, and staffing.[11,12] Adequate technology exists and further improvements will be forthcoming. Costs are modest compared with other social and medical programs.

The physician in private practice has an important role in promoting family planning. The advantages of planning and spacing pregnancies can be discussed with pregnant women before and after delivery. While nurses and social welfare personnel may attempt to educate and may refer women for family planning services, it is the medical profession that is expected to respond in a positive way. Physicians are in a position to stimulate the interest of patients in family planning and to advise the use of whatever contraceptive method is consistent with the cultural and economic background of the patient.

The cooperative efforts of the health science professions, official health agencies, and voluntary organizations can create the environment for effective programs of family planning services in the community. Various programs are emerging, including public education, in-service training of personnel, demonstration service centers, and systems of referral and follow-up. For example, Colorado has involved a broad range of community resources in a series of family planning clinics. Some of the clinics are staffed entirely by the public health department; others are staffed by public health nurses and by volunteer physicians; and still other clinics, which are held in various public buildings, are staffed entirely by volunteers. Some degree of case-finding and follow-up activity occurs in each of the arrangements. Many other states and communities have demonstrated that effective family planning services can be developed through the resources of local health and welfare agencies, hospitals and outpatient clinics, and the medical profession.

FUTURE NEEDS IN FAMILY PLANNING

Assessments of where the United States stands on solving the problems of population reveal some accomplishments and some remaining critical needs.[13,14] Although legislative enactments and fiscal appropriations testify to a national commitment to programs of family planning, there is as yet no firm national policy statement about *population growth* (i.e., whether—and how—growth should be limited). Family planning programs, in turn, are intended mainly to provide services to the poor, which overlooks the fact that, even if effective, this approach will solve only a relatively small portion of the total population problem.

Research is urgently needed to develop additional effective, safe, and acceptable methods of family planning. There is a pressing need for research on population dynamics, fertility, and sterility. In addition, further development of specific contraceptive techniques is required through research, such as vaccines that would be relatively long lasting, a type of sterilization that would be reversible, pills that could be taken less frequently than is now necessary, or injections that could be given once a month or less often.

There is a great need for more complete awareness and understanding of the stresses that future generations will experience if unchecked population increase is allowed to continue. It is difficult for one generation to be concerned with the health and welfare of future generations, and usually only a relatively small minority of persons express such concern at any particular time. A continuing program of public information and education on the problems of population growth that would have significant impact has yet to be developed. Educational systems need to make special efforts to foster and encourage the inclusion of family planning in existing courses and in the development of new courses. Special attention should be directed to the training programs for the professions of medicine, law, theology, teaching, nursing, social work, health education, and related groups. Such programs should include the study of the problems of population increase and unwanted children and the methods of alleviating such problems.

Family Planning in Other Countries

A vast complex of cultural, socioeconomic, and political factors influence population growth in a particular nation. Furthermore, these factors differ from one country to another and play an important role in determining the success or failure of particular population control measures. During recent decades, an increasing number of nations that were particularly hard pressed by overpopulation began to deal with these complicated issues. A number of governments have reached or are working toward a national policy on population. In 1962, when the United Nations was formulating a policy on technical aid in the field of fertility regulation, virtually all the Asian and Arab nations voted in favor of the proposal; opposition came largely from the European countries, which, as indicated earlier, already have low birth rates. Thus, the present trend among developing nations to effect control of their population growth is motivated by forces within these nations, rather than being due to the imposition by Western countries of the kind of behavior that has helped to achieve their own favorable population balance.

A number of international organizations offer support and assistance to the countries throughout the world that are trying to cope with a too rapidly growing population. During the 1965 World Health Assembly, the member nations of the World Health Organization unanimously approved a policy supporting research and technical aid in the field of human reproduction and fertility control. This made available to governments, on request, a vast range of reference and expert advisory services.[15]

Principal responsibility for United States assistance to the population and family planning programs of developing countries lies with the Agency for International Development. This agency works closely with a number of United States and international agencies, both private and governmental. The agency's obligations for population and family planning assistance have risen from $4.4 million in 1967 to $95.9 million in 1971. Direct help to population and family planning programs is going to 33 countries which have more than half the population of all the developing nations. Other agencies of the United States government that also have international responsibilities include the National Center for Family Planning Services, which is involved in developing family planning research and demonstration projects in foreign countries; and the Center for Population Research, which develops population research programs within, or of importance to, developing countries.

Private and voluntary organizations, which pioneered in drawing attention to the facts and problems of excessive population growth, conduct valuable international programs in family planning. Among these agencies are the International Planned Parenthood Federation, the Population Council, the Ford Foundation, the Pathfinder Fund, and the Rockefeller Foundation.

Population programs are of recent origin in many countries and are not yet apparent in some.[16,17] Existing family planning programs in developing countries vary widely in scope, and many still are not adequate to meet the needs. A number of the more comprehensive programs are so new that it is not yet possible to assess their effectiveness. Some programs operate under a handicap because they lack government sponsorship, even though they may have official approval. On balance, the problems of population growth for the world as a whole are by no means solved. Nevertheless, the serious efforts that are currently being made provide striking evidence of the fact that nations are no longer willing to endure the hardships and deprivations associated with uncontrolled population growth.

References

1. Hauser, P. M. (ed.). *The Population Dilemma*, 2nd ed. Prentice-Hall, Englewood Cliffs, New Jersey, 1969.
2. Muramatsu, M., and Harper, P. A. (eds.). *Population Dynamics*. The Johns Hopkins Press, Baltimore, 1965.
3. Berelson, B., Anderson, R. K., Harkavy, O., Maier, J., Mauldin, W. P., and Segal, S. J. (eds.). *Family Planning and Population Programs: A Review of World Developments*. University of Chicago Press, Chicago, 1966.
4. National Academy of Sciences-National Research Council. *The Growth of World Population*. Publication 1091. National Research Council, Washington, D.C., 1963.
5. Taylor, Carl E., and Hall, Marie-F. Health, population and economic development. *Science*, **157**:651–57, August 11, 1967.
6. Blake, Judith. Population policy for Americans: is the government being misled? *Science*, **164**:522–29, May 2, 1969.
7. Merrill, Malcolm H. An expanding populace in a contracting world. *JAMA*, **197**:114–19, August 1966.
8. Berelson, Bernard. Beyond family planning. *Science*, **163**:533–43, February 7, 1969.
9. Corsa, Leslie, Jr. Family planning programs in the United States: introduction. *Am J Public Health*, **56**:1–5, January 1966 (Supplement, Part II).
10. President's Committee on Population and Family Planning. *Population and Family Planning — The Transition from Concern to Action*. U.S. Government Printing Office, Washington, D.C., November 1968.
11. Program Area Committee on Population and Public Health, American Public Health Association. *Family Planning — A Guide for State and Local Agencies*. The Association, Washington, D.C., 1968.
12. U.S. Department of Health, Education, and Welfare, Office of the Assistant Secretary (Planning and Evaluation). *Family Planning Service Programs: An Operational Analysis*. U.S. Government Printing Office, Washington, D.C., May 1970.
13. Jaffe, Frederick S. Toward the reduction of unwanted pregnancy. *Science*, **174**:119–27, October 8, 1971.
14. Population Reference Bureau, Inc. *Population Activities of the United States Government*. The Bureau, Washington, D.C., August 1971.
15. World Health Organization. *Family Planning in Health Services*. Report of a WHO Expert Committee. WHO Technical Report Series No. 476, The Organization, Geneva, 1971.
16. Agency for International Development, Office of Population. *Population Program Assistance*. U.S. Government Printing Office, Washington, D.C., December 1971.
17. Berelson, Bernard (ed.). *Family-Planning Programs — An International Survey*. Basic Books, Inc., New York, 1969.

SECTION

IV

SELECTED
PUBLIC HEALTH
SUPPORTIVE
SERVICES

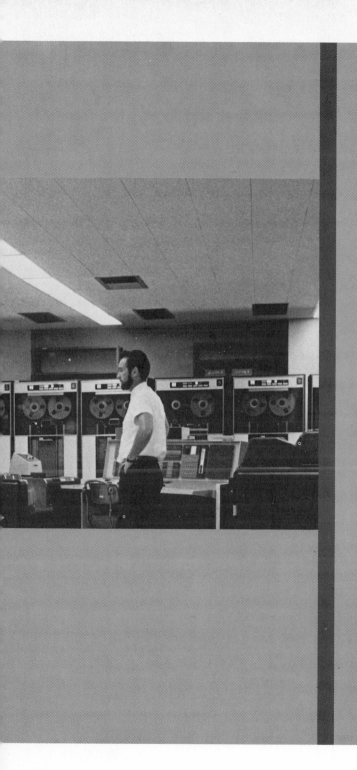

14

COMMUNITY
HEALTH
RESEARCH

CHAPTER OUTLINE

Basic Sources of Research Stimulation and Support

Settings for Community Health Research

Topics of Community Health Research

Disciplines Contributing to Community Health Research

The Payoff from Community Health Research

Community Health Research: Principles and Procedures

Definition of the Problem and Review of Existing Relevant Knowledge

Design of the Investigation

Collection of the Data

Data Processing and Analysis

Obtaining Financial Support for Community Health Research

Courtesy of Health Sciences Computing Facility, University of California, Los Angeles.

Basic Sources of Research Stimulation and Support

Most large American enterprises depend on *research and development* (R and D) to advance organizational goals. In 1971, the national outlay in the United States for R and D came to an estimated $28 billion for federal, industrial, and university activities. The search is often highly successful in reaching objectives—the U.S. space program is a good example—and results in the creation of new ideas, products, and programs that can then enter the national scene to advantage. The nation's *research* budget alone in 1971 stood at approximately $10 billion, with the federal government's share coming to about $6 billion. Major federal support for research went to engineering and the various sciences, with funding for life sciences, including health, amounting to approximately $1.5 billion and environmental sciences to more than a half-billion dollars.

As indicated in several earlier chapters, health research activities have played an important role in arriving at present-day knowledge about many diseases and conditions, including control procedures.[1] Health research continues to be looked to as a source of answers to the pressing problems of the 1970's and 1980's in connection with the environment, chronic and communicable diseases, mental health and addictions, and the organization of health services.[2-4]

Health research in the United States is carried on by universities, by independent research organizations and laboratories, by commercial organizations (sometimes large corporations with health interests), and by official and voluntary health agencies. The site of the research varies with the topic. Thus, laboratories in conducting "bench" research can be located almost anywhere, although they need in general to be near the source of their materials (biologic samples, e.g.). On the other hand, research on hospital procedures or on the relative effectiveness of two or more organizational schemes for delivering health care must be carried out at the hospital or the health service organization that is the particular subject of study.

Health research can sometimes be carried out with funds and resources available only from normal organizational operation ("use your own money"). Thus, much pharmaceutical research is conducted by ethical drug manufacturers with the corporation's own funds, the cost of the research being passed on to the consumer according to the pricing practices of the drug industry. State and local health agencies sometimes obtain funds from the legislature or other governmental body in order to undertake research on topics of high interest in a particular geographic area. Much health research is carried out *with government support* and, to a considerably smaller extent, with financial help from voluntary health associations and from foundations (see Chapter 2).

At the federal level, some health research support derives from the National Science Foundation, the Department of Defense, the Veterans Administration, and the Department of Labor (health manpower studies). The Environmental Protection Agency (EPA) is a substantial supporter of research activities, with approximately $85 million earmarked for research funding in fiscal year 1973. A wide range of studies is supported, with emphasis on (a) *processes and effects* (including health effects of many environmental factors); (b) *implementation* of environmental protection procedures (including systems analysis, economic analysis, standards research, etc.); (c) *technical research* (e.g., research in municipal technology, solid wastes, air pollution control); and (d) *environmental studies* (including research in ecosystems, technical forecasting, etc.).

The principal federal health research arm is the Department of Health, Education, and Welfare (HEW). At HEW, research activity is supported and conducted by the National Institutes of Health (NIH). As mentioned in Chapter 2, there are ten categorical institutes (including General Medical Sciences), with mandates to sponsor and carry out research activities in their respective fields. In fiscal year 1970, NIH awarded more than 10,000 individual research grants (totaling almost $500 million) and almost 900 research contracts (about $100 million) to investigators in every state in the union. As shown in Table 14-1, the National Heart and Lung Institute supported almost 1,700 grants and 130 contracts totaling $107 million; the National Cancer Institute, about 1,200 grants and 285 contracts totaling about $115 million; and the National Institute of Arthritis and Metabolic Diseases, more than 2,200 grants and 67 contracts amounting to $82 million. Size of the average grant award depends, of course, on the research job to be done, but clearly also on the nature of the field.

Research supported by the National Institutes of Health deals principally with physiologic, biochemical, pharmacologic, cytologic,

TABLE 14-1. Research Grants and Contracts Supported by Major Health Components of the U.S. Department of Health, Education, and Welfare (Fiscal 1970)

	Research Grants		Research Contracts	
	Number of Grants	Millions of Dollars	Number of Contracts	Millions of Dollars
NATIONAL INSTITUTES OF HEALTH				
National Cancer Institute	1,182	$71.4	285	$43.4
National Eye Institute	404	16.0	*	*
National Heart and Lung Institute	1,687	86.5	130	20.4
National Institute of Allergy and Infectious Diseases	1,265	49.1	132	8.3
National Institute of Arthritis and Metabolic Diseases	2,211	78.1	67	4.4
National Institute of Child Health and Human Development	884	40.1	130	7.1
National Institute of Dental Research	203	13.4	18	0.5
National Institute of Environmental Health Sciences	104	7.4	7	0.5
National Institute of General Medical Sciences	1,164	68.8	9	1.5
National Institute of Neurological Diseases and Stroke	1,422	49.1	51	7.2
National Library of Medicine	49	1.2	40	3.6
HEALTH SERVICES AND MENTAL HEALTH ADMINISTRATION				
Center for Disease Control	58	2.3		
Maternal and Child Health Service	67	5.8		
National Center for Health Services Research and Development	165	20.4		
National Institute of Mental Health	1,578	77.1		
FOOD AND DRUG ADMINISTRATION	134	4.0		

* One contract in the amount of $13,000.

SOURCE: U.S. Department of Health, Education, and Welfare, Public Health Service. *Public Health Service Grants and Awards, Fiscal Year 1970 Funds.* Part I, p. 1; and Part III, pp. 5, 417; 1971.

and clinical-medical aspects of disease. The focus is on understanding complex disease processes and in the development of treatment modes for every conceivable disease entity. This includes research involving not only traditional disciplines but new elements such as bioengineering, computer-assisted diagnosis, and new methods for testing tissue compatibility (important in all transplant procedures). Almost all institutes at NIH support epidemiologic research. Such studies involve attempts to understand the nature of disease through its geographic and demographic distributions and linkage with other biologic, physical, clinical, and social events. A number of institutes also support research that deals with behavioral aspects of disease incidence and treatment procedures.

The Health Services and Mental Health Administration (HSMHA) has a sizable research support program, not as large as at NIH since its principal thrust is the development of health service patterns and programs. In 1970, HSMHA support for research was in excess of $100 million. One relatively small research program resided in the Center for Disease Control (58 projects, $2.3 million; example, "Fetal Consequences of Rubella Immunization") and another was in the Maternal and Child Health Service (67 projects, $5.8 million; example, "Disability Among Child Amputees").

A relatively new and more sizable HSMHA research support activity is that of the National Center for Health Services Research and Development. In fiscal 1970, there were 165 projects costing $20.4 million. Research interests of this program include a broad range of topics: studies of health insurance plans, medical care utilization, social factors in recovery from disease, and systems analysis of health care institutions. A major support program of the National Center has been a network of seven regional centers for health services research located at universities and at health care institutions with suitable capability.[5]

The largest research program in HSMHA is that of the National Institute of Mental Health. In 1970, there were almost 1,600 research grants being supported at a cost of $77.1 million (plus another $35 million for intramural research). Research modalities in the various studies include biochemistry, pharmacology, psychiatry, psychology, sociology, and political science. Focus is on such diverse topics as biochemical mechanisms in drug addiction, personality inconsistency, family roles and schizophrenia, outcomes of ward therapy in hospitals, the results of psychologic treatment in prisons, and the effectiveness of mental health services.

The Food and Drug Administration maintains a health research support program which, in 1970, had 134 projects costing $4 million. These included studies on pesticides, food contamination, the role of temperature on microorganism formation, and ecologic outcomes of DDT-contaminated environment.

Settings for Community Health Research

The bulk of health research preoccupation in the past decades has been with investigations revealing basic bodily processes and with laboratory and clinical investigations concerning the etiology, course, and outcome of illness and disability. Epidemiologic studies (discussed in Chapter 9) have also maintained a strong attraction for investigators seeking clues for principles of disease causation and control. Epidemiology, as was noted earlier, often departs from clinic and laboratory and seeks scientifically sound information about disease process from field studies of defined populations.

In recent decades, interest has also turned to research activities that may be grouped under the heading of "community health research," and increasingly, health professionals are finding themselves taking part in this work. In this category the focus tends to be on factors that promote or inhibit optimal delivery of health services to populations. Several basic elements help to define the field. First, there is focus on populations or subpopulations, their health requirements (including mental health and environmental health), health-related behavior, and health attitudes. Second, there is focus on the medical and public health armamentarium (preventives, therapeutics, etc.) pertinent to the health needs and requirements of study populations. Third, there is the identification of health manpower needs and new training modalities and procedures. Fourth, there is research into the administration of programs designed to bring health care services to populations needing them, in appropriate quality and cost.[6]

Information employed in community health research derives from different sources, depending on the study in question. Some studies rely on routinely maintained records (such as are found in hospitals, clinics, health departments and social agencies, or obtained from physicians). Research use of such data requires special permission and assurances of confidentiality. In some community studies, information is obtained from questionnaires (self-administered) or from interviews. Other studies rely on physician's diagnosis, nurse's judgments, or laboratory reports, either routinely or specially obtained; some depend on social observations undertaken for purposes of the study. In some instances, important information from the decennial census about census tracts, health or hospital districts, or entire cities or counties can be utilized.

Subjects of community health studies may be patients in hospitals or nursing homes, or outpatient clients of hospitals, neighborhood health or mental health centers. They may also include members (sick or not) of group health plans or persons residing in certain health or hospital service districts or in mental health catchment areas. When an entire institution is under study ("how does a hospital really work?" and "why doesn't it work better?"), all functions and personnel may be involved, from the most highly technical to the least skilled. The study of health manpower ranges from estimation of manpower needs of whole communities or particular geographic sections, to consideration of the training, professionalization, and competence of doctors, nurses, dentists, etc.[7]

Topics of Community Health Research

The variety of research interests aimed at solutions to the health problems of the 1970's is virtually limitless. However, several key areas of community health research concern may be singled out.

In *planning community health services* a first essential is knowledge of the occurrence and distribution of disease—a contribution of descriptive epidemiology. Valuable data regarding mortality and incidence of reportable communicable diseases are routinely maintained by many local health departments, and analysis of this information by census tract is important in health planning. More recently, the National Health Survey (see Chapters 9 and 11) has supplemented these data for regions of the United States and for the country as a whole with information about chronic disease and disability. The survey regularly interviews approximately 40,000 households a year, with selected supplementary clinical examinations. These interviews permit national and regional estimates of incidence and prevalence of many conditions and disabilities not obtainable from health departments.[8]

Once the occurrence and distribution of a disease are known, such information can be supplemented by research to determine how many and what kinds of persons would be likely to utilize a proposed service, and the means of getting those who need the service actually to use it. The kinds of health services for which research-based planning is required range from the establishment of clinics to the provision of hospital beds, either for specific categories of diseases or for particular segments of the population.

The *organization, delivery, and costs of personal health services* constitute another topical area in community health research. At the broadest level is concern with understanding the most desirable options for both organization and financing of medical care. These interests lend themselves to research probing into such areas as organizational modes, costs of services, and the outcome of incentive schemes. Important research is being carried on about doctor-patient and nurse-patient relationships. Knowledge gained about patients' expectations regarding services and the roles and responsibilities of professional staffs and administrators also aids in improving the organization and delivery of service.

High interest is currently expressed in research on the individual's personal health maintenance behavior, particularly in the light of focus on prepaid health plans that count on prevention to keep subscribers healthy and to keep the health plans financially viable. Research on the utilization of health services helps to improve the development and allocation of health resources, and such data also have implications for medical education and for current developments in new forms of medical practice.

Community research in *environmental hazards,* as indicated previously, includes a host of studies in the identification, control, and eradication of air, water, and other pollutants. Studies may be made to locate pollution "hot spots" in a community or to establish criteria for safe and dangerous noise levels in workplaces, on streets, and in places where people congregate for leisure-time activities. In recent years some research emphasis has gone into the sanitation aspects of food handling, preparation, and dispensing, prompted by the expansion in automated food units as well as establishments for the quick dispensing of chicken, fish and chips, and pizza. A strong research interest is also maintained about various health factors in occupational environments and in the social and health concomitants of neighborhood and dwelling-unit quality.

Research on *health services manpower* is concerned with the supply, distribution, recruitment, and training of health workers, and includes the impact of changing patterns of health services on the requirements for health personnel. Some specific topics of investigation include the factors that affect the current distribution of health workers and the choice of field or health specialty. There is research on methods of professional training and the relationship between training programs and subsequent professional performance. Research has already begun on the acceptance and performance of personnel in the new health manpower categories (e.g., see Chapter 3 regarding the physician's assistant programs), and it is easy to forecast research into experimental training modalities for a host of health occupations.

Evaluation research has to do with the measurement of outcomes of general and specific programs and applies equally to health and mental health services. Basic questions are: How much are individual patients being helped by the specific programs being offered? Could they be helped more if certain program features were changed? The answers to these questions are not easy. Even in controlled clinical trials conducted in the laboratory it is sometimes difficult to set up satisfactory study designs and to overcome the many technical problems in measuring health status. The situation is even more complex when attempting to measure the impact of a health service on an entire community.[9,10]

Evaluation research often utilizes a series of *health indicators,* which presumably are measures that describe the health status of communities, e.g., infant death rate or life expectancy at birth. Rising or falling health indicators may help to gauge the overall effectiveness of a health program. In the mental health field, evaluation research sometimes utilizes *social indicators* (analogous to health indicators), which reveal change in the quality of social life.[11,12] Thus, for example, depending on the intensity of its communitywide preventive, educational, and consultative activities, a community mental health center could have important effects on such social indicators as school performance, crime and delinquency, alcoholism, drug use, and suicide.

Disciplines Contributing to Community Health Research

Many disciplines are involved in the conduct of community health research, and an increasing number of studies require interdisciplinary team approaches. The fields traditionally associated with research in community health include epidemiology, biostatistics, preventive medicine, public health administration, and medical care administration. However, the increasing scope and complexity of the health services have led to the recognition that the knowledge and methods of other disciplines are particularly appropriate.

Economics has obvious relevancy in research on the problems of the costs and financing of health services. Researchers from political science, law, and metropolitan and community planning have gradually become involved in the sociopolitical aspects of the organization and administration of community health services and medical care. Studies of the structure and process of governmental decision-making are also within the area of these latter disciplines, and the topics are of considerable importance in the field of community health.

The behavioral sciences—i.e., anthropology, social psychology, and particularly sociology—have become increasingly important in community health research. Within the past decade, social scientists from these disciplines have undertaken a wide variety of studies in the health field, pertaining to the social, psychologic, and cultural aspects of health problems. Medical sociology has had a particularly heavy involvement in the development of community health research methodology and has contributed to (1) the sociology of illness (social factors in disease, social factors in mental disorders); (2) the sociology of medical settings (hospitals, "asylums," patients and doctors, medical education); and (3) the sociology of medical care (utilization and organization).[13]

The Payoff from Community Health Research

Potentially, payoff is great for improvement of services from studies of the elements of health systems of nations and their regional subdivisions. However, research progress is complicated by the fact that the analysis of the delivery of community health services must sooner or later involve itself with society's larger social values in a way that, for example, classical epidemiology does only rarely. This often gives rise to resistance or apathy regarding the conduct of sociomedical research. Health delivery systems characteristically involve vested cultural, professional, and organizational interests at all levels, with these interests not always being congruent with public good.

There is also the fact of the sheer size and complexity of modern society, making difficult the development of appropriate methodologies for the study of community health phenomena. Moreover, much community health research—largely descriptive in nature —has tended to document the facts of unequal distribution of health and medical care services, namely, to tell only "bad news." Certain innovations have taken place in recent decades (e.g., the emergence of home health care services and prepaid health insurance plans), and it is becoming possible to assess their impact. Further significant contributions from community health research can be expected only when additional health service alternatives of appropriate magnitude are presented for appraisal of their impact on the public's health.

Community Health Research: Principles and Procedures

Community health research studies endeavor to adhere to the basic principles and orderly procedures that are characteristic of scientific inquiry in all fields. Even in important kinds of investigations that are not meant to confirm scientific premises (such as the National Health Survey, which gathers valuable baseline health information generally not in defense of any particular hypothesis), information is assembled through systematic observations or measurements using techniques to ensure as high a degree of accuracy and precision as possible. The data thus assembled are analyzed through a variety of appropriate statistical methods and give rise to conclusions which are tied to the observations and measurements. Throughout a rigorous investigation, special efforts are made to reduce bias that may arise from a variety of sources such as subjective or preconceived ideas or from human, mechanical, or other kinds of error. Specific methods and techniques which help to accomplish these aims have, over the years, been contributed by statistics, biomathematics, social survey methodology, and many other disciplines in the fields of the physical, biologic, and social sciences.

DEFINITION OF THE PROBLEM AND REVIEW OF EXISTING RELEVANT KNOWLEDGE

The first step in the conduct of a scientific investigation is the definition of the problem to be studied and an assessment of the knowledge that already exists on the subject. Scientific knowledge is generally built up through a series of investigations, each new endeavor utilizing what has already been learned and in turn adding to the foundation for subsequent studies. Occasionally an investigation is undertaken to replicate or retest the findings of a preceding study, and this, too, adds to the total body of knowledge. In any case, careful and thorough review of relevant, accumulated information aids in defining the problem, objectives, and methods of the investigation being undertaken. In connection with studies of conditions for which adequate therapies, preventives, or rehabilitation measures are as yet only partly known, such review of past work is sometimes a sizable intellectual task.

An important part of the initial stage of a study is the determination of the nature of the problem to be investigated, as well as its extent and significance. At this time, also, questions are formulated for which answers will be sought during the course of the investigation. These considerations provide inklings as to the nature of subsequent steps in the study and give some indication of the possible contributions to knowledge that could be expected to accrue from the effort.

DESIGN OF THE INVESTIGATION

As the body of sound knowledge on a subject grows, it becomes possible to formulate statements of relationships that might reasonably be expected to occur between particular phenomena. Such statements, or *hypotheses*, may postulate an association between phenomena, or they may even postulate a chain of causation. If the status of accumulated knowledge permits, hypotheses are formulated during the *planning stage* of an investigation, and the means for testing them thoroughly are then provided through appropriate study design. Hypotheses may also be generated *during an investigation* or as an *end product*. If existing knowledge is not sufficient to enable formulating hypotheses at the outset, the investigation should be designed to maximize the possibility of obtaining information that will lead to such formulations.

In addition to provisions for testing or developing hypotheses, there are also several other considerations in the design of an investigation; all are closely related to one another. One of the first has to do with the nature of the population that will be studied. The population may consist of individuals from a particular group (e.g., members of a health plan), a particular setting (e.g., patients in a hospital), or a particular locality (e.g., residents of a mental health catchment area). There are also countless additional ways in which a population may be defined, such as persons with or without a certain disease or with some other attribute. Once the population has been designated, the *universe* of the investigation has been established.

This leads to another consideration in design, namely, the proportion of the universe that is to be investigated. Since only rarely will it be possible to investigate the entire population, some smaller element, i.e., a *sample,* must be established according to optimally useful sampling design. A sample usually must be representative of the universe from which it is drawn in order for the results of the investigation to be applicable to the total population as it has been defined. A common sampling procedure is the *random sample* in which every individual in the defined population has an equal chance of being chosen. Other sampling procedures (all requiring technical competence for best use) include probability sampling, which often involves several steps or stages, as well as stratified sampling, systematic sampling (e.g., every *nth* case), and other methods.

Other considerations in the design of an investigation have to do with the sources and methods of data collection. As mentioned earlier, these may include clinical examinations, personal interviews, diaries, laboratory tests, clinical case records, or various kinds of official records. In some investigations, more than one source and method of data collection are used. Appropriate instruments are required, such as forms for recording the results of diagnosis, observations, or measurements; questionnaires or interview guides, etc. Other instruments, often derived from the social sciences, help to measure important attributes of the patients or other study subjects, e.g., social position, economic status, psychologic state, and social stress. Such instruments must be carefully designed and pretested—or tried out—on a population that resembles the one which will ultimately be studied. Pretest results are analyzed, preferably statistically, and modifications are made in the instruments as needed. Appropriate and detailed instructions for the use of the instruments are also required.

The frequency with which data are to be collected is a further consideration in the design of an investigation. Measurements or observations may be made at one point in time only, or they may be made repeatedly over a period of time. These elements of design are generally referred to as cross-sectional and longitudinal methods, respectively. If an investigation uses the longitudinal method, the number of times observations or measurements are to be made and the length of the time intervals between them are established as part of the design.[14]

COLLECTION OF THE DATA

The data collection phase of an investigation consists of the implementation of all aspects of the basic study design. Data collection, of course, involves whatever labor that is needed to obtain the required observations or measurements. However, it also requires special efforts to minimize as much as possible the amount of human error that otherwise can be introduced at this stage of an investigation (although, of course, it can be introduced at other stages as well). In addition, special efforts need to be made to obtain *all* of the observations or measurements that have been established as the goal of the study, i.e., a sample or a specified universe. A large proportion of missing observations or measurements at best limits the usefulness of the data, and at worst may invalidate the investigation. The goals of reducing human error and maximizing completeness of data collection pertain uniformly whether the investigation is small and has a relatively simple design, or whether it is large and complex.[15,16]

The selection and training of appropriate personnel to make the observations or measurements required by the study design are important preliminaries to the actual data collection task. Once the collection of data has begun, careful and continuous supervision of personnel is required in order to ensure that instructions are being followed and that uniform practices and procedures are being maintained. Checks on the quality and reliability of the information that is being obtained should be initiated at the outset and continued systematically. The objective of such procedures is to test for uniformity of judgments by comparing the observations and measurements that have been made independently by different individuals. Corrective action can be taken if the results of these reliability checks show anything other than inconsequential differences. Such procedures help considerably to ensure the soundness of the resulting data.

DATA PROCESSING AND ANALYSIS

Careful organization and complete analysis of the observations or measurements obtained are additional major tasks in the conduct of an investigation. The purpose of this phase of a study is to gain a thorough understanding of the information so that sound conclusions can be formulated. Analysis involves the assessment of data which have been quantified by classifying and tabulating the observations and measurements that have been made. Appropriate statistical computations and tests of the data are then performed, and the results are carefully reviewed and interpreted. The nature of this entire process should be outlined during the early planning stages of the investigation. A study is likely to encounter serious difficulty if information is collected without considerable planning at the outset as to how it will ultimately be classified, tabulated, and analyzed.

Analysis consists, in effect, of asking various relevant questions of the data. Depending, of course, on the nature of the study, such questions might include: How many persons have different diseases at a particular point in time? Is one age group more likely than another to use the health service in question? Is a particular disease more likely to be found in one geographic area than another, and if so, what factors account for its occurrence? If an investigation has set out to test hypotheses, the question asked is: Do the data confirm or reject the hypotheses? The ways in which the data are classified and the kinds of tabulations made are governed by the nature of the questions posed.[17-19]

The actual appraisal of data is made through the application of various appropriate statistical tests which are used to assess the significance or importance of differences, associations, or trends. For example, if the data indicate a relationship between two phenomena, the strength of the association can be tested statistically. If a universe has been sampled, it is important to know how much the results could be expected to vary from additional samples, if the latter were to be taken. This can be estimated statistically, and the result provides an indication of the reliability of the data, or the extent to which the results may be generalized to the entire universe. If the investigation set out to make observations or measurements of a specified universe but some were missed, the seriousness of the omissions can be determined and perhaps even compensated for statistically. Biostatistics, by applying the principles and methods of statistics to the health sciences, provides the techniques for making these and other kinds of assessments.[20-22]

Obtaining Financial Support for Community Health Research

As indicated earlier in this chapter, community health research — similar to all health research — is often carried on with the support of governmental or foundation funds. The process by

which these funds are obtained is therefore of interest to health
workers, particularly those who find themselves in research settings
after their professional or technical schooling and preparation. The
general process of research grant funding applies also to grants for
training activities or for demonstration and health service programs.

The first task is to locate a funding source (e.g., a federal agency
such as one of the institutes at NIH, an agency of HSMHA, or a
foundation) whose programmatic interests coincide with those of
the proposed project. This phase may also involve preparation of a
preliminary written statement of the project proposal, which can be
presented to and discussed with the staff of the potential granting
agency.

The second step is to develop the research idea sufficiently so
that it is plausible and creditable. This means the sponsoring organization (the hospital, clinic, or college wishing to conduct the
research project) must show that it is an appropriate place for en-
trustment with funds to do the indicated work, that the personnel
involved are properly qualified, and that they have credibility (e.g.,
know the field and have done some actual work in it). At this stage
the research design is conceptualized and thought through for general feasibility, the study population (and sampling plan, if any) is
defined, and detailed consideration is given to study goals, measurement, and analysis plans. A good job of thinking at this stage
has value, since a well-organized presentation of detailed project
plans communicates general capability and personal commitment to
the research.

The third step is the preparation of an application to be sent to
the potential granting agency by a specified deadline. Preparation
of an acceptable research, training, or demonstration application is
a demanding, time-consuming task. The organizing and writing of
the application are made easier by a thorough job of preparation in
the preceding step. It is not advisable to slight important details in
preparing an application, since missing elements in a grant application are easy to detect. The application should tell the entire story,
since it alone represents the project director to the granting agency
when the request is evaluated. It should tell briefly, but sufficiently,
the background and aims of the project, its scientific or social value,
and the preparations already made. After receiving an application, a
"site visit" is sometimes initiated by the granting agency, indicating not only that there is interest but also that there are some
questions that require answering. The visit is by representatives of
the granting agency to the applicant, and care is normally given to
preparation for it.

The fourth step takes place at the granting agency. The application is reviewed for merit and substance by agency staff and in addition, at federal granting agencies and in some foundations, by review committees and other groups who make final judgments about grant awards. The members of these review groups are selected for their competence and knowledge in fields related to the content of the project being considered. A project may be approved, and if there are no funding difficulties, the award is normally made. On the other hand, an application may be found deficient and therefore disapproved, or it may be deferred pending more information or availability of funds.

In past years, particularly 1960–1968, granting agencies were less exacting in their appraisals of applications than is true today. There has always been concern about clarity in analyzing the problem, about precision in stating the project goals and objectives, and about the level of capability of the applicant organization and project staff. Today, these matters are looked at more closely than ever before. All granting agencies have responsibility for scientifically or socially useful outcomes of the projects they sponsor, and they pass this responsibility along to the investigators whose work they support.

References

1. Fox, John P., Hall, Carrie E., and Elveback, Lila R. *Epidemiology — Man and Disease*. The Macmillan Company, New York, 1970.
2. Kessler, Irving I., and Levin, Morton L. (eds.). *The Community as an Epidemiologic Laboratory — A Casebook of Community Studies*. The Johns Hopkins Press, Baltimore, 1970.
3. Weibel, S. R., Dixon, F. R., Weidner, R. B., and McCabe, L. J. Waterborne-disease outbreaks. *J Amer Water Works Ass*, **56**:947–58, August 1964.
4. Pasamanick, B., Scarpitti, F. R., and Dinitz, S. *Schizophrenics in the Community*. Appleton-Century-Crofts, New York, 1967.
5. U.S. Department of Health, Education, and Welfare, Public Health Service, Health Services and Mental Health Administration. Conference series: Collen, Morris F. (ed.). *Proceedings of a Conference on Medical Information Systems*; Greenlick, Merwyn R. (ed.). *Proceedings of a Conference on Conceptual Issues in the Analysis of Medical Care Utilization Behavior*; and Hopkins, Carl E. (ed.). *Methodology of Identifying, Measuring and Evaluating Outcomes of Health Service Programs, Systems and Subsystems*. U.S. Government Printing Office, Washington, D.C., 1970.
6. Schulberg, Herbert C., Sheldon, Alan, and Baha, Frank (eds.). *Program Evaluation in the Health Field*. Behavioral Publications, New York, 1969.
7. Hess, I., Riedel, D. C., and Fitzpatrick, T. B. *Probability Sampling of Hospitals and Patients*. Bureau of Hospital Administration, Research Series No. 1. The University of Michigan, Ann Arbor, 1961.

8. U.S. Department of Health, Education, and Welfare, Public Health Service, National Center for Health Statistics. *Origin, Program, and Operation of the U.S. National Health Survey.* Vital and Health Statistics, Public Health Service Publication 1000, Series 1, No. 1. U.S. Government Printing Office, Washington, D.C., August 1963.

9. Suchman, Edward A. *Evaluative Research.* Russell Sage Foundation, New York, 1967.

10. Weiss, Carol H. *Evaluation Research.* Prentice-Hall, Inc., Englewood Cliffs, New Jersey, 1972.

11. Sheldon, Eleanor B., and Moore, Wilbert E. *Indicators of Social Change: Concepts and Measurements.* Russell Sage Foundation, New York, 1968.

12. Land, Kenneth C. On the definition of social indicators. *Am Sociol,* **6:**322–25, 1971.

13. Freeman, Howard E., Levine, Sol, and Reeder, Leo G. (eds.). *Handbook of Medical Sociology,* 2nd ed. Prentice-Hall, Inc., Englewood Cliffs, New Jersey, 1972.

14. Campbell, D. T., and Stanley, J. C. *Experimental and Quasi-Experimental Designs for Research.* Rand McNally & Company, Chicago, 1966.

15. Miller, Delbert C. *Handbook of Research Design and Social Measurement,* 2nd ed. David McKay Company, Inc., New York, 1970.

16. Webb, Eugene J., Campbell, Donald T., Schwartz, Richard D., and Sechrest, Lee. *Unobtrusive Measures, Nonreactive Research in the Social Sciences.* Rand McNally & Company, Chicago, 1966.

17. Densen, Paul M. Statistical reasoning. In: Sartwell, P. E. (ed.). *Maxcy-Rosenau Preventive Medicine and Public Health,* 9th ed. Appleton-Century-Crofts, New York, 1965.

18. Davis, James A. *Elementary Survey Analysis.* Prentice-Hall, Inc., Englewood Cliffs, New Jersey, 1971.

19. Tufte, E. R. (ed.). *The Quantitative Analysis of Social Problems.* Addison-Wesley Publishing Company, Reading, Massachusetts, 1970.

20. Dixon, W. J., and Massey, F. J. *Introduction to Statistical Analysis,* 3rd ed. McGraw-Hill Book Company, New York, 1969.

21. Dunn, O. J. *Basic Statistics: A Primer for the Biomedical Sciences.* John Wiley & Sons, Inc., New York, 1967.

22. Afifi, A. A., and Azen, S. P. *Statistical Analysis, A Computer Oriented Approach.* Academic Press, New York, 1972.

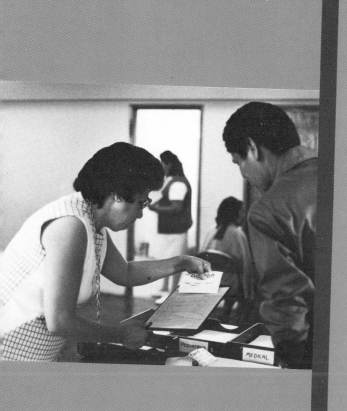

15

HEALTH
EDUCATION
IN THE
COMMUNITY

CHAPTER OUTLINE

Purpose and Growth of Health Education

Personal Health Maintenance

Health Education Manpower

The Underpinnings of Health Education

Behavioral Aspects of Health and Disease
Development and Change of Behavior

The Health Education Process

Health Information in Health Education
Analysis of Health Education Problems
Application of Health Education Methods
Evaluation in Health Education

Courtesy of California's Health, *California Department of Public Health.*
Staff photo.

436

Purpose and Growth of Health Education

Health education is the process through which individuals, social groups, and communities attend to and assimilate information about health and disease, and mobilize appropriate behavior for health-promotive ends. Important components in this process are the information itself (its reliability and unambiguity and the means for its dissemination), the health consumer (what he or she thinks, feels, and does), and the social supports and constraints that either make easy or inhibit health-promotive behavior.[1-3]

Health education activities in the United States have a history going back to the nineteenth-century founding of a number of voluntary health agencies. These organizations perceived that important aspects of their mission, still present today, were to educate the public about categoric diseases and related matters. State and local health departments quickly took up this theme, and currently health education activities are elements of health department programs everywhere in the United States.[4]

Initially health education had a narrower definition than exists today, namely, bringing health *information* to clinic patients, personnel in other agencies, and the general public. This "broadcasting" role continues to be assumed by the big voluntary health agencies ("heart and lung," "cancer," "arthritis," etc.).

A new focus, not by any means yet fully realized for many practical reasons, is to view health education as a form of *planned intervention*. In this sense there is an effort to influence largely unplanned, natural processes in such a way as to bring about improved health status. Health education thus came to abandon primary preoccupation with pamphlets and lectures and rather to rely increasingly on the theory and methodology of the behavioral sciences.

Personal Health Maintenance

Personal health maintenance is behavior on the part of the individual which is promotive of his or her own health. Personal responsibility for health has received special attention in the 1970's in the context of plans for national health insurance and health maintenance organizations. As has been mentioned previously, such plans depend for survival on promotion of preventive measures by the organization and the adoption of good health habits by the health consumer.

In 1971, the President's Committee on Health Education was created, giving White House acknowledgment to the importance of personal responsibility for health. The committee has indicated concern with (1) specific preventive action (e.g., immunization), (2) habit and attitude change (e.g., cigarette smoking, regular exercise), (3) support for community mobilization and action (e.g., pollution, noise prevention), (4) education about when to consult the doctor (especially in connection with early detection and case identification), and (5) consumer participation in development of health facilities and services in a community. Additional evidence of support for this approach was the formation of a National Health Education Foundation — private, nonprofit, and receiving no federal funds — to further the aims of preventive actions by consumers on their own behalf.

Health Education Manpower

While all health professionals in several senses stimulate health education, this activity is the particular responsibility of health educators. These numbered about 23,000 in 1970. About 3,000 *public or community health educators* are employed by state and local health departments, the Public Health Service, and various community health and health planning agencies, hospitals, clinics, industries, and others. Educational requirements are at least a B.A. or B.S. from an accredited community health education program. More advanced instruction (for the M.S. or M.P.H. degree) is offered in schools of public health (12 schools with health education programs) as well as in approximately 75 colleges and universities offering master's degrees in the health education field.

There are approximately 20,000 *school health educators* who are concerned mainly with classroom teaching and other school influences on health information and behavior. These professionals must have teaching certificates as well as background in biologic and social sciences and health education. A master's degree is now becoming a requirement in the field. There are more than 100 colleges and universities offering school and college health education instruction, with approximately 30 offering doctoral degrees.

A valuable allied professional role is played by the developing category of *health education aides.* Like other "new careers" (see Chapter 3), the health education aide or assistant can help to overcome indigenous apathy and prejudice against health agencies through demonstration and personal participation.[5,6]

The Underpinnings of Health Education

Education in the usual general sense is often regarded as good for its own sake and as an end in itself. *Health* education, however, must contribute to an outcome in which there is behavior change associated with a demonstrably improved health status of the individual, group, and community. Thus, when selecting particular health education methods in preference to others, a main consideration is the extent to which these seem likely to accomplish such an outcome. The one restriction is that the process, means, or methods should not violate the values of the community in which they are to be used. There is a relatively automatic safeguard in this connection, however, because methods that are incompatible with the values of the society are likely to fail, especially over the long run.

BEHAVIORAL ASPECTS OF HEALTH AND DISEASE

As suggested in earlier chapters, there are probably few if any diseases whose cause is known or suspected in which human behavior does not play a role, frequently a critical one. Thus, the physical proximity that people establish with one another; the dwellings they build; the way they dispose of their wastes; their use of animals for food, labor, or companionship; and their personal habits of hygiene all represent ways in which human behavior facilitates or obstructs the transmission of *communicable diseases.* The food people prefer and eat; what they drink; whether and to what extent they smoke; their daily cycles of rest, relaxation, exercise, and work; the way they relate with one another; and the way they rear their children are some of the many forms of behavior that have been implicated in the known or suspected causation of the *chronic diseases.* Moreover, as society and human behavior change, there is a constant creation of new problems or flare-up of old ones, ranging from radioactivity, air pollution, and automobile accidents to changed emotional stresses, alcoholism, and drug addiction.

It would be somewhat misleading, therefore, to surmise that there is a special phenomenon of "*health* behavior," which suggests that some forms of behavior are peculiarly associated with disease-causative or health-promotive processes, while other forms of behavior are not. Rather, it would seem more reasonable to regard *all* behavior as being *health-related* in one way or another. Health-related behavior would also include some forms of behavior that could be described as *health-directed,* that is, instances where the individual or group acts with a clear awareness of the implications for health. Examples of such health-directed behavior are the ways people behave to relieve illness or to prevent it, the kind of help they seek, the use they make of available health and medical services, and the health programs community groups might plan and implement. Individual or group decisions to give up smoking or to reduce weight for health reasons are clearly health-directed.

It should be kept in mind, however, that while human behavior plays an important role in health and disease in the individual, much or even most of this behavior is not performed principally because of the individual's concern for his health. If it were possible directly to observe the total daily patterns of behavior and associated feelings and motivations, it would probably be found that specifically health-motivated and deliberately health-directed behavior has a relatively minor role. Getting on with others in order to have the emotional comfort of belonging, eating to satisfy hunger and for enjoyment, earning a living to be able to afford the necessities and possibly some of the luxuries of life, influencing children so that they will behave in culturally acceptable ways, and playing and physical activity for the fun of it would all perhaps more accurately reflect the real world of daily behavior.

In any event, in view of the intimate relationship between health and behavior, it seems clear that effective preventive, health-promotive, diagnostic, curative, and rehabilitative action leading to the control of disease is not possible without influencing human behavior in some way.[7,8] This is true not only of the individual and the family in private life, but also of those leaders and power figures and organized groups who by their decisions and actions influence the state of health of their communities. From the remote East Indian village with its head and village elders to the mayor and councilmen of a large American city, there are groups of power figures whose function is to influence, to control in varying degrees, and to exercise vigilance over the lives of others in manifold ways. To a differing extent in various communities, groups emerge to wrestle with problems not soluble by the action of individuals alone. Thus, the control of disease and the promotion of health depend on the degree to which it is possible to influence not only the personal, private behavior of the individual and family, but also the public decisions and actions of organized groups and community leaders.

DEVELOPMENT AND CHANGE OF BEHAVIOR

No matter into which community an individual is born and in which he lives his life, maturation and learning during growth take place in a human relationship setting, surrounded by others who interact with him. In the first years, his parents or parent-substitutes take an active responsibility in rearing him in the ways of his community; and in differing degrees and at different stages, other members of his family and network of kin participate in the process. While each family will have certain unique characteristics, at the same time it is in this immediate social life-space that the individual experiences and learns the customs of perception and thought, of feeling, and of outward behavior which are characteristic of his community as a whole. These customs will be based on universal human needs, but their form and expression are subject to great cultural variability, each community having a certain uniqueness in this respect.

In addition to being a member of his community as a whole, the individual is usually a member of a class within it. This class will have its own particular variations of customs which are characteristic of the total culture, and this membership of a class will also leave its mark on the individual. Children reared as members of a higher status or income class will, for example, have a different experience of growing up from those in a lower status or income class. Such socioeconomic class differences may be more marked in some communities than in others, and upward mobility from one class to another may be more restricted.

During socialization, the complex belief, feeling, and behavior of the individual's community and social class become deeply embedded in his personality and in his view of the world. While socialization may be faster and exert more fundamental influence in the earlier years, the process of learning to live as part of one's group probably proceeds to some degree throughout life. However, regardless of the changes that the individual may exhibit from time to time, there remains a remarkable stability in the habits with which his earlier life experience endows him. This stability in individual behavior patterns is simply a reflection of a similar stability of the customs of his community as a whole.

In any community there are individuals who exercise somewhat more influence than others both in maintaining the stability of customs and in inducing change. Of these, there are the more obvious, visible formal leaders who find their place in various organized community groups. Such leaders are usually clustered in the higher status classes in the community. By and large they recognize their own roles in this respect and are usually defined by others as exercising such roles. Studies have drawn attention to the fact that, in addition, there are to a great extent less visible, less formal leaders as well.[9] Such opinion leaders, as they have been called, exercise a more informal, interpersonal influence within the families, small primary groups, and communication networks of which they are themselves members. The opinion leaders and their networks exist in all classes of a community and therefore have an important part to play in the acceptance or rejection of change through the whole range of social levels.

The Health Education Process

HEALTH INFORMATION IN HEALTH EDUCATION

Studies and experience suggest that change in health-related behavior is only under special circumstances triggered by new knowledge alone. To dispense with knowledge altogether as a determinant of change would be absurd; clearly not only does knowledge contribute to the direction change may take, but perceptual and intellectual functions cannot be abruptly separated from the emotional and motivational.

It would appear, however, that human motivation, or what people feel they want, is one of the most important determinants of behavior change. To the extent that *new knowledge* provides a relatively simple, understandable, direct solution to a *felt need*, it is likely to be successful. Thus, polio may be felt as a threat which people want reduced and for which there is a highly effective and simple solution in the form of immunization. As a consequence, countries as widely differing as the United States and the Soviet Union can report outstanding success in having their respective populations seek immunization. On the other hand, cancer is at least equally threatening but, unlike polio, there is no single, simple, effective protective measure. In this case, the dissemination of knowledge about cancer may well produce defensive and rejecting reactions among the very segments of the population who need diagnosis and care the most. There are probably a great number of smokers today who know what is being said about the relationship between smoking and lung cancer, but this seems to have made little or no impact on the cigarette smoking habit, except perhaps among special groups such as physicians and other health workers. They, incidentally, may be reacting as much to the pressures of their special image and role in the community as to the specific knowledge to which they have access.

ANALYSIS OF HEALTH EDUCATION PROBLEMS

The effectiveness of any method used in the solution of a health education problem is dependent on an analysis of the nature of the behavioral aspects of the problem in the life of members of the target group and on the nature of the change to be brought about. This analysis prior to action would include at least three components.

The first component consists of identification of the target group whose health-related behavior is the objective of the change attempt. This might be the community as a whole or any category within it such as a specific socioeconomic class, a particular group such as industrial workers of a certain kind, an age or sex group such as the elderly or adolescent boys or girls, and so on.

The second component of the analysis consists of an examination and assessment of the communication and influence networks of which the target group members are a part. This would include the more formal leaders as well as the opinion leaders who exert a special influence within these networks. Thus, obviously when dealing with young children as the target group, parents and teachers who influence their lives are important and even indispensable in developing an effective program. On the other hand, with adolescent boys the role of adults in many societies may be relatively less significant, and the leadership within the ranks of the adolescent boys themselves would have to be identified.

The third component of the analysis concerns the nature of the behavior to be changed from the special point of view of its potentiality for change. Thus, the question has be asked what the target group and relevant others know, believe, and feel about the problem, and what they may be doing about it.[10] In this connection, the underlying consideration is whether a change in knowledge through the dissemination of information is likely to be effective, or whether there are deeper emotional and motivational obstacles and resistances to be overcome. Moreover, the practical feasibility of change also has to be considered. The proposed program, for example, may be demanding a radical change in the pattern of people's lives or the use of resources and facilities that simply are not available.

APPLICATION OF HEALTH EDUCATION METHODS

In the health education process, there is a close relationship between the attempts to change behavior in the private life of the individual and the attempts, commonly known as *community organization*, to develop organized groups of community members that will undertake public action for the health of the community as a whole or of particular groups within it. Thus, community organization involves the development of formal planning and implementation of health programs as a cooperative venture between agency and community, the health education of the individual in his private life, and the provision of conditions and services that make possible and facilitate behavior change in the individual. It may, for example, be not only the means whereby a building is provided in a suitable location for use as a clinic, but also the means for educating the target group to use it.

There are numerous specific techniques which traditionally have been used in health education. These include the individual interview, group discussion, formal presentation to an audience, and the use of nonpersonal methods such as radio and television, films, posters, and pamphlets. However, the use of any of these techniques should always be based on an insight into the basic theory of how they work, and the kinds of target groups and tasks for which they may be most appropriate. There is little or no value to be derived from their routine or mechanical use.

Nonpersonal and mass methods of communication may be quite appropriate where there is already a fairly strong felt need and where there is a relatively direct, effective line of action to accomplish the desired end. When these methods are considered appropriate in respect to any specific health problem, whatever media are to be used should be systematically pretested on a small sample of the target population. This makes possible some modification of the media if they appear unlikely to achieve their purpose. Sometimes pretesting may result in their rejection altogether.

Interpersonal methods may be more appropriate wherever there is any kind of emotional resistance, where the message may be threatening, where there is no easy solution to a felt problem, or where there is no felt need. The relative power of interpersonal methods is perhaps best seen in small group techniques where, in group discussion and decision, use is made of group cohesiveness, of emotional support of the members for one another, and of relatively free self-expression to bring about change.[11] The special value of interpersonal methods is that the individual or group target of the influence attempt is able to express reactions and feelings, thus enabling the educator and others to perform mutually interacting diagnostic and educative functions concurrently.

In any single health program, however, not one but a number of health education methods tends to be used. There is often, then, an intricate planning problem in the selection of methods in terms of their specific purposes, target groups, appropriate settings, various combinations, and possible sequence.

Whatever the specific methods being used, there is a basic consideration affecting them all. This is the degree to which they can contribute to the reduction of the sociocultural distance between the health professional and the community he is serving. In the first place, the health professional has health as his overriding concern and the conscious, central objective of his daily work. However, few if any of the communities, groups, or individuals with whom the health professional deals have health as the central, deliberate concern of their daily lives. This fact assumes added significance when it is combined with the general cultural and class distance that so frequently exists between professionals and the people they serve. Similarly, a physician in private practice serving, say, mainly blue-collar workers and their families would have a real gap with which to contend owing to his higher socioeconomic status.

The health professional, therefore, has to learn to see the world through the eyes of the community. He needs to have an understanding of the community, its beliefs, felt needs, and aspirations, and of the place of the "problem" (which, incidentally, the community may not itself see as a problem) in the daily life of that community.[12]

Since this understanding is to be developed not for its own sake but in order to achieve some kind of prospective change, community organization is one important means for reducing the professional-lay distance beginning with the earliest stages of program development. Community organization involves working intimately with lay members of the community in defining and analyzing problems, in planning ways to deal with the problems, and in implementing the plans. Thus, it is important that those who do participate are at least partly drawn from the particular groups who are themselves most involved in the change. If membership of such organized groups consists predominantly or entirely of people drawn from classes or subcultures different from the target group, while they may provide power over certain resources, they may do little to reduce sociocultural distance and may even increase it. Thus, upper middle-class, Anglo-American "leadership" and community groups may have little influence among lower socioeconomic Mexican-Americans or Blacks.

The various methods of bringing about change in health-related behavior require continuing study and research, both basic and applied, particularly by behavioral scientists. The methods also need experimental innovation and testing by practitioners in the field. The evaluation of the effectiveness of ongoing programs is one important source of knowledge about health education methods.

EVALUATION IN HEALTH EDUCATION

A perennial problem, and one that is gaining increasingly serious attention today, is the evaluation of the health education component of health programs (see Chapter 14). Evaluation consists of all those procedures that provide an appraisal of the degree to which, and in what respects, the program or its health education component is achieving its stated objectives.[13,14] In this connection, it is important to have some knowledge of the change taking place independently of the program so that changes resulting predominantly from other factors are not attributed to the program itself.

Evaluation is often desirably done not only in respect to the health education component as a whole, but also in respect to its constituent parts, such as some of the specific methods being used. Thus, some methods may be included primarily to raise the level of public knowledge about a problem, others primarily to develop more favorable attitudes toward the particular agency concerned with the problem, and others to trigger action in those most personally affected by the problem. Measurement of the effectiveness of these methods in attaining their objectives is part of evaluation.

Since the objectives of health education are concerned with demonstrably health-related outcomes, the primary focus of health education evaluation should be on overt behavior change. However, evaluation may be, and perhaps too frequently is, concerned with the measurement of knowledge and of attitude change, both of which may be necessary precursors to changing overt behavior but often are not. Thus, knowledge about and attitudes toward cigarette smoking are, in themselves, from the viewpoint of health and of health education less important than the act of smoking. Health education in this case would be concerned primarily with an actual reduction, say, of the smoking adoption rate by school-age children. This change in the smoking adoption rate may conceivably be brought about by means other than changing knowledge about and attitudes toward smoking—if, indeed, the latter can bring it about at all. It is conceivable that change in the smoking adoption rate of schoolchildren might be accomplished by increasing their supervised recreation and outdoor activity time. No doubt this would and could be accompanied by changes in knowledge and attitudes about smoking, but such changes may well be incidental to the development of sports skills or the sheer exhilaration and enjoyment felt in taking part in the activities themselves.

References

1. Levin, Lowell S. Building toward the future: implications for health education. *Am J Public Health,* **59:**1983–91, November 1969.
2. System Development Corporation. *Report of a Survey of Consumers of Health Care.* Mountain States Regional Medical Program, Western Interstate Commission for Higher Education, Boulder, Colorado, May 1969.
3. Read, Donald A. (ed.). *New Directions in Health Education.* The Macmillan Company, New York, 1971.
4. Wilbur, Muriel Bliss. *Educational Tools for Health Personnel.* The Macmillan Company, New York, 1968.
5. Knittel, Robert E., Child, Robert C., and Hobgood, John. Role and training of health education aides. *Am J Public Health,* **61:**1571–80, August 1971.
6. Gales, Harriet. The community health education project: "bridging the gap." *Am J Public Health,* **60:**322–27, February 1970.
7. King, Stanley H. *Perceptions of Illness and Medical Practice.* Russell Sage Foundation, New York, 1962.
8. Knutson, Andie L. *The Individual, Society and Health Behavior.* Russell Sage Foundation, New York, 1965.
9. Katz, Elihu, and Lazarsfeld, Paul F. *Personal Influence: The Part Played by People in the Flow of Mass Communication.* The Free Press, Glencoe, Illinois, 1955.
10. Veenker, C. Harold (ed.). *Synthesis of Research in Selected Areas of Health Instruction.* School Health Education Research Monograph, Samuel Bronfman Foundation, New York, 1963.
11. SOPHE Research Committee. *Review of Research Related to Health Education.* Health Education Monographs, Supplement No. 1, New York, 1963.
12. Paul, Benjamin D. *Health, Culture and Community: Case Studies of Public Reactions to Health Programs.* Russell Sage Foundation, New York, 1955.
13. Studies and Research in Health Education. *International Conference on Health and Health Education, Philadelphia, Pennsylvania, USA, June 30–July 7, 1962.* Published by International Journal of Health Education, Geneva.
14. Klein, Susan F. Toward a framework for evaluating health education activities of a family planning program. *Am J Public Health,* **61:**1096–1109, June 1971.

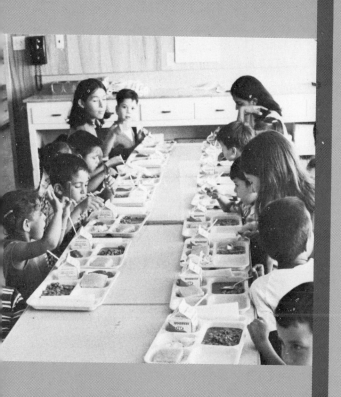

16

LABORATORY, PHARMACY, AND NUTRITIONAL SERVICES

CHAPTER OUTLINE

Courtesy of California Department of Public Health, Migrant Health Services.

Laboratory Services

Clinical (medical) laboratories have long had central roles in health services, functioning in the diagnosis and treatment of illness as well as in the prevention and control of disease. There are estimated to be between 13,000 and 14,000 clinical laboratories in the United States, *not including* the laboratories of many physicians who analyze specimens and perform other tests in their own offices.

HOSPITAL LABORATORIES

The largest group of laboratories (outside of doctors' offices) is in the hospital setting, where clinical tests are analyzed for medical management of inpatients and outpatients. Typical tests include blood chemical determinations, white blood cell count, blood grouping, hemoglobin, urinalysis, and others, all of them important in diagnosis and measuring patient progress, particularly in connection with chronic illness. Comprehensive hospital laboratory services include microbiologic testing (for diagnosis and management of infections); immunohematology (e.g., for testing transfusion and related incompatibilities); clinical physiology (medical physics — e.g., electrocardiograms, electroencephalograms); morphologic hematology (e.g., bleeding time and coagulation time determinations); immunoserology (e.g., standard blood tests for syphilis); and anatomic pathology (e.g., for examination of tissue removed in surgery).[1] Laboratory services in a functioning hospital are in great demand, require a cadre of well-trained technical staff, and represent a substantial source of income for many hospitals which sometimes charge well in excess of cost (thus subsidizing other hospital services).

PUBLIC HEALTH LABORATORIES

Public health laboratories play a substantially different role from those in hospitals, concentrating to a large extent on a microbiologic function for the diagnosis of communicable disease and for the carrying out of chemical and bacteriological tests of water, food, milk, air, drugs, etc.[2,3] Some of the larger public health (state and local) laboratories also prepare vaccines and other biologics. Newer public health laboratory services include histocompatibility tests, cytologic tests (for genetic counseling), and in some instances, the laboratory elements in multiphasic screening. Some public health laboratories are also now routinely involved in testing the quality of consumer products (e.g., testing ground meat products for adulteration).

INDEPENDENT LABORATORIES

There are a large number of independent laboratories not located in either hospitals or doctors' offices. Almost all are proprietary and many of these are owned by physicians. In 1970, a total of 2,750 were certified to provide diagnostic laboratory services for physicians in connection with Medicare patients. Not all laboratories are certified by Medicare for all testing procedures; for example, only 30 per cent were approved for tissue pathology and only half for serology. Standards have been developed for laboratories participating in Medicare, which have to do largely with preparation and background of laboratory staff.

NEW TRENDS IN THE LABORATORY FIELD

There are continually new developments in the laboratory field relating to scientific discoveries that link a laboratory test with the presence of pathologic conditions. In addition, there has been the development of automated laboratory equipment that, for example, can accomplish a number of blood chemistry determinations from a single sample and in a short time (e.g., 12-channel analyzers). Together with electronic data processing equipment, there can result easy-to-read printouts of the actual determinations, shown alongside the normal range of values from similar patients (a valuable aid in appraising a laboratory finding). A recent sequel to these advances is the "on-line" linkage of clinical laboratory equipment with a computer in such a way as to produce a record of the laboratory results while the patient is still on the premises. All of this lends itself to multiple screening of defined populations in large numbers (see Chapter 11). Such laboratory-reporting schemes are already in use in certain health-plan hospital settings and in certain health-testing, medical-care programs for low-income clients.[4-6]

LABORATORY PERSONNEL

There are an estimated 140,000 biologists, microbiologists, clinical chemists, technologists, and technicians employed in the nation's clinical laboratory services (see Table 3-2, page 74). The 2,750 Medicare-approved, independent laboratories alone (based on relatively precise information) employ 1,700 physicians and almost 12,000 technical staff.

A principal concern on the laboratory scene is the potential obsolescence of skills brought on by the rapidly changing scientific and engineering developments. A further concern is the near-extinction in recent years of provisions in universities for the preparation of professional medical microbiologists. Many graduate school microbiology programs have gone into molecular biology, a highly attractive field, and have neglected the more prosaic laboratory medical microbiology training. To some extent this trend has been compensated for by the advent of college programs which prepare individuals for intermediate and technician level jobs in laboratories (see Table 3-12, page 99).

Pharmacy Services

Pharmacy is concerned with the procuring, storage, distribution, dispensing, and administering of medicinal products. (*Pharmacology* is concerned with the discovery, standardization, manufacture, biochemical and physiologic effects, mechanisms of action, and therapeutic and other uses of these same products.) Pharmacy is a profession in transition. Where once every pharmacist compounded his own drugs, most drugs today are precompounded and the pharmacist acts as pharmaceutical repository, dispenser, and interpreter of instructions for use of prescription and other drugs. There are signs that pharmacy will play a more integral role in the health care of the future, and there are repeated calls for a considerably expanded role in what is called clinical pharmacy.[7,8]

There were, in 1971, approximately 130,000 registered pharmacists in active practice, representing a ratio of 63 pharmacists per 100,000 population (very little changed since 1965). In 1970–1971, there were 75 schools of pharmacy in 45 states and territories, with about 16,000 students enrolled and 4,800 graduates. Licensure to practice pharmacy requires graduation from an accredited pharmacy college, completion of a one-year internship (required in most states), and passing a state board examination. Customary degrees in pharmacy normally require five years of college study, resulting in the bachelor of science in pharmacy (B.S.) or the bachelor of pharmacy (B. Pharm.).

RETAIL COMMUNITY PHARMACIES

About 80 per cent (106,000) of practicing pharmacists work in retail community pharmacies, and of these not quite half are owners or partners in their drugstores, the remainder being employees. In actuality, the retail pharmacist is more than a dispenser of prescription drugs and patent medicines. In the past he was "doc, the physician of the poor," and today there is no pharmacist who is not daily asked questions about symptoms, remedies, and where to go for health-related help. Drugstores are busy places, partly because of the press of prescription business resulting from the medical-care boom, and partly from the relentless pressures of patent medicine sales. Nevertheless, the retail pharmacist, aside from over-the-counter business, often is asked or volunteers valuable information about the action and dosage of pharmaceuticals to both patient and doctor alike.

HOSPITAL PHARMACIES

In 1971, there were almost 5,000 pharmacists working in manufacturing and wholesale activities and about 6,000 in teaching and government settings. There were also approximately 12,000 pharmacists employed in hospital pharmacies. Few hospitals where pharmacotherapy is of any volume are without at least one pharmacist. Approximately two fifths of the hospitals in the United States maintain hospital pharmacies, generally serving both inpatients and outpatients.

Hospital pharmacists, like their community counterparts, maintain the pharmacy and dispense (and compound, if necessary) drug prescriptions. A most important role—increasingly utilized, but not fully so by any means—is that of the drug information specialist. Because of their training, pharmacists frequently know more about general differential drug effects than do other clinical personnel in a hospital. Advice is increasingly being sought from pharmacists about *selection* of appropriate drugs to be used in treatment, *dosage, interactions* among several drugs administered simultaneously, and the *effects* of drugs on laboratory test findings.[9]

Pharmacists can also play extraordinarily valuable roles in advice regarding the contraindication of certain drugs because of the patient's condition or because of idiosyncratic adverse drug reaction. Five per cent of hospital admissions are estimated to result from adverse drug reactions. Even more significant, an estimated 18 to 30 per cent of hospitalized patients have adverse reactions to drugs prescribed *while they are patients in the hospital,* leading to substantial extension of the hospital stay.[10]

NEW TRENDS IN PHARMACY

Persuasive arguments have been advanced for the development of the category "clinical pharmacist," for professional employment, particularly in hospitals.[11] The clinical pharmacist would take a place alongside other members of the clinical team, with particular responsibility for (a) gaining acquaintance with the patient's total condition; (b) maintaining a drug profile on each patient and regulating drug administration so as not to interfere with forthcoming diagnostic tests or dietary regimen; (c) informing the patient about drug properties and proper drug use; and (d) evaluating merits and deficits of drug products, communicating this appraisal to physicians and assisting in the choice of specific drugs. In other words, the clinical pharmacist would devote less time to the technical and mechanical aspects of drug distribution and more to direct patient care.

Needless to say, such a prospect is very appealing to many pharmacists, particularly those more recently trained, and to pharmacy students. A model clinical pharmacy training program has already been inaugurated in at least one major university and others are certain to follow. The new program involves changes in curriculum as well as new internship and residency arrangements.[12] Graduates of such programs are likely to find a growing market for their skills, since a number of hospitals and medical centers already have in one respect or another provided professional opportunities in clinical pharmacy.

Who will dispense drugs in the future? No doubt many pharmacists will continue that activity, but there is a new category of employee developing that may help solve some pressing logistical problems in the pharmacy. This is the pharmacy *aide* who works under direct supervision of a registered pharmacist. In 1970, there were already about 10,000 pharmacy aides and assistants at work in larger hospitals and in some community pharmacies. The pharmacy profession is now beginning to define education and training requirements for this new addition to the health manpower armamentarium.

Nutritional and Dietetic Services

NUTRITION AND HEALTH

Nutritional intake and nutritional status have been implicated in a wide range of health and even social problems, perhaps wider than any other set of influences in public health.[13-16] There is a substantial body of scientific and practical knowledge of immense value resulting from a century of activity in nutritional science (and related biochemistry) and principles of diet. For example, much is known about caloric intake necessary to maintain the body's energy requirements; about nutrient values—carbohydrates, proteins, fats, vitamins, minerals, and other elements—necessary for balanced dietary intake; and about the foods that are rich or poor in these nutrients—the breads, cereals, fruits and vegetables, milk and cheese, meats, butter and oils, etc. There has resulted from all this work a good understanding of the dietary requirements of individuals living in different climatic conditions (e.g., in temperate and in tropical zones); of adults who work at active or more sedentary jobs; of infants, children, and adolescents; of the elderly; and of pregnant women and new mothers.

Much is known, also, of the dietary deficiencies that lead to documented disease states, some of them of worldwide prevalence. These include protein-calorie malnutrition (PCM) where good protein is not available, manifesting itself in infants and young children as kwashiorkor. There are also the vitamin deficiency diseases (avitaminosis A, rickets, beriberi, pellagra, etc.), and the mineral defiency diseases (e.g., endemic goiter).

Over the decades there has built up a substantial store of knowledge of the psychosocial factors in food habits and diet that relate to nationality, ethnic, regional, or family custom; to education; to economic conditions, including poverty; and to personal idiosyncracy.

To be sure, many important scientific facts remain unclear, for example, the exact role—though there is plenty of speculation—that carbohydrates, sugar, and fats have in the development of cardiovascular disease, and other conditions.[17] Moreover, there is need for continued vigilance about the dangers of food additives, animal-feed stimulants, and pesticides in incidence of several diseases, including cancer, in human beings.

DIETITIANS AND NUTRITIONISTS

The armamentarium of knowledge about nutrition and the scientific search for new knowledge have given rise to the broad profession concerned with nutritional and dietetic services and with nutrition teaching and research. In the United States in 1970, there were estimated to be more than 30,000 persons employed in nutrition and dietetics. Of these, more than 95 per cent were in dietetics and the remainder (about 1,000) were nutritionists.

Half the *dietitians* in the United States (approximately 15,000) work in hospitals and in the larger nursing homes. More and more, however, dietitians are also being employed in many other settings where there are large-scale food service programs (e.g., colleges, universities, school systems, etc.) and in other public and private food-serving settings. A basic role of dietitians in these jobs is to guide the application of principles of nutrition in the selection, preparation, and serving of balanced, nutritious meals. There is also an important role in providing instruction and guidance to individuals and groups about applying principles of nutrition to food selection and preparation and to personal eating habits.

There are several recognized classifications of dietitians, including administrative dietitians, clinical (or therapeutic) dietitians, educational and research dietitians. Many dietitians are engaged as consultants to health care institutions, food processing companies, and gas and electric companies. Recommended qualifications for the professional dietitian include graduation from a suitable undergraduate program approved by the American Dietetics Association and an approved dietetic internship (or qualifying equivalent experience). Dietitians gain their educational preparation principally in about 250 home economics programs in colleges and universities. In 1968–1969, approximately 1,200 bachelor's degrees were awarded in food and nutrition or in institutional management, and there were about 225 master's degrees and 28 doctorates.

Nutritionists engage in investigations and solve problems of human nutrition for the promotion of health, and are often responsible for the nutrition component of health and medical care services. The *public health nutritionist* assesses community nutrition needs, provides nutrition counseling to patients in clinics, and furnishes up-to-date information to the public. The latter function is accomplished by teaching special classes, preparing informational material (often in several languages), and working with community agencies in planning nutrition programs.

The *teaching nutritionist* takes part in educational programs in nutrition for the preparation of professional workers, including nurses, physicians, dentists, and allied health professionals as well as dietitians and nutritionists. There is also participation in instruction (in nutritional matters) of primary and secondary school teachers. The *research nutritionist* is concerned with adding to knowledge about the interrelationship of nutrients in food and their effects on health. For example, current research into the metabolism of proteins and fatty acids is attempting to gain further understanding of factors in obesity and in heart disease as well as various other degenerative conditions.[18,19]

Nutritionists gain their education mainly from nutrition programs in departments of nutrition or biochemistry in colleges and universities. In 1968, there were 20 bachelor's graduates from such programs; 112 master's and 39 doctoral degrees were awarded.

CURRENT CONCERNS IN THE NUTRITION FIELD

In the United States, in the 1960's and continuing today, a number of new issues have arisen in the nutrition field that go well beyond traditional concerns for the nutritive value of basic foods and involve broad health and social concerns.[20] A first issue of high concern and importance is malnutrition. It is now known that malnutrition occurs in the United States, although the extent and causes are in dispute.[21] The sites of malnutrition in the United States are the central areas of cities and certain rural areas (Appalachia, the South, Southwest, West, and particular American Indian reservations). Rural groups especially affected include seasonal and migrant farm workers in addition to American Indians; urban groups particularly affected include elderly persons living on marginal incomes, and women with small children.

The long-term solutions to these problems reside in efforts to erase poverty and to raise educational levels, and thus lie outside consideration of nutrition alone. In connection with foods, however, three programs in the United States have direct import for alleviation of malnutrition. These are the food stamp program, available to persons on welfare, which are in actuality welfare "payments" earmarked expressly for food; the school lunch program, aimed at all children, including the very poor; and the food commodity program, which distributes surplus farm products. These important programs are valuable in reducing malnutrition, but have faced great problems in administration, since they are geographically very broadly based and call for close cooperation among many agencies and localities.

A second issue of concern in the nutrition field has to do with the nature of certain foods that are increasingly available for sale in America's food stores and markets. Many of the developments in food packaging and availability involve features that are genuinely appreciated by the consumer and appear to meet the national mood regarding consumer time spent in food preparation. Thus, there are convenience foods attractively packaged in a variety of forms with simple instructions for meal preparation. These foods are subject to a "hard sell" both in media and in supermarkets, but often sell themselves through their basic appeal. However, such foods are more expensive per unit measure of weight than their simpler predecessors, and thus no doubt have negative impact on the individual and family food budget.

Even more important from the viewpoint of nutrition, are the many specially prepared foods that have additives in bewildering profusion, many of which have been introduced as preservatives. There are altogether more than 1,500 chemical additives that find their way into foods stocked by American stores and markets. It has been estimated that Americans consume more than five pounds of food additives a year, aside from sodium chloride (salt), which is widely acknowledged to be overused, perhaps dangerously, in American diets. The dangers of mercury in fish have been well publicized (see Chapter 7), and attention is being directed increasingly to possible chemical hazards in meats. There is concern regarding preservatives and other chemicals sometimes added to meat and regarding hormones and other products added to feed as livestock grows. For example, American cattle for almost two decades have been fed diethylstilbestrol (DES), which causes animals to fatten more quickly on less feed. Recently, DES was implicated as a carcinogenic agent in laboratory animals. This and similar incidents highlight the need for close scrutiny of the health implications of all food additives.

A final concern has to do with the so-called empty calories presumably residing in many breakfast cereals, snack foods, and soft drinks. These are often delicious and refreshing products, subject to aggressive merchandising and sold widely, particularly to young persons. The products themselves are relatively expensive per unit weight and often include excess salt or excess sugar, the intake of which in inordinate quantities is clearly discouraged by principles of healthful nutrition. Ingestion of these calories, along with a general habit of overeating, contributes to what some consider to be America's number-one eating problem, obesity (see Chapter 11).

The issues just cited have had a forum in newspapers, magazines, and the scientific press, and drew international attention in connection with the White House Conference on Food, Nutrition and Health held late in 1969.[22] The problems remain for the decade of the 1970's, with evidence that some progress—vigilantly pressed and monitored—is under way. There is clear need for cooperation in several realms involving the food industry, consumers, governmental agencies, and voluntary organizations. There are programs afoot to expand "food delivery" services to the needy and to ensure honest labeling of food products. Such labeling would include listing on the package not only the ingredients, but also the nutrient value of the contents. There is clear need for vitalizing the Food and Drug Administration and the scientific community to study the health safety aspects of food additives. There is pressing need for information and education directed to food consumers (all Americans) and food processors—alike—to be alert to the need for nutritious, safe, and health-promoting foods. Finally, there is need for continued nutritional research, both basic and applied, which will provide the foundation for detailed knowledge of the role played by foods in the cause, prevention, and cure of disease.

References

1. Hartney, J. B. The role of the clinical laboratory in the community hospital. *Med Clin North Am*, **53:**11–23, 1969.
2. Inhorn, S. L. Future of the public health laboratory: impact of CAFOR. *Health Lab Sci*, **7:**17–20, 1970.
3. Evans, A. S. Epidemiology and the public health laboratory. *Am J Public Health*, **57:**1041–52, 1967.
4. Garfield, S. R. Multiphasic health testing and medical care as a right. *N Engl J Med*, **283:**1087–89, 1970.
5. Ahlvin, R. C. Biochemical screening—a critique. *N Engl J Med*, **283:**1084–86, 1970.
6. Yedidia, A., Bunow, M. A., and Muldavin, M. Mobile multiphasic screening in an industrial setting. *J Occup Med*, **11:**602–62, 1969.
7. Cain, R. M., and Kahn, J. S. The pharmacist as a member of the health team. *Am J Public Health*, **61:**2223–28, 1971.
8. Robles, R. R., and Winship, H. W., III. Pharmacy involvement in the neighborhood health center environment. *Am J Hosp Pharm*, **29:**68–71, 1972.
9. Tousignaut, D. R. Pharmacy. *Hospitals*, **44:**137–43, 1970.
10. Brands, A. J. *Blueprint for Pharmacists' Role in Preventive Medicine.* Drug Interaction Seminar, College of Pharmacy. Rutgers University, New Brunswick, New Jersey, 1971.
11. Sperandio, G. J., and Belcastro, P. F. The clinical pharmacist: adviser, teacher, consultant. *Mod Hosp*, **111:**100–101, November 1968.
12. Plagenz, L. Clinical pharmacy is "hot new trend." *Mod Hosp*, **111:**101–3, November 1968.
13. Scrimshaw, N., Taylor, C., and Gordon, J. Interactions of nutrition and infection. *WHO Chron*, **23:**369–74, 1969.
14. Winik, M. Nutrition and mental development. *Med Clin North Am*, **54:**1413–29, 1970.
15. U.S. Department of Agriculture, Science and Education Staff. *Human Nutrition—An Evaluation of Research in the United States.* The Department, Washington, D.C., October 1971.
16. Finch, R. Toward a comprehensive food and nutrition program. *Public Health Rep*, **84:**667–72, 1969.
17. American Heart Association. *Mass Field Trials of the Diet-Heart Question.* The Association, New York, 1969.

18. Swendseid, M. E., Tuttle, S. G., Figueroa, W. S., Mulcare, D., Clark, A. J., and Massey, F. J. Plasma amino acid levels of men fed diets differing in protein content. *J Nutr*, **88:**239–48, 1966.
19. Alfin-Slater, R. B. Carbohydrate-lipid effects on cholesterol metabolism. *J Dairy Sci*, **50:**781–86, 1967.
20. Mayer, J. Toward a national nutrition policy. *Science*, **176:**237–41, 1972.
21. Pollack, H. Hunger U.S.A. 1968; a critical review. *Am J Clin Nutr*, **22:**480–89, 1969.
22. White House Conference on Food, Nutrition and Health. *Final Report*. U.S. Government Printing Office, Washington, D. C., 1970.